DENTAL

T0198309

FIFTH EDITION

DENTAL

STEPHEN T. SONIS, DMD, DMSC
Professor of Oral Medicine
Harvard School of Dental Medicine
Distinguished Faculty in Surgery
Dana-Farber Cancer institute
Chief Scientific Officer
Biomodels, LLC
Boston, Massachusetts, United States

JENNIFER A. MAGEE DMD, MPH
Service Chief, MGH Dentistry
Department of Surgery
Massachusetts General Hospital
Assistant Professor of Oral and Maxillofacial Surgery
Harvard School of Dental Medicine
Boston, Massachusetts, United States

ELSEVIER

Elsevier
3251 Riverport Lane
St. Louis, Missouri 63043

Dental Secrets, FIFTH EDITION   ISBN: 978-0-323-93770-2
Copyright © 2024 by Elsevier, Inc. All rights reserved.

No part of this publication may be reproduced or transmitted in any form or by any means, electronic or
mechanical, including photocopying, recording, or any information storage and retrieval system, without
permission in writing from the publisher. Details on how to seek permission, further information about the
Publisher's permissions policies and our arrangements with organizations such as the Copyright Clearance
Center and the Copyright Licensing Agency, can be found at our website: www.elsevier.com/permissions.

This book and the individual contributions contained in it are protected under copyright by the Publisher
(other than as may be noted herein).

Notice

Practitioners and researchers must always rely on their own experience and knowledge in evaluating and
using any information, methods, compounds or experiments described herein. Because of rapid advances
in the medical sciences, in particular, independent verification of diagnoses and drug dosages should be
made. To the fullest extent of the law, no responsibility is assumed by Elsevier, authors, editors or contributors for any injury and/or damage to persons or property as a matter of products liability, negligence or
otherwise, or from any use or operation of any methods, products, instructions, or ideas contained in the
material herein.

Previous editions copyrighted 2015, 2003, 1998, and 1994.

Content Strategist: Lauren Boyle
Content Development Specialist: Himanshi Chauhan
Publishing Services Manager: Deepthi Unni
Project Manager: Sindhuraj Thulasingam
Design Direction: Bridget Hoette

Printed in India

Last digit is the print number: 9   8   7   6   5   4   3   2   1

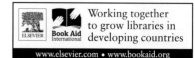

Working together
to grow libraries in
developing countries

www.elsevier.com • www.bookaid.org

In memory of my father, H. Richard Sonis, DDS,
with admiration and gratitude.

To my grandfather, Richard Magee,
who inspired my love of learning and service
to others.

PREFACE TO THE FIFTH EDITION

The first edition of *Dental Secrets* was published almost 30 years ago. Since then, there have been three subsequent editions, with the last one released in 2015. It has been heartening to see that interest and enthusiasm for the Q&A short answer format found in this book is still of considerable value to students, residents, and practitioners and justified an updated edition.

Besides new contributors and fresh content, the most notable change to this version of *Dental Secrets* is the addition of Dr. Jennifer Magee as my coeditor. Dr. Magee adds the perspective of a practicing general dentist coupled with an outstanding history as an innovative and broad-thinking teacher.

Dr. Magee and I would like to thank Dr. Kathryn Forth and Dr. Mona Meshkin for their review and feedback on the book's content.

The science and practice of dentistry continues to evolve, which is both exciting and challenging for those of us who want to ensure that we provide optimum care for our patients. "Life-long learning" is not just a catchy phrase. Hopefully, this book will help achieve that objective.

And, as always, *Dental Secrets* is written for those who like to learn by those who love to teach.

Stephen Sonis
Boston, Massachusetts
March 2023

CONTRIBUTORS

Sama Abdul-Aziz, DMD
Program Director, Attending Dentist
Division of Dentistry
Massachusetts General Hospital
Boston, Massachusetts
United States

Helene Sharon Bednarsh, BS, RDH, MPH
Dental Director
New England AIDS Education and Training Center
Department of Family Medicine and Community Health
UMASS Chan Medical School
Worcester, Massachusetts
United States

Isabelle Chase, DDS, FRCD(C)
Director, Postdoctoral Pediatric Dentistry
Pediatric Dentistry
Boston Children's Hospital, Boston
Massachusetts
United States
Assistant Professor
Department of Developmental Biology
Harvard School of Dental Medicine
Boston, Massachusetts
United States

Chia-Yu Chen, DDS, DMSc
Instructor
Oral Medicine, Infection, and Immunity
Harvard School of Dental Medicine
Boston, Massachusetts
United States

Amanda C. Colebeck, DDS, MS, FACP
Maxillofacial Prosthodontist
Dentistry/Oral Oncology and Maxillofacial
  Prosthetics
Erie County Medical Center
Buffalo, New York
United States

Eve Cuny, BA, MS
Executive Associate Dean
Administration
University of the Pacific Arthur A. Dugoni School of
  Dentistry
San Francisco, California
United States
Professor
Diagnostic Sciences
University of the Pacific Arthur A. Dugoni School of
  Dentistry
San Francisco, California
United States

Bernard Friedland, BChD, MSc, JD
Associate Professor
Oral Medicine, Infection, and Immunity
Harvard School of Dental Medicine
Boston, Massachusetts
United States

Jennifer L. Frustino, DDS, PhD
Director of Oncology Research
Dentistry/Oral Oncology and Maxillofacial
  Prosthetics
Erie County Medical Center
Buffalo, New York
United States

Winna G. Gorham, DMD, MS
Private Practice
Endodontics
Endodontic Care, PC
Boston, Massachusetts
United States

Mark A. Green, MD, DDS
Surgeon
Plastic and Oral Surgery
Boston Children's Hospital
Boston, Massachusetts
United States
Instructor
Department of Oral Surgery
Harvard School of Dental Medicine
Boston, Massachusetts
United States

David M. Kim, DDS, DMSc
Associate Professor
Oral Medicine, Infection, and Immunity
Harvard School of Dental Medicine
Boston, Massachusetts
United States

Paul A. Levi Jr., DMD, PhD
Instructor
Periodontology
Harvard School of Dental Medicine
Boston, Massachusetts
United States

Pamela J. Linder, DMD
Director of Hospital and Special Needs Dentistry
Oral and Maxillofacial Surgery and
  Hospital Dentistry
Indiana University School of Dentistry
Indianapolis, Indiana
United States

James MacLaine, BDS, FDS Orth RCSEd
Director of Craniofacial Orthodontics
Department of Dentistry
Boston Children's Hospital
Boston, Massachusetts
United States
Instructor
Department of Developmental Biology
Harvard School of Dental Medicine
Boston, Massachusetts
United States

Jennifer Anne Magee, DMD, MPH
Service Chief, MGH Dentistry
Department of Surgery
Massachusetts General Hospital
Boston, Massachusetts
United States
Assistant Professor of Oral and Maxillofacial Surgery
Harvard School of Dental Medicine
Boston, Massachusetts
United States

Reshma S. Menon, BDS, DMSc
Assistant Professor
Diagnostic Sciences
Tufts University School of Dental Medicine
Boston, Massachusetts
United States

Bonnie L. Padwa, DMD, MD
Professor of Oral and Maxillofacial Surgery
Department of Oral and Maxillofacial Surgery
Harvard School of Dental Medicine
Boston, Massachusetts
United States
Oral Surgeon-in-Chief
Department of Plastic and Oral Surgery
Boston Children's Hospital
Boston, Massachusetts
United States

Edward S. Peters, DMD, SM, ScD
Professor
Epidemiology
University of Nebraska Medical Center
Omaha, Nebraska
United States

Gustavo Machado Santaella, DDS, MS, PhD
Assistant Professor
Diagnosis and Oral Health
University of Louisville School of Dentistry
Louisville, Kentucky
United States

Deborah P. Saunders, DMD
Medical Director
Dental Oncology
Health Sciences North
Sudbury, Ontario
Canada
Associate Professor
Northern Ontario School of Medicine
Sudbury, Ontario
Canada

Jeffry Rowland Shaefer, DDS, MS, MPH
Assistant Professor
Oral and Maxillofacial Surgery
Harvard School of Dental Medicine
Boston, Massachusetts
United States
Director Massachusetts General Hospital Orofacial Pain
    Residency
Department of Surgery
Massachusetts General Hospital
Boston, Massachusetts
United States

**Adam Omar Shafik, DDS, Diplomate of American Board
of Orofacial Pain**
Clinical Assistant Professor
Oral and Maxillofacial Surgery
Loma Linda University
Loma Linda, California
United States

Stephen T. Sonis, DMD, DMSc
Chief Scientific Officer
Biomodels
Biomodels, LLC
Watertown, Massachusetts
United States
Senior Surgeon
Oral Medicine/Surgery
Brigham and Women's Hospital
Boston, Massachusetts
United States
Distinguished Faculty
Surgery
Dana-Farber Cancer Institute
Boston, Massachusetts
United States
Professor
Oral Medicine
Harvard University
Boston, Massachusetts
United States

Nathaniel Treister, DMD, DMSc
Division Chief
Division of Oral Medicine and Dentistry
Brigham and Women's Hospital
Boston, Massachusetts
United States
Associate Professor
Department of Oral Medicine, Infection, and
    Immunity
Harvard School of Dental Medicine
Boston, Massachusetts
United States

Alessandro Villa, DDS, PhD, MPH
Professor
Translational medicine
Florida International University, Herbert Wertheim College
   of Medicine
Miami, Florida
United States
Chief of Oral Medicine, Oral Oncology and Dentir
Miami Cancer Institute
Miami, Florida
United States

Sook-Bin Woo, DMD MMSc FDSRCS (Edin)
Professor
Oral Medicine, Infection, and Immunity
Harvard School of Dental Medicine
Boston, United States
Director
Center for Oral Pathology
StrataDx Inc
Lexington, Massachusetts
United States

Athanasios Zavras, DDS, MS, DMSc
Professor, Chair and Assistant Dean
Department of Public Health and Community Service
Tufts University School of Dental Medicine
Boston, Massachusetts
United States

CONTENTS

PATIENT MANAGEMENT: THE DENTIST-PATIENT RELATIONSHIP

Sama Abdul-Aziz, Jennifer A. Magee

CHAPTER 1

ESTABLISHING THE DENTIST-PATIENT RELATIONSHIP

1. **What is the Guild Model of the dentist-patient relationship?**
   In the Guild Model the dentist has all the expertise, knowledge, training, and experience. The patient is a passive recipient to the dentist. The dentist is the only active party in the decision-making process. The patient's values and biopsychosocial factors are excluded from consideration as the dentist is the sole decision-maker. Furthermore, as the patient is assumed to be uninformed, it does not equip the patient with the knowledge to make positive changes to improve health and prevent further disease in the future. The Guild Model is criticized because this model fails to satisfy the patient's right to autonomy, a main principle of dental ethics. Having professional expertise does not eclipse a patient's autonomous choice regarding treatment.

2. **What is the Agent Model of the dentist-patient relationship?**
   Whereas in the Guild Model the dentist is the sole decision-maker, in the Agent Model the patient becomes the main decision-maker. The patient's values and needs dictate all aspects of the care. The dentist acts as the patient's "agent" and is tasked to meet all the patient's desires. The dentist's expertise and experience are excluded from the decision-making process. The Agent Model is criticized because this model runs the risk of not satisfying principles of dental ethics such as nonmaleficence. A patient's requests and autonomy should not dictate the care in such a way that could jeopardize the patient's oral and overall health. It is the role of the dentist to educate and adequately inform the patient. The patient cannot consent to substandard care, even if this is what the patient is requesting.

3. **What is the Commercial Model of the dentist-patient relationship?**
   In the Commercial Model, dentistry is a commodity and the relationship between dentist and patient is that of a seller and buyer. The dentist and patient are competitors in a free market. The patient's priority is to receive a dental service for as little monetary value as possible, while the dentist is hoping to offer the service for as much as possible. The Commercial Model is criticized as there is no ethical component to the relationship. The emphasis is on what the patient is willing to pay for a service rather than the dental needs, potentially resulting in no impetus for the patient to improve their health.

4. **What is the Interactive Model of the dentist-patient relationship?**
   The Interactive Model is the ideal relationship model. The dentist and patient are equal parties in care. The dentist and patient both bring value to the decision-making process. For this model to be successful, the dentist and patient must both actively contribute and fulfill their roles. The patient must disclose their medical and dental histories and conditions, specify concerns such as dental phobia and financial limitations, and state their values. The dentist must consider the patient's individual circumstances while applying professional expertise. This model allows for individualized care that provides ethical and successful care delivery. By creating a relationship of trust, the patient feels that they have more control and are empowered to improve their health.

5. **When is the dentist-patient relationship established?**
   The dentist-patient relationship can be established at any time once the provider says or does anything that the patient interprets as professional advice. In a dentist-patient relationship, each party must fulfill their role. For example, the dentist is expected to practice ethically, maintain patient confidentiality, and comply with local rules and regulations. The patient is expected to maintain appointments, follow proper medical advice, and maintain an acceptable model of behavior. If a relationship is not beneficial, the termination of the dentist-patient relationship may be indicated. However, if the dentist terminates the dentist-patient relationship, the dentist must ensure the patient's well-being by providing a notice and basis for termination, facilitating the transfer of care, and being available for emergency care. Otherwise, termination of the relationship constitutes patient abandonment. The dentist cannot terminate the relationship based on race, sexual orientation, disability, or other discriminatory characteristics.

6. **Is the dentist obligated to treat all patients seeking their care?**
   While the dentist-patient relationship is often established during the first encounter with the patient, there are instances when the dentist will not be treating the patient subsequently. This is especially the case if the patient

has needs that exceed the scope of care that the dentist can provide. However, if the dentist-patient rapport does not result in a trusting relationship, it is best to be upfront with the patient and consider termination of care. In either case, the dentist must document the reasons for the decision, inform the patient, and provide appropriate referrals.

PATIENT INTERVIEW

7. **What is the basic goal of the initial patient interview?**
To establish a therapeutic dentist-patient relationship in which accurate data are collected, presenting problems are assessed, and effective treatment is suggested, all the elements of the medical and dental history relevant to treating the patient's dental needs should be elicited. The patient should feel heard and validated, which leads to a feeling of safety and trust.

8. **What are the major sources of clinical data derived during the interview?**
The clinician should be attentive to what the patient verbalizes (i.e., the chief complaint), manner of speaking (how things are expressed), and nonverbal cues that may be related through body language (e.g., posture, gait, facial expression, or movements). While listening carefully to the patient, the dentist can observe associated mannerisms such as gestures, fidgeting movements, excessive perspiration, or patterns of irregular breathing that might indicate underlying health conditions such as anxiety.

9. **Why is open-ended questioning useful as an interviewing format?**
Broad and open-ended questions are a good way to begin an interview. Open-ended questions can also be used to bridge to a new topic. Questions that do not have specific yes or no answers give patients more latitude to express themselves and help build rapport. More information allows the dentist to have a better understanding of patients and their problems. Throughout the interview, the clinician listens for any cues that indicate the need to pursue further questioning and obtain more information about expressed fears, concerns, or conditions. Typical questions in the open-ended format include the following:
- "What brings you here today?"
- "Are you having any problems?"
- "Please tell me more about it."

10. **What useful nonverbal communication skills can the dentist employ during the patient interview?**
The adept use of face, voice, and body facilitates the classic "bedside manner," including the following:

Eye Contact: Looking at the patient without overt staring establishes rapport.
Facial Expression: A smile or nod of the head in affirmation shows warmth, concern, and interest.
Vocal Characteristics: The voice is modulated to create a calm tone, emphasize meaning, and help the patient understand important issues.
Body Orientation: Facing patients when communicating signals attentiveness. Turning away may seem like rejection. The dentist should be at the same eye level as the patient when communicating.
Forward Lean and Proximity: Leaning forward tells a patient that the dentist is interested and wants to hear more, thus making it easier for the patient to comment. Proximity infers intimacy, whereas distance signals less attentiveness. In general, 4 to 6 feet is considered a social consultative zone.

A verbal message of low empathetic value may be altered favorably by maintaining eye contact, leaning forward with the trunk, and having appropriate distance and body orientation. However, even a verbal message of high empathetic content may be reduced to a lower value when the speaker does not have eye contact, turns away with a backward lean, or maintains too far a distance. For example, do not tell the patient that you are concerned while washing your hands with your back to the dental chair.

11. **During the interview, what cues alert the dentist to search for more information about a statement made by the patient?**
Most people express information that they do not fully understand by using generalizations, deletions, and distortions in their phrasing. For example, the comment, "I am a horrible patient," does not give much insight into the patient's intent. By probing further, the dentist may discover specific fears or behaviors that have led the patient to make the opening generalization. The dentist should be alert to such cues and use the interview to clarify and work through the patient's comments. As the interview proceeds, trust and rapport are built as a mutual understanding develops and the patient's negative emotions decrease.

12. **How can the dentist help the patient relate more information or talk about a certain issue in greater depth?**
Giving full attention while listening demonstrates to the patient that you are physically present and comprehend what the patient relates. Reflection after active listening, where the provider restates what the patient has told them, is beneficial to ensure that the patient's concerns have been heard and understood by both parties.

Active listening is important during an assessment and following an open-ended question. Reflections after active listening can come in many forms. Simple reflection offers a short summary of what is happening and can be only slightly modified from what was said. Complex reflection communicates the nuance of a situation and conveys to the patient that the dentist understands the patient's emotions such as those of frustration, anxiety, or desperation. A common reaction to a dentist's accurate and careful reflection is patient elaboration, allowing the dentist to learn more information about the patient and further enhance rapport.

13. **When is closed-ended questioning useful in an interviewing format?**
If after open-ended questioning there is still important information that patient has not disclosed, close-ended questions can be utilized. Close-ended questions help concrete data collection. This can be especially useful when gathering pieces of information that the patient may not realize is important to the dentist to form a diagnosis such as the nature of the pain or systemic symptoms associated with the pain or infection. However, the dentist should not rely solely on close-ended questions and should provide context to a series of close-ended questions prior to beginning the questioning, such as saying, "I am going to ask you a series of questions to better understand the severity of your pain." In the event of a medical emergency, close-ended questioning should be utilized as it is the most efficient mode of gathering specific information.

14. **Discuss the insecurities that patients might encounter while relating their personal histories and how to effectively manage these insecurities.**
Patients may feel the fear of rejection, criticism, shame, or even humiliation from the dentist because of the state of their oral health. Patients may react to the dentist with irrational comments. Patients who perceive the dentist as judgmental are likely to become defensive, uncommunicative, or even hostile. Anxious patients are more observant of any signs of displeasure or negative reactions by the dentist. The role of effective communication is extremely important with such patients. Communication founded on the basic concepts of empathy and respect gives the most support to patients. Understanding their point of view (empathy) and recognizing their right to their own opinions and feelings (respect), even if different from the dentist's personal views, help deal with and avert potential conflicts.

15. **Why is it important for dentists to be aware of their own feelings when dealing with patients?**
Although the dentist tries to maintain an attitude that is attentive, friendly, and even sympathetic toward a patient, the dentist needs an appropriate degree of objectivity in relation to patients and their problems. Dentists who find that they are not listening with some degree of emotional neutrality to the patient's information should be aware of any personal feelings of anxiety, sadness, indifference, resentment, or even hostility that may be aroused by the patient. Recognition of any aspects of the patient's behavior that arouse such emotions helps dentists understand their own behavior and prevent possible conflicts in clinical judgment and treatment plan suggestions. It is important to strive to be as neutral and nonjudgmental as possible so that the patient can feel safe and trusting.

16. **What are professional boundaries?**
Professional boundaries are mutually understood, unspoken physical and emotional limits of the professional relationship between the patient and dentist. The discussion of highly personal and intimate topics in the patient interview and clinical encounter can result in blurring of these boundaries, which can have unintended consequences. It is the responsibility of the dentist to maintain the professional boundary between them and the patient.

17. **How can strategies be used when responding to a patient's request for personal information?**
Initially, a patient's request for personal information may appear to be a threat to the professional boundary. Within reason, it is important for the dentist not to take these questions personally. Often, the patient is expressing genuine interest in getting to know their dentist better. In responding to these requests, the dentist should respond calmly and in a matter-of-fact manner. The dentist can redirect the patient back to the clinical visit. Often times, the patient's question may reflect insecurity or confusion. If this is suspected, the dentist should probe further and determine the underlying reason for the question.

18. **What type of language or phrasing is best avoided in patient communications?**
Certain words or descriptions that are routine in the technical terminology of dentistry may be offensive or frightening to patients. The words *cutting, drilling, bleeding, injecting,* or *clamping* may be anxiety-provoking terms to some patients. Furthermore, being too technical in conversations with patients may result in poor communication and provoke rather than reduce anxiety. It is beneficial to choose terms that are neutral yet informative. One may prepare a tooth rather than cut it or dry the area rather than suction all the blood.

19. **During the clinical interview, how may one address patient fears?**
Common elements of fear include fear of the unknown, fear of loss of control, fear of physical harm, and fear of helplessness. It is important to acknowledge the prevailing element contributing to the patient's fear and establish trust with the patient to help dissipate these fears. Preparatory explanations that address the element of fear the patient presents with are effective and convey to the patient that the dentist is caring and attentive to the patient's

specific needs. The goals in a situation in which patient presents with an already formed negative predisposition are to enhance communication, develop trust and rapport, and start a new chapter in this patient's dental experience.

20. **What is the spectrum of cultural competence?**
Cultural competence ranges from cultural destructiveness to cultural humility, as described as follows:

Cultural Destructiveness: Attitudes and practices that are destructive to a cultural group. Everyone is expected to fit into the same cultural pattern and those that do not are excluded or forced to assimilate and differences are seen as barriers.
Cultural Blindness: Does not acknowledge cultural differences.
Cultural Awareness: Acknowledges that each individual functions within a culture of their own and that everyone's identity is shaped by their culture.
Cultural Sensitivity: Understands that there are cultural differences and accepts different cultural values, attitudes, and behaviors.
Cultural Competency: The capacity to work effectively with people from different cultures by integrating elements of the other culture's vocabulary, values, attitudes, and norms.
Cultural Humility: A process of self-reflection and self-critique as a life-long commitment to understanding and addressing biases and how they impact behaviors and interactions, on the personal, institutional, and community level.

21. **What techniques can be used to deliver culturally competent care?**
The dentist is responsible for striving to provide culturally competent care. It is important for the dentist to be aware of their own prejudice, biases, and emotions during each patient encounter and to strive to be as neutral and nonjudgmental as possible so that the patient can feel safe and trusting.
    The dentist must be constantly taking active steps to strive for providing culturally competent care. The dentist must aware be of cultural differences and avoid making assumptions. Gender-neutral pronouns should always be used, including when describing the patient's family members as "spouse/partner" and "parent" during the patient interview. The dentist should perform cultural assessments to identify how the patient's culture may be affecting their care preference and decision-making and approach situations with an open mind without prejudice or bias. If there is a language barrier, the dentist should provide interpretation services. Patients should be spoken to nontechnical medical and dental jargon.

DENTAL FEAR AND ANXIETY

22. **How common is dental-related anxiety?**
It is estimated that about 75% to 80% of individuals in the United States have some anxiety about dental treatment. Approximately 5% to 10% of US adults are considered to experience dental phobia to such a degree that complete avoidance of care ensues unless there is an emergency toothache or abscess. This can be extremely stressful for the patient and provider. Women tend to be more phobic than men and younger individuals more than older adults. Unless this cycle of avoidance is treated by a knowledgeable and caring dentist, a patient may never seek anything beyond emergent care, resulting in deteriorating oral health.

23. **How are dental fears learned?**
Usually, dental-related fears are learned directly from a traumatic experience in a dental or medical setting. The experience may be real or perceived by the patient as a threat, but a single event may lead to a lifetime of fear when any element of the traumatic situation is reexperienced. The situation may have occurred many years before, but the intensity of the recalled fear may persist. Associated with the incident is the behavior of the doctor in the past. Thus, for defusing learned fear, the behavior of the present doctor is paramount.
    Fears also may be learned indirectly as a vicarious experience from family members, friends, or even the media. Cartoons and movies often portray the pain and fear of the dental setting. How many times have dentists seen the negative reaction of patients to the term *root canal,* even though they may not have had one?
    Past fearful experiences often occur during childhood, when perceptions are out of proportion to events, but memories and feelings persist into adulthood, with the same distortions. Feelings of helplessness, dependency, and fear of the unknown are coupled with pain, and a possible uncaring attitude on the part of the dentist creates a conditioned response of fear when any element of the past event is reexperienced. Such events may not even be available to conscious awareness.

24. **How is a phobia different than a fear?**
A phobia is an irrational fear of a situation or object. The reaction to the stimulus is often greatly exaggerated in relation to the reality of the threat. The fears are beyond voluntary control, and avoidance is the primary coping mechanism. Phobias may be so intense that severe physiologic reactions interfere with daily functioning. In the dental setting, acute syncopal episodes may result.

Almost all phobias are learned. The process of dealing with true dental phobia may require a long period of individual psychotherapy and adjunctive pharmacologic sedation. However, relearning is possible, and establishing a good doctor-patient relationship is paramount.

25. **What is anxiety and how is it related to fear?**
Anxiety is a subjective state commonly defined as an unpleasant feeling of apprehension or impending danger in the presence of a real or perceived stimulus that the person has learned to associate with a threat to well-being. The feelings may be out of proportion to the real threat, and the response may be grossly exaggerated. Such feelings may be present before the encounter with the feared situation and may linger long after the event. Associated somatic feelings include sweating, tremors, palpitations, nausea, difficulty with swallowing, and hyperventilation.

Fear is usually considered an appropriate defensive response to a real or active threat. Unlike anxiety, the response is brief, the danger is external and readily definable, and the unpleasant somatic feelings pass as the danger passes. Fear is the classic fight-or-flight response and may serve as an overall protective mechanism by sharpening the senses and ability to respond to the danger. The fear response does not usually rely on unhealthy actions for resolution, but the state of anxiety often relies on noncoping and avoidance behaviors to deal with the threat.

26. **How is stress related to pain and anxiety? What are the major parameters of the stress response?**
When a person is stimulated by pain or anxiety, the result is a series of physiologic responses dominated by the autonomic nervous system, skeletal muscles, and endocrine system. These physiologic responses define stress. In what is termed an *adaptive response,* the sympathetic responses dominate—increases in pulse rate, blood pressure, respiratory rate, peripheral vasoconstriction, skeletal muscle tone, and blood sugar; decreases in sweating, gut motility, and salivation. In an acute maladaptive response, the parasympathetic responses dominate, and a syncopal episode may result—decreases in pulse rate, blood pressure, respiratory rate, and muscle tone; increases in salivation, sweating, gut motility, and peripheral vasodilation, with overall confusion and agitation. In chronic maladaptive situations, psychosomatic disorders may evolve. It is important to control anxiety and stress during dental treatment. The medically compromised patient requires appropriate control to avoid potentially life-threatening situations.

27. **What is the relationship between pain and anxiety?**
Many studies have shown the close relationship between pain and anxiety. The greater the person's anxiety, the more likely it is that they interpret the response to a stimulus as painful. In addition, the pain threshold is lowered with increasing anxiety. People who are debilitated, fatigued, or depressed respond to threats with a higher degree of undifferentiated anxiety and thus are more reactive to pain.

28. **What is the relationship between gag reflex and anxiety?**
The gag reflex is a basic physiologic protective mechanism that occurs when the posterior oropharynx is stimulated by a foreign object; normal swallowing does not trigger the reflex. A psychogenic gag reflex may be induced without a tactile stimulation of the trigger areas but by visual, auditory, or olfactory stimuli or by thinking about these stimuli. When overlying anxiety is present, especially if anxiety is related to the fear of being unable to breathe, the gag reflex may be exaggerated. The comorbidity between gag reflex and dental anxiety may be evidence that gagging behavior is an expression of dental anxiety.

29. **How can learned fears be eliminated or unlearned?**
Because fears of dental treatment are learned, relearning or unlearning is possible. A comfortable experience without the associated fearful and painful elements may eliminate the conditioned fear response and replace it with an adaptive and more comfortable coping response. Through the interview process, the secret is to uncover which elements have resulted in the maladaptation and subsequent response of fear, eliminate them from the present dental experience by reinterpreting them for the adult patient, and create a more caring and protected experience. During the interview, the exchange of information and insight gained by the patient decrease levels of fear, increase rapport, and establish trust in the doctor-patient relationship. The clinician only needs to apply an expert operative technique to treat most fearful patients.

30. **Why is understanding the patient's perception of the dentist so important in the control of fear and stress?**
According to studies, patients perceive the dentist as both the controller of what the patient perceives as dangerous and as the protector from that danger. Thus, the dentist's behavior and communications assume increased significance. The patient's ability to tolerate stress and cope with fears depends on their ability to develop and maintain a high level of trust and confidence in the dentist. To achieve this goal, patients must express all the issues that they perceive as threatening, and the dentist must explain what he or she can do to address patients' concerns and protect them from the perceived dangers. This is the purpose of the clinical interview. The result of this exchange should be increased trust and rapport and a subsequent decline in fear and anxiety.

31. **What remarks may be given to a patient before beginning a procedure to manage a patient's fear?**
Opening comments by the dentist to inform the patient about what to expect during a procedure—for example, pressure, noise, pain—may reduce the patient's fear of the unknown and sense of helplessness. Control through knowing is increased with these preparatory communications.

32. **How may the dentist further address the issue of loss of control?**
A simple instruction that allows patients to signal by raising a hand if they wish to stop or speak returns a sense of control. Also, patients can be given the choice of whether to lie back or sit up.

33. **What is PTSD and what are the symptoms?**
Posttraumatic stress disorder (PTSD) is an anxiety disorder that develops after a traumatic event, such as sexual or physical abuse, serious accident, assault, war combat, or natural disaster. Symptoms include intrusive memories, avoidance behaviors, mood disorders, and high levels of physiologic arousal.

34. **What is trauma-informed care?**
Trauma-informed care is the practice of approaching each patient as if they are a survivor of a former trauma. Trauma can present as PTSD, panic attacks, and uncontrollable anxiety. Trauma-informed care acknowledges that a patient with a history of trauma can be triggered by the intimate nature of a dental appointment. A trauma-informed care approach to all patient care allows for a more empathetic and individualized care model, without the patient having to reveal the history of trauma. It also allows dentists to acknowledge that perceived irrational behavior from the patient may be trauma based that has not been disclosed to the dentist.

35. **How do traumatic events create behaviors later in life?**
Past traumatic events, whether remembered or suppressed in the subconscious, may trigger behavioral responses that occur when similar or even vicarious events occur in the present. These events may be through direct experience, such as an accident, combat wound, or sexual abuse, or associated with observation of such events. The triggered behavior in the patient may be generalized fear and anxiety, and even extreme panic.

36. **Why is it important for dental providers to be sensitive to a patient's history of trauma?**
Patients with a history of trauma who come for dental treatment may feel very vulnerable and can sometimes find the experience retraumatizing. This is because of the intimate nature of a dental appointment where the patient can be alone with the dentist, is placed in a horizontal position, is being touched by the dentist, who is hierarchically more powerful, is having objects placed in the mouth, is unable to swallow, and is anticipating or feeling pain. Many patients with a history of trauma avoid going to the dentist, often cancel or reschedule appointments, have stress-related dental issues, and experience heightened distress while undergoing procedures.

37. **How might a dentist know if a patient suffers from PTSD or has a history of trauma?**
Often these patients are reluctant to admit this, so careful attention during the patient interview can provide the dentists with clues and ways to gently probe for information. Depending on the situation, it can be a good idea to ask during the patient interview, "Have you ever suffered from posttraumatic stress disorder?", framing the question to the patient so that they understand that their answer can allow the dentist to create a more positive environment for the patient. Alternatively, the dentist could inquire about any triggers or concerns that the patient has for the upcoming dental care, which demonstrates that the dentist is aware that aspects of the care may be difficult for some people, based on their individual past experiences. This can serve to open a more meaningful dialogue and strengthen a trusting dentist-patient relationship.

38. **What are some special considerations when treating patients with a history of trauma?**
Like treating other anxious patients, dentists want to practice active listening, show compassion, and try to give the patient as much control in the situation as possible. The dentist may offer an initial appointment just to talk, place the chair in an upright position, keep the door open, have an assistant present, check in frequently to see how the patient is doing, offer reassurance, and explain the procedures.

Also, the dentist can offer soothing music, blanket, or body covering (e.g., an x-ray lead apron). It is important that the patient has been instructed to stop the dentist whenever their anxiety level is getting too high, and the dentist responds immediately when the signal to stop is given.

If the patient is unable to tolerate being in the dental chair because their anxiety is uncontrollably high, the dentist might want to refer this patient to a professional who specializes in the treatment of anxiety disorders. Counseling and antianxiety medications can be helpful and, in some cases, may be a prerequisite to dental work being carried out.

39. **How can the patient interview be tailored for a self-identified fearful patient?**
The dentist should recognize a patient's anxiety by acknowledging what the patient says or observing the patient's demeanor. Recognition, which is verbal and nonverbal, may be as simple as saying, "Are you nervous about being here?" This indicates the dentist's concern, acceptance, supportiveness, and intent to help. The dentist

can facilitate patient's cues as they tell their story and help them go from generalizations to specifics, especially to past origins, if possible. The dentists listen for generalizations, distortions, and deletions of information or misinterpretation of events as the patient talks. As the patient is allowed to speak freely, their anxiety decreases as they tell their story, describing the nature of their fear and the attitude of previous doctors. Trust and rapport between doctor and patient also increase as the patient is allowed to speak to someone who cares and listens. As the dentist gives feedback to the patient, this interpretation of the information helps the patient learn new strategies for coping with their feelings and adopting new behaviors by confronting past fears. Thus, a new set of feelings and behaviors may replace maladaptive coping mechanisms. Finally, the dentist makes a commitment to protect the patient—a commitment that the patient may have perceived as absent in past dental experiences. Strategies include allowing the patient to stop a procedure by raising a hand or simply assuring a patient that you are ready to listen at any time.

40. **What are common avoidance behaviors associated with anxious patients?**
Generally, putting off making appointments, followed by cancellations, and failing to appear are routine events for anxious patients. The avoidance of care can be of such magnitude that personal suffering is endured from tooth ailments, with emergency consequences.

41. **Who do dentists often consider their most "difficult" patient?**
Surveys have repeatedly shown that dentists often view the anxious patient as their most difficult challenge. Almost 80% of dentists report that they themselves become anxious with an anxious patient. The ability to carefully assess a patient's emotional needs will help the clinician improve his or her ability to deal effectively with an anxious patient. Furthermore, because anxious patients require more chair time for procedures, are more reactive to stimuli, and associate more sensations with pain, effective anxiety management yields more effective practice management.

42. **What are the major practical considerations in scheduling identified anxious dental patients?**
Autonomic arousal increases in proportion to the length of time before a stressful event. A patient left to anticipate the event with negative self-statements and perhaps frightening images for a whole day or for a long time in the waiting area is less likely to have an easy experience. Thus, it is considered prudent to schedule patients earlier in the day and keep the waiting period after the patient's arrival as short as possible. In addition, the dentist's energy is usually optimal earlier in the day for dealing with more demanding situations.

43. **What do patients describe as qualities and behaviors of a dentist who makes them feel relaxed and lowers their anxiety?**
   - Explains procedures before starting
   - Gives specific information during procedures
   - Verbally supports the patient and gives reassurance
   - Helps the patient redefine the experience to minimize threat
   - Gives the patient some control over procedures and pain
   - Attempts to teach the patient to cope with distress
   - Provides distraction and tension relief

44. **What qualities do patients describe as making them feel satisfied with their dentist and dental experience?**
   - Was friendly
   - Assured me that they would prevent pain
   - Worked quickly, but did not rush
   - Had a calm manner
   - Gave me moral support
   - Reassured me that they would alleviate pain
   - Asked if I was concerned or nervous
   - Made sure I was numb before starting
   - Offered me time to raise questions or concerns

PATIENT EDUCATION

45. **What is the paternalistic model for communicating clinical findings and discussing treatment plans with the patient?**
The paternalistic model creates a dynamic where the dentist assumes the role of the parent and relates to the patient as an immature, inexperienced individual. The patient becomes acquiescent to the directives of the dentist, who has the clinical information and knows what the best treatment is. In this style, the dentist uses their clinical knowledge and values in the decision process, giving the patient little or no autonomy. In essence, the dentist becomes the patient's guardian. This model is like the Guild Model for the patient interview and is discouraged.

46. **What is the informative model for communicating clinical findings and discussing treatment plans with the patient?**
The informative model assumes that the patient is very inquisitive, perhaps even scientific, in their thoughtful analysis of presented information. The objective of the dentist is to provide all the relevant clinical findings and treatment choices to the patient. The patient then can make the decision about what dental treatment he or she wishes to receive. This model gives the patient autonomy to choose based on their values. The dentist only presents the factual objective information and does not include personal values in the decision process. The patient relies on the dentist's clinical knowledge and technical expertise to execute the desired therapy.

47. **What is the interpretive model for communicating clinical findings and discussing treatment plans with the patient?**
The interpretive model creates a cooperative interaction between the dentist and patient in which the patient's values are elucidated and then the appropriate treatment choices are developed that meet the patient's desires. The dentist does not dictate the patient's values but tries to help the patient articulate and understand them. The dentist becomes a counselor, helping create patient autonomy through self-understanding by the patient.

48. **What is the deliberative model for communicating clinical findings and discussing treatment plans with the patient?**
The deliberative model creates a dentist's role as teacher and partner by helping the patient choose the best health-related values that can be realized for the patient's health. After presenting the clinical findings, the dentist explains the values related to the treatment options and expresses their opinions about why some choices are more worthwhile to overall health. The dentist's expression of these values is presented here, but only to help patients in developing their own self-awareness of their choices about health-related issues. Having a dialogue with the patient becomes the goal, with mutual respect preserved.

49. **What is the opportune time to teach new health information to patients?**
Patients are most receptive to learning new health behaviors when there is an immediate need for the new skill or behavior. For example, a patient with gingival bleeding at a furcation site wants to know how to resolve the problem and is most receptive to learning how to use a proxy brush.

50. **What is a strong motivational tool to use for communicating health improvement issues?**
Positive feedback while instructing often yields the greatest acceptance and minimizes patient resistance to compliance. Fear of tooth loss, for example, may not weigh as much in communicating the consequences of not brushing as creating a desire for a healthy smile and teeth that last a lifetime.

51. **In introducing new ideas about oral hygiene, what considerations help maximize compliance?**
People learn best when information is presented in the context of their own personal experience. Additionally, patients come from all levels of educational backgrounds. Whenever possible, avoid medical or dental jargon and find ways to explain otherwise complex topics with simplified language and analogies. By understanding what a patient values, a dentist can educate and counsel the patient in a way that resonates with the patient.

52. **Does self-esteem play a role in adopting new behaviors such as flossing and regular brushing?**
Yes, it absolutely plays a role. Most adults want to learn concepts that enhance or maintain their self-esteem. Enhancing their physical appearance is directly related to the acceptance of new health behaviors.

53. **List four important elements in maximizing the long-term retention of information given by the dental team to patients..**
Repetition of key ideas enhances patient learning and compliance. A patient may recall only one-third of a conversation after 24 hours and even less after 30 days. By artfully repeating ideas and concepts at the initial presentation, recall is maximized.
Interest and direct relevance of information to the patient's specific needs yield the greatest learning experience. A patient with a loose tooth is concerned about why the problem occurred and how to prevent tooth loss. This concern may outweigh issues related to the general concepts of periodontal disease and the outcome of needing full dentures.
Context of the information presented should be within the personal experience of the patient to maximize acceptance and understanding.
Emotion relates to the patient's feelings about dental issues. Understanding relevant emotional history enhances doctor-patient rapport and the patient's trust and acceptance of the suggestions made by the dental team.

54. **When is reassurance most valuable in the clinical session?**
Positive supportive statements to the patient that they are going to do well or be all right are an important part of treatment. At some point, everyone may have doubts or fears about the outcome. Reassurance given too early, such as before a thorough examination of the presenting symptoms, may be interpreted by some patients as

insincerity or as trivializing their problem. The best time for reassurance is after the examination when a tentative diagnosis is reached. The support is best received by the patient at this point.

55. **When is the best time to inform patient of possible negative outcomes and side effects of treatment?**

The best time to discuss treatment outcomes, such as postoperative sensitivity following a restorative procedure and difficulty in becoming accustomed to a new complete denture, is prior to treatment being initiated. By providing this information in advance, the patient not only is making an informed decision about the subsequent treatment but has the correct expectations. Tempering expectations is an important aspect of patient management and helps allow for a positive patient experience. It is much more challenging to inform the patient of a treatment complication after it has occurred, and this occurrence can erode a patient's trust.

ACKNOWLEDGMENT

The authors gratefully acknowledge the contributions of previous chapter authors.

BIBLIOGRAPHY

Bochner S. *The Psychology of the Dentist-Patient Relationship.* New York, NY: Springer-Verlag; 1998.

Corah N. Dental anxiety: assessment, reduction and increasing patient satisfaction. *Dent Clin North Am.* 1988;32:779–790.

Cross T, Bazron B, Dennis K, Isaacs M. *Towards a Culturally Competent System of Care.* Vol 1. Washington, DC: CASSP Technical Assistance Center, Center for Child Health and Mental Health Policy, Georgetown University Child Development Center; 1989.

Rubin JG, Slovin M, Krochak M. Dental phobia and anxiety. *Dent Clin North Am.* 1988;32:647–840.

Dixon Sarah A, Branch Morris A. *Post Traumatic Stress Disorders (PTSD) and Dental Practice, Clinical Update.* vol. 30. Bethesda, MD: Naval Postgraduate Dental School; 2008.

Dworkin SF, Ference TP, Giddon DB. *Behavioral Science in Dental Practice.* St. Louis, MO, Mosby.

Friedman N. Psychosedation. Part 2: Iatrosedation. In: McCarthy FM, ed. *Emergencies in Dental Practice.* 3rd ed. Philadelphia, PA, WB Saunders; 236–265.

Friedman N, Cecchini JJ, Wexler M, et al. A dentist-oriented fear reduction technique: the iatrosedative process. *Compend Cont Educ Dent.* 1989;10:113–118.

Gelboy MJ. *Communication and Behavior Management in Dentistry.* London: Williams & Watkins; 1990.

Gerber MR. *Trauma-Informed Healthcare Approaches: A Guide to Primary Care.* Springer; 2019.

Gregg JM. Psychosedation. Part 1: The nature and control of pain, anxiety, and stress. In McCarthy FM, ed. *Emergencies in Dental Practice.* 3rd ed Philadelphia, PA, W.B. Saunders, pp. 220–235.

Jacquot J: *Trust in the dentist-patient relationship (website),* 2005. http://www.jyi.org/?s=trust+in+the+dentist-patient+relationship. Accessed April 4, 2014.

Jepsen CH: Behavioral foundations of dental practice. In Williams A, editor: *Clark's Clinical Dentistry,* vol 5. Philadelphia, PA, J.B. Lippincott, pp. 1–18.

Krochak M, Rubin JG. An overview of the treatment of anxious and phobic dental patients. *Compend Cont Educ Dent.* 1993;14:604–615.

Liu M: *The dentist/patient relationship: The role of dental anxiety (website),* 2011. http://scholarship.claremont.edu/cmc_theses/277. Accessed April 4, 2014.

Magee J. Trauma informed approach to dental care. *J Mass Dent Soc.* 2019:12–16.

Wirth FH: Knowing your patient. Part I: The role of empathy in practicing dentistry (website). http://www.spiritofcaring.com/public/218print.cfm?sd=75. Accessed May 2, 14.

CHAPTER 2

TREATMENT PLANNING AND ORAL DIAGNOSIS

Stephen T. Sonis, Nathaniel Treister

TREATMENT PLANNING

1. **What are the objectives of pretreatment evaluation of a patient?**
   1. Establishment of a diagnosis
   2. Determination of underlying medical conditions that may modify the oral condition or require modification of dental treatment plan
   3. Discovery of concomitant illnesses
   4. Prevention of medical emergencies associated with dental treatment
   5. Establishment of rapport with the patient

2. **What are the essential elements of a patient history?**
   1. Chief complaint
   2. History of the present illness (HPI)
   3. Past medical history
   4. Social history
   5. Family history
   6. Review of systems
   7. Dental history

3. **Define the chief complaint..**
   The chief complaint is the reason that the patient seeks care, as described in the patient's own words.

4. **What is the history of the present illness?**
   The history of present illness (HPI) is a chronologic description of the patient's symptoms and should include information about duration, location, character, and previous treatment.

5. **What elements need to be included in the medical history?**
   - Current status of the patient's general health
   - Medications
   - Hospitalizations and surgeries
   - Allergies

6. **What areas are routinely investigated in the social history?**
   - Present and past occupations
   - Smoking, alcohol, or drug use
   - Occupational hazards
   - Marital status and relevant sexual history

7. **Why is the family history of interest to the dentist?**
   The family history often provides information about diseases of genetic origin or diseases that have a familial tendency. Examples include clotting disorders, atherosclerotic heart disease, psychiatric diseases, and diabetes mellitus.

8. **How is the medical history usually obtained?**
   The medical history is obtained with a written/electronic questionnaire supplemented by a verbal history. The verbal history is imperative because patients may leave out or misinterpret questions on the written form. For example, some patients may take daily aspirin and yet not consider it a "true" medication. Similarly, patients who are treated with an annual infusion of zoledronic acid or denosumab for osteoporosis may not consider this a medication. The verbal history also allows the clinician to pursue positive answers on the written form and, in doing so, establish rapport with the patient.

9. **What techniques are used for physical examination of the patient? How are they used in dentistry?**
   Inspection, the most commonly used technique, is based on visual evaluation of the patient. Palpation, which involves touching and feeling the patient, is used to determine the consistency and shape of masses in the mouth,

jaws, or neck. Percussion, which involves differences in sound transmission of structures, has little application to the head and neck. Auscultation, the technique of listening to differences in the transmission of sound, is usually accomplished with a stethoscope. In dentistry, auscultation may be used to listen to changes in sounds emanating from the temporomandibular joint, as well as during routine blood pressure measurement.

10. What are the patient's vital signs?
    - Blood pressure
    - Respiratory rate
    - Pulse
    - Temperature

11. What are the normal values for the vital signs?
    - Blood pressure: 120 mm Hg/80 mm Hg
    - Respiratory rate: 16 to 20 respirations per minute
    - Pulse: 72 beats per minute
    - Temperature: 98.6°F or 37°C

12. What is a complete blood count (CBC)?
    A CBC consists of measurements of the patient's hemoglobin, hematocrit, white blood cell count, differential white blood cell count, and platelet count.

13. What are the normal ranges of a CBC?

Hemoglobin:	Men, 14-18 g/dL Women, 12-16 g/dL	Differential white blood count: Neutrophils, 50%-70%
Hematocrit:	Men, 40%-54% Women, 37%-47%	Lymphocytes, 30%-40% Monocytes, 3%-7%
White blood count:	4,000-10,000 cells/mm^3	Eosinophils, 0%-5%
Platelet count:	150,000-400,000 cells/mm^3	Basophils, 0%-1%

14. What is the most effective blood test to screen for diabetes mellitus?
    The most effective screening test for diabetes mellitus is fasting blood glucose. The glycosylated hemoglobin test (HGbA1c, usually just called A1c) can be ordered without fasting and effectively assesses glucose levels over a 90-day period. A1c is typically used to monitor patients, rather than for diagnostic screening.

15. What is a normal A1C? A normal fasting blood glucose?
    An A1C below 5.7% is considered to be normal. Whereas pre-diabetes is considered with levels between 5.7% and 6.4%, and diabetes with levels of 6.5% and above. Fasting blood glucose (FBG) levels up to 99 mg/dL are considered to be normal. FBGs of 100 mg/dL to 125 mg/dL are associated with pre-diabetes and above 125 mg/dL, diabetes.

ORAL DIAGNOSIS

16. What is the technique of choice for the diagnosis of a soft tissue lesion in the mouth?
    With a few exceptions, a biopsy is the diagnostic technique of choice for soft tissue lesions of the mouth that can't otherwise be easily diagnosed based on clinical features alone.

17. Is there any alternative diagnostic technique to biopsy for the evaluation of suspected malignancies of the mouth?
    Exfoliative cytology may be used for the diagnosis of oral lesions. Because of its high false-negative rate, it has never been particularly effective. A commercial laboratory has kit that includes the use of a brush to obtain a cell sample and then a specific processing and evaluation procedure that increases the sensitivity of the assay. Biopsy remains the most reliable way to make a diagnosis.

18. When is immunofluorescence of value in oral diagnosis?
    Immunofluorescent techniques are used in the diagnosis of autoimmune vesiculobullous diseases that affect the mouth, including pemphigus vulgaris and mucous membrane pemphigoid. Immunofluorescence can also be used in the diagnosis and typing of herpes simplex virus (HSV) infection.

19. When is it appropriate to use microbiologic culturing in oral diagnosis?
    1. **Bacterial infection.** Because the majority of oral infections are sensitive to treatment with penicillin, routine bacteriologic culture of primary dental infections is not generally indicated (or cost effective). However, cultures are indicated for patients who are immunocompromised or myelosuppressed for two reasons: (1) they are at significant risk for sepsis; and (2) the oral flora often change in these patients. Cultures should be obtained for infections that are refractory to the initial course of antibiotics before changing antibiotics.
    2. **Viral infection.** Immunocompromised patients who present with mucosal ulcerations may be manifesting signs of a herpes simplex infection. In most routine situations, HSV PCR is typically ordered as it is a simple

and inexpensive test that provides rapid results. Viral culture for HSV diagnosis is generally reserved for situations in which there is suspicion for acyclovir resistance and drug susceptibility testing is necessary. Routine culturing for typical secondary herpes infections (herpes labialis) is not warranted for healthy patients. Once a specimen is obtained (in appropriate viral medium), it should be kept on ice and transported to the laboratory as quickly as possible because viral specimens are highly temperature-sensitive.

3. **Fungal infection.** Candidiasis is the most common fungal infection affecting the oral mucosa. Because its appearance is often varied, especially in immunocompromised patients, fungal cultures may be of value. Similar to use of viral culture, fungal culture is indicated in cases of antifungal drug resistance so that drug susceptibility testing can be performed. It must be noted that a positive fungal culture does not confirm infection, but only the presence of fungal organisms.

20. **How do you obtain access to a clinical laboratory?**
It is easy to obtain laboratory tests for your patients, even if you do not practice in a hospital. Community hospitals provide almost all laboratory services that your patients may require. Usually, the laboratory provides order slips and culture tubes. Simply indicate the test needed, and send the patient to the laboratory. Patients who need a test at night or on a weekend can generally be accommodated through the hospital's emergency department. Commercial laboratories also may be used, and they also supply order forms. If you practice in a medical building with other physicians, find out which laboratory they use. If they use a commercial laboratory, a pick-up service for specimens may be provided.

21. **Which laboratory tests should be used to assess a patient who may be at risk for a deficiency in hemostasis?**
The basic laboratory tests for a possible deficiency in hemostasis that may lead to excess/uncontrolled bleeding following an invasive dental procedure should include assessments of platelet count and clotting factors of the internal and external pathways. The three essential tests are a complete blood count (CBC), which includes platelet count, prothrombin time (typically expressed as the international normalized ratio, or INR), and partial thromboplastin time.

22. **What positive responses in the medical history should suggest to you that a patient may have a problem with hemostasis?**
- Family history of a bleeding problem, such as hemophilia
- Taking medications that can cause thrombocytopenia, such as cancer chemotherapy
- History of a disease that may cause thrombocytopenia
- Taking medications known to cause prolonged bleeding, such as aspirin, warfarin, or vitamin E
- History of liver disease

23. **What are the causes of halitosis?**
Halitosis may be caused by local factors in the mouth, or by extraoral or systemic factors. Local factors include food retention, periodontal infection, caries, acute necrotizing gingivitis, mucosal infection, and salivary gland hypofunction. Extraoral and systemic causes of halitosis include smoking, alcohol ingestion, pulmonary or bronchial disease, metabolic defects, diabetes mellitus, sinusitis, and tonsillitis.

24. **Which bacteria are associated with halitosis?**
Gram-negative anaerobes are associated with halitosis.

25. **Which gases are associated with halitosis?**
Volatile sulfur compounds—in particular, hydrogen sulfide, methyl mercaptan, and dimethyl sulfide—are associated with halitosis.

26. **What are the most commonly abused substances in the United States?**
- Alcohol
- Cannabis
- Cocaine
- Phencyclidine (PCP)
- Heroin
- Methamphetamines
- Prescription medications
  1. Narcotic analgesics
  2. Tricyclic antidepressants
  3. Sedative-hypnotics
  4. Stimulants
  5. Anxiolytic agents
  6. Diet aids

27. **What are the common causes of lymphadenopathy?**
- Infectious and inflammatory diseases of all types—oral conditions that can cause lymphadenopathy in the head and neck region include herpes infections, dental infection, pericoronitis, aphthous or traumatic ulceration, and acute necrotizing ulcerative gingivitis

- Immunologic diseases, such as rheumatoid arthritis, systemic lupus erythematosus, and drug reactions
- Malignant disease, such as Hodgkin disease, non-Hodgkin lymphoma, leukemia, and metastatic disease from solid tumors
- Hyperthyroidism
- Lipid storage diseases, such as Gaucher disease and Niemann-Pick disease
- Other conditions, including sarcoidosis, amyloidosis, and granulomatosis

28. **How can one differentiate between lymphadenopathy associated with an inflammatory process and lymphadenopathy associated with tumor?**
    - Onset and duration. Inflammatory nodes tend to have a more acute onset and course than nodes associated with malignancy.
    - Identification of an associated infected site. An identifiable site of infection associated with an enlarged lymph node is probably the source of the lymphadenopathy. Effective treatment of the site should result in resolution of the lymphadenopathy.
    - Symptoms. Enlarged lymph nodes associated with an inflammatory process are usually tender to palpation. Nodes associated with cancer are not.
    - Progression. Continuous enlargement over time is associated with cancer.
    - Fixation. Inflammatory nodes are usually freely movable, whereas nodes associated with tumor are hard and fixed.
    - Lack of response to antibiotic therapy. Continued nodal enlargement in the face of appropriate antibiotic therapy for a presumed bacterial infection should be viewed as suspicious for malignancy.
    - Distribution. Unilateral nodal enlargement is a common presentation for malignant disease. In contrast, bilateral enlargement is often associated with systemic processes.

29. **What is the most appropriate technique for lymph node diagnosis?**
    The most appropriate technique for lymph node diagnosis is biopsy or needle aspiration. Needle aspiration is preferred as it is less invasive, but it is more technique sensitive.

30. **What are the most frequent causes of intraoral swelling?**
    The most frequent causes of intraoral swelling are infection and neoplasm (benign or malignant).

31. **Why do humans get parotitis?**
    A viral or bacterial infection is the most common cause of parotitis in humans. Viruses causing parotitis include mumps, coxsackie, cytomegalovirus, and influenza. *Staphylococcus aureus,* the most common bacterial cause of parotitis, results in the production of pus within the gland. Other bacteria, such as *Actinomyces,* streptococci, and gram-negative bacilli, may also cause suppurative parotitis. Risk factors for bacterial parotitis include salivary hypofunction, obstruction (sialolithiasis), and malnutrition.

32. **Why does Polly get parotitis?**
    Polly gets it from too many crackers.

33. **What are common causes of xerostomia?**
    - Dehydration
    - Medications
    - Radiation therapy (head and neck)
    - Sjögren syndrome
    - Advanced age

34. **What is the presentation of a patient with a tumor of the parotid gland? How is the diagnosis made?**
    The typical patient with a parotid gland tumor presents with a firm, fixed mass in the region of the gland. Involvement of the facial nerve is common and results in facial palsy. Fine-needle biopsy is a commonly used technique for diagnosis. However, the small sample obtained by this technique may be limiting and an open biopsy may be necessary. Computed tomography (CT) and magnetic resonance imaging (MRI) are also often helpful for evaluating suspected tumors.

35. **What are the major risk factors for oral and oropharyngeal cancers?**
    Human papilloma virus (HPV) is now the most common etiologic factor associated with new cancers of the oral cavity and oropharynx and is associated with about 70% of new cases in the United States. Tobacco and alcohol use remain significant risk factors, especially for cancers of the mouth.

36. **What is the most common location of squamous cell carcinoma of the tongue?**
    The most common location is the lateral or ventral edge of the posterior tongue.

37. **Summarize the impact of early detection on the survival rates for cancers of the oral cavity and oropharynx**
    The survival rate for oral and oropharyngeal cancers is directly related to how advanced the tumor is at the time of diagnosis. Whereas localized tumors (early stage) have an excellent overall survival rate of 85%, that rate drops

to under 70% for patients with local spread of their cancer and plummets to 40% for patients with metastatic disease.

38. How is oral cancer staged?
Tumor staging is a system whereby cancers are clinically defined and categorized based on the parameters of *t*umor size, involvement of local *n*odes, and *m*etastases (TNM).

39. What is staging for cancer? What are the criteria for staging cancers of the mouth?
Staging is a method of defining the clinical status of a cancer diagnosis in order to determine the extent of disease, likely future clinical behavior, and most appropriate therapy. Thus, it is related to prognosis and is helpful for providing a basis for treatment planning. The staging system used for oral cancers is called the TNM system. It is based on three parameters: T = size of the tumor on a scale from 0 (no evidence of primary tumor) to 3 (tumor > 4 cm in greatest diameter); N = involvement of regional lymph nodes on a scale from 0 (no clinically palpable cervical nodes) to 3 (clinically palpable lymph nodes that are fixed; metastases suspected); and M = presence of distant metastases on a scale from 0 (no distant metastases) to 1 (clinical or radiographic evidence of metastases to nodes other than those in the cervical chain).

40. How can toluidine blue stain be used in oral diagnosis?
Because toluidine blue is a metachromatic nuclear stain, it has been reported to be preferentially absorbed by dysplastic and cancerous epithelium. Consequently, it has been used as a technique to screen oral lesions and to determine the best site for obtaining a biopsy. The technique has a reported false-positive rate of 9% and a false-negative rate of 5%.

41. What are the two most common clinical presentations of oral cancers?
The two most common clinical presentations of oral cancer are a nonhealing ulcer or an area of leukoplakia, often accompanied by erythema.

42. What percentage of keratotic white lesions in the mouth are dysplastic or cancerous?
Keratotic white lesions are generally regarded as leukoplakia. The term has had inconsistent interpretations, but is now considered simply to be a nonscrapable, keratotic plaque. The risk of such lesions being dysplastic or cancerous is between 5% and 15% (although there is some evidence to suggest that the risk may be higher). The risk is higher in smokers.

43. What is a simple way to differentiate clinically between necrotic and keratotic white lesions of the oral mucosa?
Necrotic lesions of the mucosa, such as those caused by burns or candidal infections, scrape off when gently rubbed with a moist tongue blade. Conversely, because keratotic lesions result from epithelial changes, scraping fails to dislodge them.

44. How long should one wait before obtaining a biopsy of an oral ulcer?
Almost all ulcers caused by trauma or aphthous stomatitis heal within 14 days of presentation. Consequently, any ulcer that is present for 2 weeks or longer should be biopsied.

45. What is the differential diagnosis of ulcers of the oral mucosa?
- Traumatic ulcer
- Aphthous stomatitis
- Oral lichen planus
- Mucous membrane pemphigoid
- Pemphigus vulgaris
- Cancer
- Tuberculosis
- Recrudescent HSV infection
- Chancre of syphilis
- Noma
- Necrotizing sialometaplasia
- Deep fungal infection
- Cytomegalovirus (CMV) infection

46. Why is it a good idea to aspirate a pigmented lesion before obtaining a biopsy?
Because pigmented lesions may be vascular in nature, prebiopsy aspiration is prudent to prevent unanticipated hemorrhage.

47. What are the major causes of pigmented oral and perioral lesions?
Pigmented lesions are caused by endogenous or exogenous sources. **Endogenous sources** include melanoma, endocrine-related pigmentation (e.g., as in Addison disease), perioral pigmentation associated with intestinal polyposis or Peutz-Jeghers syndrome, and varices (i.e., "varix" of lip vermilion). **Exogenous sources** of pigmentation include heavy metal poisoning (e.g., lead), amalgam tattoos, and changes caused by chemicals or

medications. A common example of medication-related changes is black hairy tongue associated with antibiotics, particularly tetracycline, or bismuth-containing compounds, such as Pepto-Bismol.

48. **Do any diseases of the oral cavity also present with lesions of the skin?**
Numerous diseases can cause simultaneous lesions of the mouth and skin—these are referred to as mucocutaneous disorders (and may involve other mucosal sites, such as female genitalia). Among the most common are lichen planus, erythema multiforme, lupus erythematosus, bullous pemphigoid, and pemphigus vulgaris.

49. **What is the appearance of the skin lesion associated with erythema multiforme?**
The skin lesion of erythema multiforme looks like an archery target, with a central erythematous bull's eye and a circular peripheral area. Hence, the lesions are called bull's-eye or target(oid) lesions.

50. **A 25-year-old woman presents with a chief complaint of spontaneously bleeding gingiva. She also notes malaise. On oral examination, you find that her hygiene is excellent. Would you suspect a local or systemic basis for her symptoms? What tests might you order to make a diagnosis?**
Spontaneous bleeding, especially in the presence of good oral hygiene, is most likely of systemic origin. Gingival bleeding is among the most common presenting signs of acute leukemia, which should be high on the differential diagnosis. A CBC and platelet count should provide data to help establish a preliminary diagnosis. Definitive diagnosis most likely requires a bone marrow biopsy. Such a patient should be referred to their primary care physician or an emergency room for further evaluation and management.

51. **A 45-year-old overweight man presents with suppurative periodontitis. As you review his history, he tells you that he is always hungry, drinks water almost every hour, and awakens four times each night to urinate. Which systemic disease is most likely a cofactor in his periodontal disease? What test(s) might you order to help you with a diagnosis?**
The combination of polyuria, polyphagia, polydipsia, and suppurative periodontal disease should raise a strong suspicion of undiagnosed or poorly controlled diabetes mellitus. A fasting blood glucose test is the most efficacious screen.

52. **A 60-year-old woman presents with a complaint of numbness of the left side of her mandible. Four years ago, she had a mastectomy for treatment of breast cancer. What diagnosis must be considered? What is the first step that you take to confirm it?**
The mandible is not an infrequent site for metastatic breast cancer. As the metastatic lesion grows, it puts pressure on the inferior alveolar nerve and causes paresthesia. Radiographic evaluation of the jaw is a reasonable first step to make a diagnosis. If the oncologist has suspicion in a patient without history of metastatic disease, a positron emission tomography (PET)/CT will be ordered that would demonstrate "PET avidity" or increased activity in the area of concern.

53. **Which endocrine disease may present with pigmented lesions of the oral mucosa?**
Pigmented lesions of the oral mucosa may suggest Addison disease.

54. **What drugs may cause gingival hyperplasia?**
- Phenytoin
- Cyclosporine
- Nifedipine

55. **What is the most typical presentation of the oral lesions of tuberculosis? How do you make a diagnosis?**
The oral lesions of tuberculosis are thought to result from organisms brought into contact with the oral mucosa by sputum originating at the site of infection in the lung. A nonhealing ulcer, which is impossible to differentiate clinically from carcinoma, is the most common presentation in the mouth. Ulcers are typically located on the lateral borders of the tongue and may have a purulent center. Lymphadenopathy also may be present. Diagnosis is made by histologic examination and demonstration of organisms in the tissue.

56. **What are the typical oral manifestations of a patient with pernicious anemia?**
Pernicious anemia is caused by a vitamin B_{12} deficiency caused by a lack of intestinal absorption. The most common oral manifestation is a smooth, dorsal surface of the tongue denuded of papillae that may be associated with sensitivity and burning. Angular cheilitis is a frequent accompanying finding.

57. **What is angular cheilitis? What is its cause?**
Angular cheilitis, or cheilosis, is fissuring or cracking at the corners of the mouth. The condition typically occurs because of a localized mixed infection of bacteria and fungi. Angular cheilitis most frequently results from a change in the local environment caused by excessive saliva because of loss of the vertical dimension between the maxilla and mandible. In addition, several systemic conditions, such as deficiency anemias and long-term immunosuppression, predispose to the condition.

58. **What is the classic oral manifestation of Crohn disease?**
Mucosal lesions with a cobblestone appearance are associated with Crohn disease. These lesions may include non-specific, irregular, deep linear ulcerations, often in the mandibular buccal vestibules. Oral manifestations of Crohn disease may also include aphthous-like lesions, orofacial granulomatosis, and angular cheilitis.

59. **List the oral changes that may occur in a patient receiving radiation therapy for treatment of a tumor on the base of the tongue..**
    - Xerostomia
    - Cervical, interproximal and incisal edge caries
    - Osteoradionecrosis
    - Mucositis
    - Trismus

60. **A patient presents for extraction of a carious tooth. In taking the history, you learn that the patient is undergoing chemotherapy for treatment of a breast carcinoma. What information is critical before proceeding with the extraction?**
Because cancer chemotherapy nonspecifically affects the bone marrow, the patient is likely to be myelosuppressed after treatment. Therefore, you need to know the patient's white blood cell count and platelet count before initiating treatment. Because antiresorptive therapy (e.g., zoledronic acid, denosumab) may constitute part of the supportive care regimen, the patient might be at risk for developing medication-related osteonecrosis of the jaw. Communication with the patient's oncologist is critical to determine the best time to perform the extraction to minimize the risk of post-operative bleeding or infection.

61. **What oral findings have been associated with use of the diuretic hydrochlorothiazide?**
Lichen planus has been associated with hydrochlorothiazide.

62. **Some patients believe that topical application of an aspirin to the mucosa next to a tooth will help to manage acute odontogenic pain. How may you detect this form of therapy by looking in the patient's mouth?**
Because of its acidity, topical application of aspirin to the mucosa frequently causes a chemical burn, which appears as a white necrotic lesion in the area corresponding to aspirin placement.

63. **What are the possible causes of oral burning symptoms?**
    1. Dry mouth
    2. Nutritional deficiencies
    3. Diabetes mellitus
    4. Psychogenic factors
    5. Medications
    6. Acid reflux from the stomach
    7. Hormonal imbalances
    8. Allergy
    9. Chronic infections (especially fungal)
    10. Blood dyscrasias
    11. Anemia
    12. Iatrogenic factors
    13. Inflammatory conditions such as lichen planus

64. **What is the most important goal in the evaluation of a taste disorder?**
The most important goal in evaluating a taste disorder is the elimination of any underlying neurologic, olfactory, or systemic disorder as a cause of the condition.

65. **What drugs often prescribed by dentists may affect taste or smell?**
    1. Metronidazole
    2. Benzocaine
    3. Ampicillin
    4. Tetracycline
    5. Sodium lauryl sulfate toothpaste
    6. Codeine

66. **What systemic conditions may affect smell and/or taste?**
    1. Bell's palsy
    2. Multiple sclerosis
    3. Head trauma
    4. Cancer
    5. Chronic renal failure
    6. Cirrhosis

7. Niacin deficiency
8. Adrenal insufficiency
9. Cushing syndrome
10. Diabetes mellitus
11. Sjögren syndrome
12. Radiation therapy to the head and neck
13. Viral infections
14. Hypertension
15. Dysesthesias

67. **What is burning mouth syndrome?**

Burning mouth syndrome, also referred to as glossodynia or stomatodynia, is characterized by unprovoked oral burning that most commonly affects the tongue, anterior aspects of the lips, and anterior hard palate. It is a diagnosis of exclusion in which the mucosa appears normal and is not associated with any underlying disease. Other frequently associated symptoms include xerostomia and dysgeusia. While many treatments appear to be effective, the highest level of evidence supports use of topical or systemic clonazepam. Clinical trials demonstrate a high placebo response among patients suffering with the condition.

68. **What questions should a clinician consider before ordering a diagnostic test to supplement a clinical examination?**

- What is the likelihood that the disease is present, given the history, clinical findings, and known risk factors?
- How serious is the condition? What are the consequences of a delay in diagnosis?
- Is an appropriate diagnostic test available? How sensitive and accurate is it?
- Are the costs, risks, and ease of administering the test justified?

69. **Distinguish among the accuracy, sensitivity, and specificity of a particular diagnostic test..**

The **accuracy** is a measure of the overall agreement between the test and a gold standard. The more accurate the test, the fewer false-negative or false-positive results. In contrast, the **sensitivity** of the test measures its ability to show a positive result when the disease is present. The more sensitive the test, the fewer false-negatives. The **specificity** of the test measures the ability to show a negative finding in people who do not have the condition; the more specific the test, the fewer false-positives.

70. **What is meant by FNA? When is it used?**

No, FNA is not an abbreviation for the Finnish Naval Association. It refers to a diagnostic technique termed *fine-needle aspiration,* in which a 22-gauge needle on a syringe is used to aspirate cells from a suspicious lesion for pathologic analysis. Otolaryngologists use the technique to aid in the diagnosis of cancers of the head and neck. It can be particularly valuable for the diagnosis of submucosal tumors, such as lymphoma, salivary gland tumors, and parapharyngeal masses that are not easily accessible for routine surgical biopsy. Like many techniques, the efficacy of FNA depends on the skill of the operator and experience of the interpreting cytopathologist.

71. **Which systemic diseases have been associated with alterations in salivary gland function?**

1. Cystic fibrosis
2. Human immunodeficiency virus (HIV) infection
3. Diabetes mellitus
4. Affective disorder
5. Metabolic disturbances (e.g., malnutrition, dehydration, vitamin deficiency)
6. Renal disease
7. Cirrhosis
8. Thyroid disease
9. Autoimmune disease (e.g., Sjögren syndrome, myasthenia gravis, graft-versus-host disease, IgG4-related disease)
10. Sarcoidosis
11. Autonomic dysfunction
12. Alzheimer disease
13. Cancer

72. **What is PCR? Why is it an important technique in oral diagnosis?**

Polymerase chain reaction (PCR) is a technique developed by researchers in molecular biology for the enzymatic amplification of selected DNA sequences. Because of its exquisite sensitivity and relatively low cost compared with other techniques (e.g., cell culture), PCR is frequently used for the diagnosis of viral diseases of the head and neck, particularly herpes simplex virus (HSV). PCR testing has been an important component of COVID screening.

73. **What conditions and diseases may cause blistering (vesiculobullous lesions) in the mouth?**

- Viral disease
- Lichen planus
- Pemphigoid

- Pemphigus vulgaris
- Erythema multiforme

74. What are the most common sites of intraoral cancer?

The posterior lateral and ventral surfaces of the tongue are the most common sites of intraoral cancer. The soft palate, posterior third of the tongue, and tonsillar pillars are common sites of oropharyngeal cancer.

BIBLIOGRAPHY

Furness S, Bryan G, McMillan R, Worthington HV. Interventions for the management of dry mouth: non-pharmacological interventions. *Cochrane Database Syst Rev.* 2013;9:CD009603.

Harahap M. How to biopsy oral lesions. *J Dermatol Surg Oncol.* 1989;15:1077–1080.

Heslop G, Oliver CL. Modern approach to the neck mass. *Surg Clin North Am.* 2022;102(2S):e1–e6.

Jones JH, Mason DK. *Oral Manifestations of Systemic Disease.* 2nd ed. Philadelphia: Baillière Tindall-WB Saunders; 1980.

Lamster IB. Preface. Primary health care in the dental office. *Dental Clin North Am.* 2012;56:ix–xi.

Matthews, Banting DW, Bohay RN. The use of diagnostic tests to aid clinical diagnosis. *J Can Dent Assoc.* 1995;61:785–791.

Memon MA, Memon HA, Muhammad FE, et al. Aetiology and associations of halitosis: a systematic review. *Oral Dis.* 2022. https://doi.org/10.1111/odi.14172. Online ahead of print.

Rose LF, Steinberg BJ. Patient evaluation. *Dent Clin North Am.* 1987;31:53–73.

Sollecito TP, Stoopler ET. Clinical approaches to oral mucosal disorders. *Dent Clin North Am.* 2013;57:ix–xi.

Warnakulasuriya S, Kerr AR. Oral cancer screening: past, present, and future. *J Dent Res.* 2021;100(12):1313–1320.

CHAPTER 3

MANAGEMENT OF MEDICALLY COMPLEX PATIENTS

Alessandro Villa, Deborah P. Saunders

A SHORT HISTORY OF MEDICINE
2000 BC "Here, eat this root."
1000 BC "That root is heathen. Say this prayer."
1850 AD "That prayer is superstition. Drink this potion."
1940 AD "That potion is snake oil. Swallow this pill."
1985 AD "That pill is ineffective. Take this antibiotic."
2000 AD "That antibiotic is artificial. Here, eat this root."

—Authors Unknown

DISORDERS OF HEMOSTASIS

1. **What questions should be asked to screen a patient for potential bleeding problems?**
   The best screening procedure for a bleeding disorder is a thorough medical history. If the review of the medical history indicates a bleeding problem, a more detailed history is needed. The following questions may be asked:
   a. Is there a family history of bleeding problems?
   b. Is there excessive bleeding after tooth extractions or other surgeries?
   c. Has there been excessive bleeding after trauma, such as minor cuts and falls?
   d. Does the patient bruise easily or have frequent nosebleeds?
   e. Is the patient taking any medications that affect bleeding, such as acetylsalicylic acid, commonly prescribed anticoagulants (e.g., warfarin [Coumadin], enoxaparin [Lovenox], dabigatran [Pradaxa], rivaroxaban [Xarelto], and apixaban [Eliquis], heparin), herbal medications, chemotherapy, or antibiotics?
   f. Does the patient have any known illnesses that are associated with bleeding (e.g., hemophilia, leukemia, renal disease, liver diseases, cardiac diseases)?
   g. Has the patient ever had spontaneous episodes of bleeding from anywhere in the body?

2. **What laboratory tests should be ordered if a bleeding problem is suspected?**
   - Platelet count: normal values = 150,000 to 450,000 cells/mm^3
   - Prothrombin time (PT): normal value = 10 to 13.5 seconds
   - International normalized ratio (INR): normal value = 1 to 2 (only useful for those patients on known anticoagulant medications)
   - Activated partial thromboplastin time (aPTT): normal value = 25 to 36 seconds
   - Thrombin time (TT): normal value = 9 to 13 seconds
   - Bleeding time: normal value ≤9 minutes (bleeding time is a nonspecific predictor of platelet function and has limited utility in dentistry)

   Normal values may vary from one laboratory to another. It is important to check the normal values for the laboratory that you use. If any of the tests are abnormal, the patient should be referred to a hematologist for evaluation before treatment is performed.

3. **What are the clinical indications for use of 1-deamino-8-D-arginine vasopressin (DDAVP) in dental patients?**
   DDAVP (desmopressin) is a synthetic antidiuretic hormone that controls bleeding in patients with type I von Willebrand's disease, platelet defects secondary to uremia related to renal dialysis, and immunogenic thrombocytopenic purpura (ITP). DDAVP can be delivered intravenously, subcutaneously, or as a nasal spray. DDAVP should not be used in patients younger than 2 years; caution is necessary in older patients and patients receiving intravenous fluids. It should be avoided or used with extreme care in patients with cardiovascular disease and pregnant women. In consultation with a patient's hematologist, it can be used to reduce the risk of excessive bleeding after surgical procedures.

4. **What is hemophilia A?**
   Hemophilia A is an X-linked inherited bleeding disorder characterized by a deficiency of clotting factor VIII.

5. **What is hemophilia B?**
   Hemophilia B is an X-linked inherited bleeding disorder characterized by a deficiency of clotting factor IX.

6. **How is bleeding in hemophilias managed?**
In general, bleeding in hemophilia A and hemophilia B patients requires factor replacement (factor VIII for hemophilia A and factor IX for hemophilia B) and should be coordinated by the patient's hematologist. The dose and duration of factor replacement treatment depend on patient's related factors and the type of the procedure. Preoperative factor levels should be at least 40% to 50% of normal to reduce the risk of postoperative bleeding.

Adjunctive treatment with ε-aminocaproic acid (Amicar) and tranexamic acid can reduce the amount of factor replacement treatment needed.

7. **How does bleeding typically manifest in a patient with thrombocytopenia compared with a patient with hemophilia?**
Patients with severe thrombocytopenia typically present with mucosal bleeds. Patients with hemophilia typically present with deep hemorrhage in weight-bearing joints.

8. **When do you use ε-aminocaproic acid or tranexamic acid?**
ε-Aminocaproic acid (Amicar) and tranexamic acid are antifibrinolytic agents that inhibit the activation of plasminogen. They are used to prevent clot lysis in patients with hereditary clotting disorders.

Aminocaproic acid is available as oral solution 25% (236.5 mL), oral tablets (500 mg, 1000 mg), and intravenous solution 250 mg/mL. The oral solution can be swished and swallowed, or soaked in gauze for management of postoperative bleeding.

Tranexamic acid is available via IV administration and it also comes in a mouth rinse formulation (4.8%), which can be used as a local hemostatic agent (10 mL, up to four times daily). The mouth rinse is not currently available for use in the United States.

9. **What is the minimal acceptable platelet count for an oral surgical procedure?**
The normal platelet count is 150,000 to 450,000 cells/mm^3. In general, the minimal count for an oral surgical procedure is 50,000 platelets. However, emergency procedures may be done with as few as 30,000 platelets if the dentist is working closely with the patient's hematologist and uses excellent techniques of tissue management. Patients with severe thrombocytopenia (<20,000 cells/mm^3) are at significant risk for spontaneous bleeding and often require platelet transfusions.

10. **For a patient taking warfarin (Coumadin), a dental surgical procedure can be done without undue risk of bleeding if the PT is below what value?**
Warfarin affects clotting factors II, VII, IX, and X by impairing the conversion of vitamin K to its active form. The normal PT for a healthy patient is 10.0 to 13.5 seconds. The normal INR is 1 to 2. Oral procedures with a risk of bleeding should not be attempted if the PT is more than 1.5 times normal (>18 seconds). Caution must be taken when the INR is greater than 2. Patients taking warfarin usually have a normal therapeutic INR in the 2 to 3 range, and simple dental prophylaxis can usually be accomplished with an INR in this range. Simple extractions or other minor surgical procedures can also usually be accomplished in the 2 to 3.5 range, using careful surgical technique. When the INR is 3.5 or above, surgery should be deferred, and the patient's physician should be consulted. Consider tapering the dose of warfarin to bring the patient into the 2 to 3 range.

11. **Is the bleeding time a good indicator of perisurgical and postsurgical bleeding?**
The bleeding time is used to test for platelet function. However, studies have shown no correlation between blood loss during cardiac or general surgery and prolonged bleeding time. The best indicator of a bleeding problem in the dental patient is a thorough medical history. The bleeding time should be used in patients with no known platelet disorder to help predict the potential for bleeding.

12. **Should oral surgical procedures be postponed in patients taking aspirin (acetylsalicylic acid)?**
Aspirin irreversibly acetylates cyclooxygenase, an enzyme that assists platelet aggregation. The effect is not dose dependent and lasts for the 7- to 10-day life span of the platelet. Dental procedures in the absence of a positive medical history for bleeding should not be postponed because of aspirin therapy. Bleeding may be exacerbated in a patient with mild platelet defect.

13. **Are patients taking nonsteroidal medications likely to bleed from oral surgical procedures?**
Nonsteroidal anti-inflammatory drugs (NSAIDs) produce a transient inhibition of platelet aggregation that is reversed when the drug is cleared from the body. Patients with a preexisting platelet defect may have increased bleeding.

14. **If a patient presents with spontaneous gingival bleeding, which diagnostic tests should be ordered?**
A patient who presents with spontaneous gingival bleeding without a history of trauma, tooth brushing, flossing, or eating should be assessed for a systemic cause. The causes of gingival bleeding include inflammation secondary to periodontal disease, platelet defect, factor deficiency, hematologic malignancy, and metabolic disorder. A thorough medical history should be obtained, and the following laboratory tests should be ordered: (1) PT/INR, (2) PTT, and (3) complete blood count (CBC).

15. Should oral surgical procedures be postponed in patients taking direct-acting oral anticoagulants (dabigatran, apixaban, rivaroxaban)?

    These drugs differ from traditional oral anticoagulant therapy (e.g., warfarin) and require little to no routine monitoring. According to the current evidence, there is no need to modify direct-acting oral anticoagulant regimen prior to most dental procedures. Bleeding is usually controlled by local hemostatic measures.

INDICATIONS FOR PROPHYLACTIC ANTIBIOTICS

16. For what cardiac conditions is prophylaxis for endocarditis recommended in patients receiving dental care?
    - Prosthetic cardiac valves or prosthetic material used for cardiac valve repair
    - Previous, relapse, or recurrent infective endocarditis
    - Cardiac transplant recipients who develop cardiac valvulopathy
    - Congenital (present from birth) heart disease (CHD) such as:
      - Unrepaired cyanotic congenital CHD, including palliative shunts and conduits
      - Completely repaired congenital heart defect with prosthetic material or device, whether placed by surgery or by transcatheter during the first 6 months after the procedure
      - Repaired CHD with residual defects at the site of or adjacent to the site of a prosthetic patch or prosthetic device
      - Surgical or transcatheter pulmonary artery valve or conduit placement such as Melody valve and Contegra conduit

17. What cardiac conditions do not require endocarditis prophylaxis?
    - Implantable electronic devices such as a pacemaker or similar devices
    - Septal defect closure devices when complete closure is achieved
    - Peripheral vascular grafts and patches, including those used for hemodialysis
    - Coronary artery stents or other vascular stents
    - CNS ventriculoatrial shunts
    - Vena cava filters
    - Pledgets

18. What are the antibiotics and dosages recommended by the American Heart Association (AHA) for the prevention of endocarditis from dental procedures?

    The AHA updates its recommendations every few years to reflect new findings. The dentist has an obligation to be aware of the latest recommendations. The patient's well-being is the dentist's responsibility. Even if a physician recommends an alternative prophylactic regimen, the dentist is liable if the patient develops endocarditis and the latest AHA recommendations were not followed.
    - Standard regimen for adults:
      - Amoxicillin, 2.0 g orally 30-60 minutes before procedure
    - For adult patients unable to take oral medication:
      - Ampicillin (2 g IM or IV) OR Cefazolin or ceftriaxone 1 g IM or IV
    - For adult patients allergic to amoxicillin and penicillin:
      - Cephalexin 2 g OR azithromycin or clarithromycin 500 mg OR doxycycline 100 mg OR cefazolin or ceftriaxone 1 g IM or IV

19. For which dental procedures is antibiotic prophylaxis recommended in patients identified as being at risk for endocarditis?

    Prophylaxis is for all dental procedures that involve manipulation of the periapical region of the teeth, or gingival tissue, or perforation of the oral mucosa.

20. Should a patient who has had a coronary bypass operation be placed on prophylactic antibiotics before dental treatment?

    No evidence indicates that coronary artery bypass graft surgery introduces a risk for endocarditis. Therefore, antibiotic prophylaxis is not needed.

21. What precautions should you take when treating a patient with central line devices such as a Hickman peripherally inserted central catheter (PICC) or Port-a-Cath (manufacturer: Smiths Medical, Dublin, OH)?

    Antibiotic prophylaxis is not routinely recommended to prevent catheter-related infections associated with an invasive oral procedure in these patients.

22. Should a patient with a prosthetic joint be placed on prophylactic antibiotics before dental treatment?

    The most recent guidelines concerning the use of prophylactic antibiotics before dental treatment in patients with prosthetic joints are evidence-based. Research fails to demonstrate an association between dental procedures and prosthetic joint infections. The guidelines state that there is insufficient evidence to recommend routine antibiotic prophylaxis for dental procedures in patients with joint replacements. Therefore, dental practitioners might consider discontinuing the practice of routinely prescribing prophylactic antibiotics for patients with hip and knee prosthetic joint implants undergoing dental procedures. According to the American Dental Association, in patients "where antibiotics are deemed necessary, it is most appropriate that the orthopedic surgeon recommend the appropriate antibiotic regimen and, when reasonable, write the prescription."

23. **Is it necessary to prescribe prophylactic antibiotics for a patient on renal dialysis or affected by end-stage renal disease (ESRD)?**
Antibiotic prophylaxis for preventing infective endocarditis in ESRD or hemodialysis is not indicated. However, patients affected by ESRD are at higher risk of infective endocarditis and patients in hemodialysis may develop infections of the vascular access (endarteritis) with possible secondary bacteremia. Dental providers should follow medication recommendations from the patient's nephrologist (including antibiotic prophylaxis).

TREATMENT OF HIV-POSITIVE PATIENTS

24. **What do ART and HAART stand for as they relate to HIV (human immunodeficiency virus) treatment?**
ART stands for antiretroviral treatment. HAART stands for highly active antiretroviral treatment. The choice of treatment regimen depends on a patient's individual needs. The primary goals of treatment are to reduce the HIV viral load to an undetectable level for a prolonged period and reduce the virus mutation rates, which lead to drug resistance.

25. **What are the common oral manifestations of HIV disease?**
There are several oral manifestations of HIV infection, which in some cases may be related to disease progression or poor response to therapy. The most common HIV-associated conditions include the following:
- Oral candidiasis
- Oral hairy leukoplakia
- Linear gingival erythema
- Necrotizing ulcerative gingivitis
- Kaposi's sarcoma
- Human papillomavirus (HPV)-associated squamous papilloma, verruca vulgaris, and condyloma acuminatum
- HSV and VZV mucosal and cutaneous lesions
- Major aphthous ulcers
- Neutropenic ulcers
- Diffuse parotid enlargement

26. **What are the classifications of the most commonly used drugs to treat HIV infection?**
- Non-nucleoside reverse transcriptase inhibitors (NNRTIs). NNRTIs disable a protein needed by HIV to make copies of itself. Examples include efavirenz (Sustiva), etravirine (Intelence), and doravirine (Pifeltro).
- Nucleoside reverse transcriptase inhibitors (NRTIs). NRTIs incorporate into the DNA of the HIV virus and stop transcription. These drugs may be used in combination with other ART. Examples include abacavir (Ziagen), the combination drugs emtricitabine plus tenofovir (Truvada), and lamivudine plus zidovudine (Combivir).
- Protease inhibitors (PIs). PIs block the activity of the protease enzyme, which is a protein that HIV needs to make copies of itself. Examples include atazanavir (Reyataz), darunavir (Prezista), fosamprenavir (Lexiva), tipranavir (Aptivus) and ritonavir (Norvir).
- Fusion inhibitors. Fusion inhibitors block the entry of HIV into CD4 cells. An example includes enfuvirtide (Fuzeon).
- Integrase Strand Transfer Inhibitor (INSTIs). Integrase inhibitors disable the HIV integrase enzyme that HIV uses to insert its genetic material into CD4 cells. An example is cabotegravir (Vocabria).
- Other classes of ART include: CCR5 antagonists, attachment inhibitors, post-attachment inhibitors, and pharmacokinetic enhancers.

27. **What are the drugs that typically comprise the initial antiretroviral regimen (AVR) used to treat HIV infection?**
The AVR is continually changing according to the latest research. The goal of therapy is to provide an effective, safe, tolerable regimen to achieve sustained virologic control. Naive adults and adolescents usually receive two nucleoside reverse transcriptase inhibitors (NRTIs) administered in combination with a third active ARV drug from one of three drug classes: an integrase strand transfer inhibitor (INSTI), a non-nucleoside reverse transcriptase inhibitor (NNRTI), or a protease inhibitor (PI) with a pharmacokinetic (PK) enhancer. There are several other possible drug combinations that may be selected depending on the patient age, comorbidities, cost, and potential adverse effects.

28. **A patient with HIV infection requires an oral surgical procedure to remove several teeth after severe bone loss caused by HIV-related localized periodontitis. What precautions should be taken?**
Most patients with HIV on an antiretroviral regimen (AVR) tolerate routine dental care and procedures, including dental surgery. AVR may be associated with increased bleeding, glucose intolerance, or hyperlipidemia.

Consultation with the primary care provider and a CBC should be obtained before any oral surgical procedure. In patients with thrombocytopenia (platelet count <60,000 cells/mL) the procedure should be done only after consultation with the patient's physician and with the knowledge that bleeding may be increased. The patient may require platelet transfusions to control postoperative bleeding. If the absolute neutrophil count is <500 cells/mL, an antibiotic prophylaxis is required.

In the absence of any coagulopathy caused by thrombocytopenia or hemophilia, an otherwise healthy HIV-positive patient who presents for a dental extraction typically may undergo the procedure. However, the practitioner must proceed with caution. A careful medical history must be taken, and consultation with the patient's physician should be completed, as needed. If no underlying blood dyscrasia is present, the patient may safely undergo extractions without further precautions.

29. **Are there any contraindications to restorative dentistry procedures in patients with HIV infection?**
    If the patient is not neutropenic or thrombocytopenic, there are no contraindications to preventive and restorative dental care. They should be placed on a 3- to 6-month recall to maintain optimal oral health and followed closely for opportunistic infections and HIV-related oral conditions.

30. **What is a normal CD4 count? At what level is a patient at risk for infections? When should a patient begin antiretroviral treatment?**
    A normal CD4 count is from 500 to 1000 cells/mm^3. When the CD4 count is less than 350 cells/mm^3, the patient is considered to be at risk for acquiring an opportunistic infection. A CD4 count of less than 200 cells/mm^3 is one of the criteria for a diagnosis of acquired immunodeficiency syndrome (AIDS).

    Treatment with antiretroviral therapy (ART) is recommended for everyone with HIV and should be started as soon as possible after HIV is diagnosed. ART reduces mortality as well as serious acquired immunodeficiency syndrome (AIDS)- and non-AIDS-related complications. ART should be initiated in most individuals with HIV and detectable viremia, regardless of their CD4 count.

CARDIOVASCULAR DISEASE

31. **What is the appropriate response if a patient with a history of cardiac disease develops chest pain during a dental procedure?**
    - Discontinue treatment immediately and place the patient in a semi-reclined position.
    - Obtain and record vital signs (blood pressure, pulse, respiration), and question the patient about the pain. Chest pain from ischemia may be retrosternal or more diffused. Patients often describe the pain as crushing, pressure, or heavy; it may radiate to the shoulders, arms, neck, or back.
    - Administer oxygen.
    - If the patient has a history of angina and takes nitroglycerin, give the patient his or her own nitroglycerin or a tablet from your emergency cart. Continue to monitor the patient's vital signs. If the pain does not stop after 3 minutes, give the patient a second dose. If after three doses in a 10-minute period the pain does not subside, contact the medical emergency service and have the patient transported to an emergency department to rule out a myocardial infarction.
    - If the patient does not have a history of heart disease but has persistent chest pain for longer than 2 minutes, the medical emergency service should be contacted and the patient transported to a hospital emergency department for evaluation.
    - If the patient is not allergic to aspirin, administer one tablet of aspirin (325 mg) orally. The aspirin acts as an antithrombotic agent.

32. **At what blood pressure should elective dental care be postponed?**
    Elective dental care should be postponed if the systolic blood pressure is ≥160 mm Hg or higher and/or the diastolic pressure is 100 mm Hg or higher. Refer the patient to a physician for follow-up. If the patient is also symptomatic, refer to the emergency room for immediate care.

33. **Can or should emergency dental treatment be administered to a patient with uncontrolled hypertension?**
    Emergency dental treatment can be used to treat problems such as pain, infection, or bleeding. The dentist must compare the benefit of such treatment with the risks. The patient must be managed in consultation with a physician and be carefully monitored with intraoperative blood pressure readings, at a minimum. Other measures such as electrocardiographic monitoring, IV lines, and nitrous oxide sedation can also be used. In addition to treatment of the dental emergency, great care must be taken to reduce the patient's stress and anxiety.

34. **What are the dental treatment considerations for patients with unstable angina or a history of myocardial infarction (MI) within the past 30 days?**
    Elective dental treatment should be avoided in a patient with unstable angina or who has had an MI within the past 30 days. If care is absolutely necessary, the patient's physician should be consulted to help develop a

plan. Care should be limited to management of pain, infection, and/or bleeding. If possible, refer the patient to a hospital-based dental clinic.

35. **Can a patient with stable (mild) angina and a past history of MI be treated safely in the dental office?**
   This patient is at intermediate risk for having perioperative complications from dental procedures. Dental treatment can be completed with some treatment modifications, such as short morning appointments, comfortable chair position, recording of pretreatment vital signs, having nitroglycerin readily available, use of oral sedation as needed, use of nitrous oxide–oxygen sedation if needed, excellent local anesthesia (limiting the amount of epinephrine to no more than two cartridges containing 1:100,000 epinephrine), and excellent postoperative pain management.

36. **Can nonsteroidal anti-inflammatory drugs (NSAIDs) such as ibuprofen be administered safely to patients who have had a history of MI?**
   A recent study has shown that the use of NSAIDs including celecoxib patients with a history of MI increases the risk for another MI. This is true even if it is a relatively short course (e.g., 7 days) of NSAID treatment. Therefore, NSAIDs should be used with caution in patients who have had a previous MI, if at all, and perhaps limited to less than 7 days of use.

37. **How do you differentiate between stable and unstable angina?**
   Unstable angina is characterized by a change in the pattern of pain. The pain occurs with less exertion or at rest, lasts longer, and is less responsive to medication. Dental care for such patients must be postponed and the patient referred to his or her physician immediately for care. Patients are at increased risk for MI. If emergency dental care is necessary before the patient is stable, it should be attempted only with cardiac monitoring and sedation.

38. **Should a retraction cord that contains epinephrine be used in a patient with cardiovascular disease?**
   The concentration of epinephrine in an impregnated cord is high, and systemic absorption occurs. An impregnated cord may be used cautiously in patients who have cardiovascular disease (congestive heart failure, atrial fibrillation) or with poorly controlled hypothyroidism.

39. **Should vasoconstrictors be avoided in any patients with cardiovascular disease?**
   In a patient at major risk of developing perioperative cardiovascular complications, vasoconstrictors should be used only in consultation with the patient's physician. The result of this consultation may dictate that vasoconstrictors be avoided. This high-risk category includes the following conditions: acute or recent MI (between 7 and 30 days prior); decompensated heart failure; and significant arrhythmias (e.g., AV block, ventricular-related arrhythmia). Some studies have shown that very modest quantities of a vasoconstrictor are safe in these high-risk patients when accompanied by oxygen, sedation, nitroglycerin, and adequate pain control. Recent evidence showed that the use of 1 to 2 cartridges of local anesthetics with 1:80,000, 1:100,000, or 1:200,000 epinephrine in patients with controlled hypertension and/or coronary heart disease is safe.

40. **Is it safe to treat a patient who has undergone heart transplantation in an outpatient dental office?**
   During the first 3 months after heart transplantation, elective dental treatment should be avoided. Various systemic complications and infections are common during this period because the patient is receiving an intensive course of immunosuppressive medications. Emergency dental treatment can be provided in consultation with the patient's physician. If treatment is required during these first 3 months, antibiotic prophylaxis should be administered. Emergency dental treatment should be completed only after consultation with the patient's cardiologist.
   In the stable post-transplantation period (usually after 3–6 months, but the timing is determined in consultation with the physician), heart transplant patients can receive elective dental treatment. The use of prophylactic antibiotics during this period is determined on an individual basis based on the patient's level of immunosuppression, whether he or she has shown evidence of rejection, and other factors.

METABOLIC DISORDERS

41. **What precautions do you need to take in treating a patient with insulin-dependent diabetes mellitus (IDDM)?**
   The major concern for the dental practitioner treating the patient with IDDM is hypoglycemia. It is important to question the patient about changes in insulin dosage, diet, and exercise routine before undertaking any outpatient dental treatment. A decrease in dietary intake or increase in the normal insulin dosage or exercise may place the patient at risk for hypoglycemia. Morning dental appointments are usually indicated for patients with IDDM.

42. **What are the symptoms of hypoglycemia?**
   1. Tachycardia
   2. Palpitations
   3. Sweating
   4. Tremulousness

5. Nausea
6. Hunger
   The symptoms may progress to coma and convulsions without intervention.

43. **What should the dentist be prepared to do for the patient who has a hypoglycemic reaction?**
    The dental practitioner should have some form of sugar readily available, such as packets of table sugar, candy, or orange juice. Also available are 4- to 5-g tablets of glucose. It is recommended that a hypoglycemic patient take 15 g of fast-acting carbohydrates (glucose), which is approximately 3 to 4 tablets. If a patient develops symptoms of hypoglycemia, the dental procedure should be discontinued immediately; if conscious, the patient should be given some form of oral glucose.

    If the patient is unconscious, the emergency medical service should be contacted. Glucagon, 1 mg, can be injected IM, or 50 mL of 50% glucose solution can be given by rapid IV infusion. The glucagon injection should restore the patient to a conscious state within 15 minutes, and then some form of oral sugar can be given.

44. **Is the diabetic patient at greater risk for infection after an oral surgical procedure? It is important to minimize the risk of infection in diabetic patients. They should have aggressive treatment of dental caries and periodontal disease and be placed on frequent recall examinations and oral prophylaxis..**
    After oral surgical procedures, endodontic procedures, and treatment of suppurative periodontitis, diabetic patients with an HbA1c of >7% should be placed on antibiotics to prevent infection secondary to delayed healing. Antibiotics of choice are amoxicillin, 500 mg 3 times daily, or clindamycin, 300 mg 3 times daily for 7 to 10 days.

45. **When is it necessary to increase the dose of corticosteroids in dental patients who have primary or secondary adrenal insufficiency?**
    Guidelines on the use of supplemental corticosteroids state that only those patients who have primary adrenal insufficiency and who are undergoing surgical procedures require supplementation with additional corticosteroids. They do not require supplementation for routine dental procedures.

    Patients who have secondary adrenal insufficiency only require their usual dose of corticosteroid on the morning of the procedure.

    If supplementation is needed for those patients with primary adrenal insufficiency, the following guidelines apply:

Procedure	*Target Dose*
Routine dentistry	None
Minor surgery	25 mg hydrocortisone preoperatively on day of surgery
Moderate surgical stress	50–75 mg hydrocortisone on day of surgery and up to 1 day after
Major surgical stress	100–150 mg/day of hydrocortisone, given for 2–3 days

46. **What are the clinical symptoms of hypothyroidism? What dental care can be safely provided?**
    The clinical symptoms of hypothyroidism are weakness, fatigue, intolerance to cold, changes in weight, constipation, headache, menorrhagia, and dryness of the skin. Dental care should be deferred until after a medical consultation in a patient with or without a history of thyroid disease who experiences a combination of these signs and symptoms. If the patient is myxedematous, he or she should be treated as a medical emergency and referred immediately for medical care. It is important not to prescribe opiates for the palliative treatment of the myxedematous patient, who may be unusually sensitive and die after being given a normal dose of an opiate.

ALLERGIC REACTIONS

47. **What would you prescribe for the patient who develops a mild soft tissue swelling of the lips under the latex rubber dam?**
    The patient probably has had a contact allergic reaction from the latex. If the reaction is mild (slight swelling, with no extension into the oral cavity) and self-limiting, the patient should be given 50 mg of oral diphenhydramine and observed for at least 2 hours for a possible delayed reaction. If the reaction is moderate to severe, the patient should be given 50 mg of diphenhydramine IM or IV and closely monitored. Emergency services should be contacted to transport the patient to the emergency department for treatment and observation. Allergic patients should be instructed to inform their health care providers of their latex allergy and referred to an allergist. Dentists are encouraged to use nonlatex rubber dams and gloves whenever possible.

48. **What should you do if a patient for whom you prescribed the prophylactic antibiotic amoxicillin approximately 1 hour previously reports urticaria, erythema, and pruritus (itching)?**
    If the reaction is delayed (>1 hour) and limited to the skin, the patient should be given 50 mg of diphenhydramine IM or IV and then observed for 1 to 2 hours before being released. If no further reaction occurs, the patient should be given a prescription for 25 to 50 mg of diphenhydramine to be taken every 6 hours until symptoms are gone.

If the reaction is immediate (<1 hour) and limited to the skin, 50 mg of diphenhydramine should be given immediately IM or IV. The patient should be monitored, and emergency services contacted to transport the patient to the emergency department. If other symptoms of allergic reaction occur, such as conjunctivitis, rhinitis, bronchial constriction, or angioedema, 0.3 mL of aqueous 1:1000 epinephrine should be given by subcutaneous (SC) or IM injection. The patient should be monitored until emergency services arrive. If the patient becomes hypotensive, an IV line should be started with Ringer's lactate or 5% dextrose in water.

49. **What are the signs and symptoms of anaphylaxis? How should it be managed in the dental office?**

Anaphylaxis is characterized by bronchospasm, hypotension or shock, and urticaria or angioedema. It is a medical emergency in which death may result from respiratory obstruction, circulatory failure, or both. With the first indication of anaphylaxis, 0.3 to 0.5 mL of 1:1000 aqueous epinephrine should be injected SC or IM, and emergency services should be contacted. The injection of epinephrine may be repeated every 20 to 30 minutes, if necessary, for as many as three doses. Oxygen at a rate of 4 L/min must be delivered with a face mask. The patient must be continuously monitored, and an IV line containing Ringer's lactate or normal saline should be infused at 100 mL/hr. If the patient becomes hypotensive, the IV infusion should be increased. If airway obstruction occurs because of edema of the larynx or hypopharynx, a cricothyrotomy must be performed. If the airway obstruction is caused by bronchospasm, an albuterol or terbutaline nebulizer should be used or IV aminophylline, 6 mg/kg, infused over 20 to 30 minutes.

HEMATOLOGY AND ONCOLOGY

50. **What are the normal values for a CBC?**

White blood cell count		Hemoglobin (Hgb)	
≥18 years 12–17 years	4,000–10,000/mL	≥18 years	
	4,500–13,000/mL	Male	13.5–18.0 g/dL
6 months–11 years	4,500–13,500/mL	Female	11.5–16.4 g/dL
Red blood cell count		12–17 years	12.0–16.0 g/dL
≥18 years		6 months–11 years	10.5–14.0 g/dL
Male	4.5–6.4 M/mL		
Female	3.9–6.0 M/mL		
12–17 years	4.1–5.3 M/mL	**Platelet count (PLT)**	
6 months–11 years	3.7–5.3 M/mL	8 days and older	150,000–450,000/mL
		Up to 7 days	150,000–350,000/mL
Hematocrit (Hct)			
≥18 years	40%–54%		
Male			
Female	36%–48%		
12–17 years	36%–39%		
6 months–11 years	34%–45%		

51. **What precautions should be taken when providing dental care to a patient with sickle cell anemia?**

1. Patients with sickle cell disease should not receive dental treatment during a crisis, except for the relief of dental pain and treatment of acute dental infections. Dental infections should be treated aggressively; if facial cellulitis develops, the patient should be admitted to the hospital for treatment.

2. Patients who are short of breath and in whom Hb levels are less than 11 g/dL, have an abnormal heart rate, or have an oxygen saturation less than 91% (as determined by pulse oximetry) are considered medically unstable, and routine treatment should be deferred until their health status improves.

3. Patients with G6PD deficiency exhibit an increased incidence of drug sensitivity with sulfonamides (sulfamethoxazole), aspirin, and chloramphenicol being the prime offenders. Penicillin, streptomycin, and isoniazid also have been linked to hemolysis in these patients. Dental infection may accelerate the rate of hemolysis in patients with this type of anemia. The drugs listed previously should not be used in these patients.

4. The patient's physician should be consulted about the patient's cardiovascular status. Myocardial damage secondary to infarctions and iron deposits is common.

5. Patients with sickle cell anemia are at increased risk for bacterial infections when surgical procedures are performed. Although there is no evidence to support their use, prophylactic antibiotics are often administered before any dental surgical procedure to prevent the possibility of wound infection and/or osteomyelitis. It is not recommended for routine, nonsurgical procedures. The same prophylactic antibiotic regimen used for the prevention of endocarditis should be followed. After a surgical procedure, antibiotics (amoxicillin, 500 mg three times daily, or clindamycin, 300 mg three times daily) should be considered for 7 to 10 days postoperatively.

52. **What hematologic disorders are characterized by a so-called hair-on-end appearance of bone on radiographic surveys?**
Thalassemia major and sickle cell anemia are characterized in this way.

53. **Can local anesthetic with a vasoconstrictor be used for a patient with sickle cell disease?**
Because of the possibility of impairing local circulation, the use of vasoconstrictors in patients with sickle cell disease is controversial. It is recommended that the planned dental procedure dictate the choice of local anesthetic. If the planned procedure is a short routine procedure that can be performed without discomfort by using an anesthetic without a vasoconstrictor, the vasoconstrictor should not be used. However, if the procedure requires long profound anesthesia, 2% lidocaine with 1:100,000 epinephrine is the anesthetic of choice.

54. **Can nitrous oxide be used to help manage anxiety in patients with sickle cell anemia?**
Nitrous oxide can be safely used in patients with sickle cell anemia as long as the concentration of oxygen is greater than 50%, the flow rate is high, and the patient can ventilate adequately.

55. **Can a dental infection cause a crisis in a patient with sickle cell anemia?**
Appropriate restorative and preventive dental care are important because oral infection can precipitate a crisis.

56. **What are the oral symptoms of acute leukemia?**
More than 65% of patients with acute leukemia have oral symptoms. The symptoms result from myelosuppression caused by the overwhelming numbers of malignant cells in the bone marrow and/or large numbers of circulating immature cells (blasts). Platelet deficiency–associated mucosal bleeding, petechiae, easy bruising, easy bleeding, and increased susceptibility to infection and poor wound healing due to the decreased number of mature, normal, functioning WBCs.
   1. Symptoms from thrombocytopenia—gingival oozing, petechiae, hematoma, and ecchymosis.
   2. Symptoms from neutropenia—recurrent or unrelenting bacterial infections, lymphadenopathy, oral ulcerations, pharyngitis, and gingival infection. Infections often develop in the presence of neutropenia as the result of invasion by unusual oral pathogens.
   3. Symptoms from circulating immature cells (blasts)—gingival hyperplasia from blast infiltration.
   Patients with these signs or symptoms should be evaluated to rule out a hematologic malignancy. The dentist should consider carefully whether the symptoms can be explained by local factors or are disproportionate to these factors. If a hematologic malignancy is suspected, a CBC with a differential white cell count should be ordered.

57. **Which leukemia is typically referred to as the leukemia of childhood?**
Acute lymphocytic leukemia almost always occurs in children. The condition can be successfully treated, with a 50% to 70% 5-year survival.

58. **Is it safe to extract a tooth in a patient who is receiving chemotherapy?**
The major organ system affected by cytotoxic chemotherapy is the hematopoietic system. When a patient receives chemotherapy, the white cell count and platelets may be expected to decrease in about 7 to 10 days. If the patient's absolute neutrophil count (calculated by multiplying the white cell count by the number of neutrophils in the differential count and dividing by 100) drops below 500 neutrophils, the patient is considered neutropenic and at high risk for infection. Neutropenia is graded as mild, moderate, or severe. Moderate neutropenia is when the counts are between 1000 and 500, and this places the patient at moderate risk of infection. If the platelet count drops below 50,000/μL, the patient is at risk for bleeding.
   If possible, dental procedures should be scheduled 2 weeks before planned chemotherapy or after the counts begin to recover, usually 14 days for white cells and 21 days for platelets. Dental treatment should be attempted only after consultation and in coordination with the patient's oncology team and after the patient has had a CBC. For urgent dental care in the event of acute dental infection, consultation and blood work should be ordered and necessary treatment carried out based on the risks and benefits of leaving or removing the foci of infection during times of neutropenia and/or thrombocytopenia.

59. **Which precautions should be taken in treating a patient who has undergone bone marrow transplantation for a hematologic malignancy?**
Dental care should be done only in consultation with the patient's oncology team. As a rule, elective dental treatment should be postponed for 6 months after transplantation. However, emergency dental treatment can be carried out. If dental care must be done before the recommended postponement, a CBC should be checked, and if the results are acceptable (platelets >50,000/μL and neutrophils >500 cells/mm^3), the patient should be premedicated using the same regimen as for the prevention of endocarditis.

60. **What should be done if a patient has enlarged lymph nodes?**
Lymphadenopathy may be secondary to a sore throat, upper respiratory infection, or the initial presentation of a malignancy. A thorough history and clinical examination help determine the cause of the lymphadenopathy.
   Patients with lymphadenopathy and an identifiable inflammatory process should be reexamined in 2 weeks to determine whether the lymphadenopathy has responded to treatment. If persistent, patients should be referred to a specialist for further evaluation and management.

If no inflammatory process can be identified or the lymphadenopathy does not resolve after treatment, the patient should be referred to a physician for further evaluation and possible biopsy (Table 3-1).

KIDNEY DISEASE

61. **Which precautions should be taken before beginning treatment of a patient on dialysis?**
Patients typically receive dialysis three times/week, usually on a Monday, Wednesday, Friday schedule or Tuesday, Thursday, Saturday schedule. Dental treatment for a patient on dialysis should be done on the day between dialysis appointments to avoid bleeding difficulties (patients receive the anticoagulant, heparin, on dialysis days). Premedication prophylaxis per se is not needed with peritoneal dialysis. However, in some cases, the patient will need to be premedicated prior to invasive dentistry if there is an indwelling catheter for anticipated long-term peritoneal dialysis. Patients with an AV shunt do not need to be premedicated.

62. **Which adjustments in the dosage of oral antibiotics should you make for a patient on renal dialysis who has a dental infection?**

Penicillin	500 mg orally every 6 hours; dose after hemodialysis
Amoxicillin	500 mg orally every 24 hours; dose after hemodialysis
Ampicillin	250 mg to 1 g orally every 12–24 hours; dose after hemodialysis
Erythromycin	250 mg orally every 6 hours; not necessary to dose after hemodialysis
Clindamycin	300 mg every 6 hours; not necessary to dose after hemodialysis

63. **Which regional lymph nodes are most commonly involved in the presentation of early Hodgkin's disease?**
Hodgkin's disease typically presents with cervical, subclavicular, axillary, or mediastinal lymph node involvement and, less commonly, with inguinal and abdominal lymph node involvement.

64. **Which pain medications can be safely prescribed for patients on dialysis? Codeine is safe to use in dialysis but may produce more profound sedation. The dose should be titrated, beginning with 50% of the normal dose for patients on dialysis and 50% to 75% of the normal dose for patients with severely decreased renal function..**
Acetaminophen is nephrotoxic in overdoses. However, it may be prescribed in patients on dialysis at a dose of 650 mg every 8 hours. For patients with decreased renal function, the regimen should be 650 mg every 6 hours.

Aspirin should be avoided in patients with severe renal failure and patients on renal dialysis because of the possibility of potentiating hemorrhagic diathesis.

Meperidine (Demerol) should not be prescribed for patients on renal dialysis. The active metabolite, normeperidine, accumulates and may cause seizures.

Table 3-1. Clinical Presentations of Lymphadenopathy

PARAMETER	INFLAMMATORY PROCESS	GRANULOMATOUS DISEASE OR NEOPLASIA
Onset	Acute	Progressive enlargement
Pain on palpation	Tender	Neoplasia, asymptomatic
		Granulomatous, painful
Symmetry	Bilateral for systemic infections	Usually unilateral
	Unilateral for localized infections	
Consistency	Firm, movable	Firm, non-movable

From Sonis ST, Fazio RC, Fang LS. *Principles and Practice of Oral Medicine.* 2nd ed. Philadelphia: WB Saunders; 1995, pp 269–271.

65. **Which changes do you expect to see in the dental radiographs of a patient on renal dialysis?**
The most common changes are decreased bone density with a ground glass appearance, increased bone density in the mandibular molar area compatible with osteosclerosis, loss of lamina aura, subperiosteal cortical bone resorption in the maxillary sinus and mandibular canal, and brown tumor.

66. **What is uremic stomatitis?**
Uremic stomatitis is an ulcerative condition of the oral mucosa that develops in patients with chronic renal failure. It is thought to be caused by ammonia metabolites. Uremic stomatitis is an uncommon complication of uremia due to advent of renal dialysis that may occur as a result of advanced renal failure with the presence of markedly elevated BUN level around 150 to 300 mg/dL. Clinically, it presents as white plaques distributed predominantly

on the buccal mucosa, floor of the mouth, and dorsal or ventral surface of the tongue. Patients usually complain of pain, dysgeusia, and burning sensation with the lesions, and the clinician may detect an odor of ammonia or urine in the patient's breath. The clinical appearance occasionally mimics oral hairy leukoplakia. Uremic stomatitis can be classified into four types such as erythemopultaceous, ulcerative, hemorrhagic, and hyperkeratotic. Differential diagnosis should be mainly performed from vesiculobullous, microbial infections, vitamin deficiencies, lichen planus, oral hairy leukoplakia, and chronic hyperplastic candidiasis. The treatment consists mainly of hemodialysis, and increased oral hygiene with antiseptic mouthwashes and antimicrobial/antifungal agents if necessary.

67. **What is a common oral complication of renal transplant patients who are on chronic doses of cyclosporine?**
Gingival hyperplasia is a common oral complication.

68. **Which other medications are known to cause gingival hyperplasia?**
Phenytoin (Dilantin), verapamil, nifedipine (Procardia), and amlodipine (Norvasc) are known to cause gingival hyperplasia. Phenytoin is an anticonvulsant. Verapamil, nifedipine, and amlodipine are calcium channel blockers.

69. **What precautions should be taken when treating a patient after renal transplantation?**
After renal transplantation, patients receive immunosuppressive drugs and have an increased susceptibility to infection. Dental infections should be treated aggressively. As with other post-transplantation patients, elective dental treatment should be deferred during the first 3 months after renal transplantation. If emergency dental treatment is needed during the first 3 months, prophylactic antibiotics should be administered but should only be given thereafter on an individual case basis in consultation with the patient's physician. Erythromycin should not be prescribed for any patient taking cyclosporine. mTOR inhibitor-associated stomatitis (mIAS), a frequent, early-onset side effect of this drug class, can be dose limiting and diminish patient's quality of life. This can be effectively treated at most times with topical steroid therapy.

70. **Which antibiotic should be avoided in a patient taking cyclosporine?**
Cyclosporine is used to prevent organ rejection in renal, cardiac, and hepatic transplantation and to prevent graft-versus-host disease in patients who have received a bone marrow transplant. Erythromycin should not be prescribed for patients taking cyclosporine. Erythromycin increases the levels of cyclosporine by decreasing its metabolism.

PULMONARY DISEASE

71. **What precautions should be taken in treating a patient with chronic obstructive pulmonary disease (COPD)?**
Caution must be taken in prescribing drugs with antiplatelet activity (aspirin and NSAIDs) to patients with COPD and a history of hemoptysis. Hemoptysis has been reported after the use of aspirin in patients with COPD.

72. **Which antibiotic should not be prescribed for patients with COPD who take theophylline?**
Erythromycin should not be prescribed for patients taking theophylline because it decreases the metabolism of theophylline and may cause toxicity.

73. **Which intervention is appropriate for a dental patient who has had an asthma attack in the office?**
The medical history should provide an indication of the severity of the asthma and the medications that the patient takes for an asthma attack. The symptoms of an acute asthma attack are shortness of breath, wheezing, dyspnea, anxiety, and, with severe attacks, cyanosis. As with all medical emergencies, the first two steps are to discontinue treatment and remain calm and not increase the patient's anxiety. Patients should be allowed to position themselves for optimal comfort and then placed on low-flow (2–3 L/min) O_2 when oxygen saturation falls under 95%. If patients have their own nebulizer, they should be allowed to use it. If the patient does not have a nebulizer, he or she should be given a metaproterenol or albuterol nebulizer from the emergency cart or case and take two inhalations.

If the symptoms do not subside or increase in severity, emergency services should be contacted. The patient must be closely monitored and given 0.3 to 0.5 mL of a 1:1000 solution of epinephrine SC or IV aminophylline, 5.6 mg/kg, in 150 mL of 5% dextrose in half-normal saline or normal saline infused over 30 minutes. (To calculate the patient's weight in kilograms, divide the patient's weight in pounds by 2.2.) The dose of epinephrine may be repeated every 30 minutes for as many as three doses. Epinephrine should not be used in patients with severe hypertension, severe tachycardia, or cardiac arrhythmias. Aminophylline should not be used in patients who have had theophylline in the past 24 hours.

74. **Can nitrous oxide be used safely to sedate a patient with COPD?**
Nitrous oxide–oxygen inhalation sedation should be used with caution in patients with mild to moderate chronic bronchitis. It should not be used in patients with stage III or IV COPD because the nitrous oxide may accumulate in air spaces of the diseased lung. If this sedation modality is used in a patient with chronic bronchitis, flow rates

should be reduced to no greater than 3 L/min, and the clinician should anticipate induction and recovery times with nitrous oxide approximately twice as long as those in a healthy patient.

LIVER DISEASE

75. **Which laboratory blood tests should be ordered for a patient with alcoholic hepatitis?**
    Alcoholic hepatitis is the most common cause of cirrhosis, which is one of the most common causes of death in the United States. There are a number of concerns in treating the patient with alcoholic hepatitis:
    1. Increased risk of perioperative and postoperative bleeding, secondary to a decrease in vitamin K-dependent coagulation factors.
    2. Qualitative and quantitative effects of alcohol on platelets.
    3. Anemia secondary to dietary deficiencies and/or hemorrhage.
    4. Before attempting a surgical procedure, the minimal laboratory tests that should be ordered are PT/INR, PTT, CBC, and bleeding time.
       A CBC with differential and determinations of AST and ALT, bleeding time, thrombin time, and prothrombin time are needed to identify the patient for potential problems. When a patient has not been seen by a physician within the past several months, screening laboratory tests should be ordered, including a CBC with differential and determinations of AST and ALT, platelet count, thrombin time, and prothrombin time before invasive procedures are undertaken.

76. **What precautions should be taken with patients on anticonvulsant medications?**
    It is important to obtain a detailed history of the seizure disorder to determine whether the patient is at risk for seizures during dental treatment. Important information includes the type and frequency of seizures, date of the last seizure, prescribed medications, last blood test to determine therapeutic ranges, and activities that tend to provoke seizures. For patients taking valproic acid or carbamazepine, periodic tests for liver function should be performed. Blood counts for patients taking carbamazepine and ethosuximide should be done by the patient's physician. Liver function test results and blood counts should be checked before any oral surgical procedure is planned (Table 3-2).

77. **Which emergency procedures should be taken for a patient having a seizure?**
    It is important to determine whether the patient has a history of seizure disorders. Any patient who has a seizure in the dental office without a history of seizures must be treated as a medical emergency. The emergency medical service should be contacted as the dentist proceeds with management. There are two stages of a seizure, the ictal phase and postictal phase. The management of each is described here.
    1. Place the patient in a supine position, away from hard or sharp objects to prevent injury; a carpeted floor is ideal. If the patient is in the dental chair, it is important to protect the patient by moving equipment out of the way as far as possible.

Table 3-2. Seizure Medications and Precautions for the Dental Practitioner

MEDICATION	ADVERSE REACTIONS	INTERACTIONS
Valproic acid (Depakote), bleeding with heparin	Prolonged bleeding time, leukopenia, thrombocytopenia	Increased risk of aspirin and NSAIDs or warfarin; additive depression of central nervous system (CNS) with other depressants, including narcotic analgesics and sedative-hypnotics
Carbamazepine (Tegretol)	Aplastic anemia, agranulocytosis, thrombocytopenia, leukopenia, leukocytosis	Erythromycin increases levels of carbamazepine; may cause toxicity
Phenytoin (Dilantin)	Aplastic anemia, agranulocytosis, leukopenia, thrombocytopenia sedative-hypnotics	Additive depression of CNS with other depressants, including narcotics and sedative-hypnotics
Phenobarbital		Additive depression of CNS with other depressants, including narcotics and sedative-hypnotics; may increase risk of hepatic toxicity of acetaminophen
Primidone	Blood dyscrasias, orthostatic hypotension	Additive depression of CNS with other depressants, including narcotics and sedative-hypnotics
Ethosuximide	Aplastic anemia, granulocytosis, leukopenia	Additive depression of CNS with other depressants
Clonazepam	Anemia, thrombocytosis, leukopenia	Additive depression of CNS with other depressants

2. The airway must be maintained, and vital signs monitored during the tonic stage. If suctioning equipment is available, it should be ready with a plastic tip for suctioning secretions to maintain the airway. The patient may experience periods of apnea and develop cyanosis. The head should be extended to establish a patent airway, and oxygen should be administered. Vital signs, pulse, respiration, and blood pressure must be monitored throughout the seizure.
3. If the ictal phase of the seizure lasts more than 5 minutes, emergency services should be called. Tonic-clonic status epilepticus is a medical emergency. If the dentist is trained to do so, an IV line should be initiated, and a dose of 25 g (50 mL) of 50% dextrose should be given immediately in case the seizure is caused by hypoglycemia. If there is no response, the patient should be given 10 mg of diazepam IV over a 2-minute period.
4. Once the seizure activity has stopped and the patient enters the postictal phase, it is important to continue to monitor the vital signs and, if necessary, to provide basic life support. If respiratory depression is significant, emergency services should be called, the airway maintained, and respiration supported. Blood pressure may be initially depressed but should recover gradually.
5. If the patient recovers from the postictal phase without basic life support or other complications, the patient's physician should be contacted and the patient, if stable, should be discharged from the dental office, accompanied by a responsible adult.

78. **Which dental considerations must be considered in treating patients with seizure disorders?**
Patients taking phenytoin are at risk for gingival hyperplasia. Tissue irritation from orthodontic bands, defective restorations, fractured teeth, plaque, and calculus accelerate the hyperplasia.

    The dental practitioner should consider the patient's seizure status. A rubber dam with dental floss tied to the clamp should be used for all restorative dental procedures to enable the rapid removal of materials and instruments from the patient's oral cavity. Fixed prosthetics, when indicated, should be fabricated, rather than removable prosthetics. If removable prosthetics are indicated, they should be fabricated with metal for all major connectors. Acrylic partial dentures should be avoided because of the risk of breaking and aspiration during seizure activities. Unilateral partial dentures are contraindicated. Temporary crowns and bridges should be laboratory-cured for strength.

79. **Is general anesthesia contraindicated for patients with a seizure disorder?**
No, it is not contraindicated. However, general anesthesia lowers the seizure threshold, and precautions must be taken to ensure that serum levels of the antiseizure drug are within therapeutic range.

80. **What are the common causes of unconsciousness in dental patients?**
The most common cause of loss of consciousness in the dental office is syncope. The signs and symptoms are diaphoresis, pallor, and loss of consciousness. Place the patient in the supine position with the feet elevated, monitor vital signs, and administer oxygen, 3 to 4 L/min via a nasal cannula.

RADIATION THERAPY

81. **What are the risk factors for the development of osteoradionecrosis?**
Bone exposed to high radiation therapy is hypovascular, hypocellular, and hypoxic tissue. Osteoradionecrosis develops because the radiated tissue is unable to repair itself. The risk for osteoradionecrosis increases as the dose of radiation increases from 5400 cGy to over 8000 cGy. Tissues receiving less than 5400 rad are at low risk for necrosis. In addition, the risk increases with poor oral health. Oral surgical procedures after radiation therapy place the patient at high risk for developing osteoradionecrosis. Soft tissue trauma from dentures and oral infections from periodontal disease and dental caries also put the patient at risk. Modifiable risk factors for ORN include active periodontal disease, dry mouth, dental caries leading to necrotic pulp, uncontrolled diabetes, and smoking.

82. **How should the dentist prepare the patient for radiation therapy of the head and neck?**
    1. The dentist should consult with the oncology team to determine which oral structures will be in the field of radiation, as well as the maximal radiation dose. If teeth are in the field and the dose is greater than 5400 cGy, periodontally involved teeth and teeth with periapical lucencies should be extracted at least 2 weeks before radiation therapy begins.
    2. The dentist should prepare the patient for postradiation xerostomia—provide custom fluoride trays and prescribe 0.4% stannous fluoride gel to be used for 3 to 5 minutes twice daily. Alternatively, a prescription strength toothpaste of 1.1% sodium fluoride 5000 PPM can be used.
    3. It is advantageous to recommend a calcium phosphate toothpaste as well to be used on alternative times of bi-daily brushing. This optimizes the uptake of fluoride in a patient with salivary hypofunction.
    4. Patients should be encouraged to use a 0.5% sodium bicarbonate 0.9% saline rinse multiple times a day for the management of dry mouth. This equates to 1 tsp baking soda and 1 tsp salt in 4 cups water.
    5. The patient must be placed on a 2- to 3-month recall schedule. On recall, the teeth must be carefully examined for root caries, and instruction in oral hygiene should be reviewed.

83. **How is medication-related osteonecrosis of the jaw defined?**
Medication-related osteonecrosis of the jaw (MRONJ) is defined as exposed bone or bone that can be probed through one or more intraoral or extraoral fistulae in the maxillofacial region and that does not heal within 8 weeks, occurring in a patient who has received a bone-modifying agent (BMA) or an angiogenic inhibitor agent and has no history of head and neck radiation.

84. **What are the risk factors for the development of medication-related osteonecrosis of the jaw?**
Members of the multidisciplinary team should address modifiable risk factors for MRONJ with the patient as early as possible. These risk factors include poor oral health, invasive dental procedures, ill-fitting dentures, uncontrolled diabetes mellitus, and tobacco use.

85. **How should the coordination of care for cancer patients scheduled to receive bone-modifying agents in a nonurgent setting take place?**
For cancer patients scheduled to receive a BMA in a non-urgent setting, oral care assessment (including a comprehensive dental, periodontal, and oral radiographic exam when feasible to do so) should be undertaken prior to initiating therapy (Table 3-3). Based on the assessment, a dental care plan should be developed and implemented. The care plan should be coordinated between the dentist and the oncologist to ensure that medically necessary dental procedures are undertaken prior to the initiation of the BMA. Follow-up by the dentist should then be performed on a routine schedule (e.g., every 6 months) once therapy with a BMA has commenced.

ACKNOWLEDGMENT

The authors gratefully acknowledge the contribution of the previous chapter author.

Table 3-3. Descriptions of Complete, Partial, and Minimal Dental Evaluation Protocols Based on the Type of Dental and/or Periodontal Pathology

DENTAL PATHOLOGY	COMPLETE	PARTIAL	MINIMAL, INCOMPLETE, OR NO CLEARANCE
Caries	Restore all teeth	Mild/moderate caries were restored if time permitted	Intervention only if symptomatic
Severe caries/pulp involvement/dental abscess	Root canal treatment or extract		
Apical periodontitis	Retreat	Symptomatic lesions and lesions ≥5 mm should be endodontically treated	
	Apicoectomy	Asymptomatic lesions and lesions <5 mm should be observed	
	Extract		
Advanced periodontal disease	Extract teeth with	Extract teeth with	
	Probing depth ≥6 mm	Probing depth ≥8 mm	
	Furcation I, II, III; Mobility III	Mobility III	
	Severe inflammation	Severe inflammation	
Partially erupted third molars	Extract	Asymptomatic teeth were observed	
		Partially erupted third molars with purulence of pericoronitis were extracted	

Note: The proper protocol should be selected by the oncologist and dentist according to the patient's medical status.
From Hong C.H.L., Hu S., Haverman T., et al. A systematic review of dental disease management in cancer patients. *Support Care Cancer.* 2017; 26:155–174.

BIBLIOGRAPHY

Aronoff GR, Bennett WM, Berns JS, et al. *Drug Prescribing in Renal Failure: Dosing Guidelines for Adults and Children.* 5th ed. Philadelphia: American College of Physicians; 2007.

Baddour LM, Bettmann MA, Bolger AF, et al. Nonvalvular cardiovascular device-related infections. *Circulation.* 2003;108:2015–2031.

Cintron G, Medina R, Reyes AA, Lyman G. Cardiovascular effects and safety of dental anesthesia and dental interventions in patients with recent uncomplicated myocardial infarction. *Arch Intern Med.* 1986;146:2203–2204.

Dajani AS, Taubert KA, Wilson W, et al. Prevention of bacterial endocarditis. Recommendations by the American Heart Association. *JAMA.* 1997;277:1794–1801.

Deeks SG, Smith M, Holodniy M, Kahn JO. HIV-1 protease inhibitors: a review for clinicians. *JAMA.* 1997;277:145–153.

Dodson TB. HIV status and the risk of post-extraction complications. *J Dent Res.* 1997;76:1644–1652.

Ganda K. *Dentist's Guide to Medical Conditions, Medications and Complications.* Hoboken, NJ: John Wiley & Sons; 2013.

Holroyd SV, Wynn RL, Requa-Clark B, eds. *Clinical Pharmacology in Dental Practice.* 4th ed. St. Louis: Mosby; 1988.

Ifudu O. Care of patients undergoing hemodialysis. *N Engl J Med.* 1998;339:1054–1062.

Kang DO, An H, Park GU, et al. Cardiovascular and bleeding risks associated with nonsteroidal anti-inflammatory drugs after myocardial infarction. *J Am Coll Cardiol.* 2020;76(5):518–529.

Kaplovitch E, Dounaevskaia V. Treatment in the dental practice of the patient receiving anticoagulation therapy. *J Am Dent Assoc.* 2019;150(7):602–608.

Kilmartin C, Munroe CO. Cardiovascular diseases and the dental patient. *J Can Dent Assoc.* 1986;6:513–518.

Krasner AS. Glucocorticoid-induced adrenal insufficiency. *JAMA.* 1999;282:671.

Liao CY, Wu CC, Chu PL. Uremic stomatitis. *QJM.* 2017;110(4):247–248.

Lind SE. The bleeding time does not predict surgical bleeding. *Blood.* 1991;77:2547–2552.

Little JW. Managing dental patients with joint prostheses. *J Am Dent Assoc.* 1994;125:1374–1379.

Little JW, Miller C, Rhodus NL. *Dental Management of the Medically Compromised Patient, E-Book.* Elsevier Health Sciences; 2017.

Magnac C, de Saint Martin J, Pidard D, et al. Platelet antibodies in serum of patients with human immunodeficiency virus (HIV) infection. *AIDS Res Hum Retroviruses.* 1990;6:1443–1449.

Malamed SF. *Medical Emergencies in the Dental Office, E-Book.* St. Louis: Elsevier Health Sciences; 2022.

Napeñas JJ, Oost FC, DeGroot A, et al. Review of postoperative bleeding risk in dental patients on antiplatelet therapy. *Oral Surg Oral Med Oral Pathol Oral Radiol.* 2013;115(4):491–499.

NIH. *HIV Treatment: The Basics* (website). https://hivinfo.nih.gov/understanding-hiv/fact-sheets/hiv-treatment-basics. Accessed January 12, 2023.

NIH. *Guidelines for the Use of Antiretroviral Agents in Adults and Adolescents with HIV (website).* https://clinicalinfo.hiv.gov/en/guidelines/hiv-clinical-guidelines-adult-and-adolescent-arv/whats-new-guidelines. Accessed January 12, 2023.

Niwa H, Sato Y, Matsuura H. Safety of dental treatment in patients with previously diagnosed acute myocardial infarction or unstable angina pectoris. *Oral Surg Oral Med Oral Pathol Oral Radiol Endod.* 2000;89:35–41.

Papadakis MA, McPhee SJ, Rabow MW, McQuaid KR, eds. *Current Medical Diagnosis & Treatment 2022.* New York, NY; McGraw Hill; 2022.

Pastan S, Bailey J. Dialysis therapy. *N Engl J Med.* 1998;338:1428–1437.

Reznick DA. Oral manifestations of HIV disease. *Top HIV Med JT.* 2005;13(5):143–148.

Saag MS, Gandhi RT, Hoy JF, et al. Antiretroviral drugs for treatment and prevention of HIV infection in adults: 2020 recommendations of the International Antiviral Society—USA Panel. *JAMA.* 2020;324(16):1651–1669.

Salem M, et al. Perioperative glucocorticoid coverage. A reassessment 42 years after emergence of a problem. *Ann Surg.* 1994;219:416–425.

Sams DR, Thornton JB, Amamoo PA. Managing the dental patient with sickle cell anemia: a review of the literature. *Pediatr Dent.* 1990;12:317–320.

Schjerning Olsen AM, Fosbøl EL, Lindhardsen J, et al. Duration of treatment with nonsteroidal anti-inflammatory drugs and impact on risk of death and recurrent myocardial infarction in patients with prior myocardial infarction: a nationwide cohort study. *Circulation.* 2011;123:2226–2235.

Smith HB, McDonald DK, Miller RI. Dental management of patients with sickle cell disorders. *J Am Dent Assoc.* 1987;114:85.

Sollecito TP, Abt E, Lockhart PB, et al. The use of prophylactic antibiotics prior to dental procedures in patients with prosthetic joints: Evidence-based clinical practice guideline for dental practitioners—a report of the American Dental Association Council on Scientific Affairs. *J Am Dent Assoc.* 2015;146(1):11–16.e8.

Sonis ST, Fazio RC, Fang LS. *Principles and Practice of Oral Medicine.* 2nd ed. Philadelphia: WB Saunders; 1995.

Spolnik KJ. Dental radiographic manifestations of end-stage renal disease. *Dent Radiogr Photogr.* 1981;54:21–31.

Troulis M, Head TW, Leclerc JR. Dental extractions in patients on an oral anticoagulant: a survey of practices in North America. *J Oral Maxillofac Surg.* 1998;56:914–917.

Vallerand AH, Sanaoksi CA, Deglin JH. *Davis's Drug Guide for Nurses.* 13th ed. Philadelphia: FA Davis Co; 2013.

Watters W, Rethman MP, Hanson NB, et al. Prevention of orthopaedic implant infection in patients undergoing dental procedures. *J Am Acad Orthop Surg.* 2013;21(3):180–189. https://doi.org/10.5435/JAAOS-21-03-180.

Wilson WR, Gewitz M, Lockhart PB, et al. Prevention of viridans group Streptococcal infective endocarditis: a scientific statement from the American Heart Association [published correction appears in *Circulation.* 2021;144(9):e192] [published correction appears in *Circulation.* 2022;145(17):e868]. *Circulation.* 2021;143(20):e963–e978.

Wilson W, Taubert KA, Gewitz M, et al. Prevention of infective endocarditis: guidelines from the American Heart Association: a guideline from the American Heart Association Rheumatic Fever, Endocarditis, and Kawasaki Disease Committee, Council on Cardiovascular Disease in the Young, and the Council on Clinical Cardiology, Council on Cardiovascular Surgery and Anesthesia, and the Quality of Care and Outcomes Research Interdisciplinary Working Group. *Circulation.* 2007;116(15):1736–1754.

World Health Organization. *Consolidated Guidelines on the Use of Antiretroviral Drugs for Treating and Preventing HIV Infection: Recommendations for a Public Health Approach.* World Health Organization; 2016.

Yarom N, Shapiro CL, Peterson DE, et al. Medication-related osteonecrosis of the jaw: MASCC/ISOO/ASCO clinical practice guideline. *J Clin Oncol.* 2019;37(25):2270–2290.

CHAPTER 4

ORAL PATHOLOGY

Sook-Bin Woo, Reshma S. Menon

DEVELOPMENTAL CONDITIONS
TOOTH-RELATED PROBLEMS

1. True or false: Dental fluorosis increases pitting and porosity of the enamel and therefore increases the risk of dental caries.
   It is true that fluorosis causes increased pitting and porosity because fluoride increases retention of amelogenin, which results in hypomineralization of the enamel. This causes an unaesthetic chalky white or even brown discoloration of the enamel, which may be pitted and fissured. However, because this enamel is more caries-resistant, the risk of dental caries is lower.

2. Name the three main forms of amelogenesis imperfecta.
   Hypoplastic: Inadequate deposition of enamel matrix. Whatever is deposited calcifies normally. The teeth have thin enamel that may be pitted.
   Hypomaturation: Adequate deposition of enamel, but the enamel crystal does not mature normally. The result is soft pigmented enamel that chips easily.
   Hypocalcified: Inadequate mineralization. The result is enamel that gets lost a few years after eruption.

3. Describe the different types of dentinogenesis imperfecta.
   Dentinogenesis imperfecta (DI) is a condition caused by abnormal dentin formation and several types exist. The classic type leads to opalescent teeth in the primary and permanent dentition. The teeth are bluish-brown and translucent. Enamel is lost early, and the exposed dentin undergoes rapid attrition.

Osteogenesis imperfecta with opalescent teeth	Dentin dysplasia Type I
Dentinogenesis imperfecta	Dentin dysplasia Type II

4. Describe the two main types of dentin dysplasia.
   Type I, radicular type. The roots are poorly formed, short, and distorted or even absent, with poorly formed crescent-shaped pulp chambers and absent pulp canals. Periapical lucencies develop early and teeth exfoliate prematurely.
   Type II, coronal type. The crowns contain large pulp chambers that are thistle- or flame-shaped, that extend into the root. Pulp stones often develop. Primary teeth look like those of dentinogenesis imperfect with early obliteration of the pulp.

5. What is the difference between fusion and concrescence? Between twinning and gemination?
   Fusion is a more complete process than concrescence and involves fusion of the entire length of two teeth (enamel, dentin, and cementum) to form one large tooth, with one less tooth in the arch, or fusion of the root only (dentin and cementum), with the maintenance of two clinical crowns. Concrescence involves fusion of cementum only.
   Twinning is more complete than gemination and results in the formation of two separate teeth from one tooth bud (one extra tooth in the arch). In gemination, separation is attempted, but the two teeth share the same root canal.

6. What is a Turner tooth?
   A Turner tooth is a solitary, usually permanent tooth with signs of enamel hypoplasia or hypocalcification. This phenomenon is caused by trauma or infection in the overlying deciduous tooth that damages the ameloblasts of the underlying tooth bud and thus leads to localized enamel hypoplasia or hypocalcification.

7. What are "bull teeth"?
   Bull teeth, also known as taurodonts, have long anatomic crowns, large pulp chambers, and short roots, resembling teeth found in bulls. They are most dramatic in permanent molars but may affect teeth in either dentition. They occur more frequently in certain syndromes, such as Klinefelter syndrome.

8. **What is the difference between dens evaginatus and dens invaginatus?**
Dens evaginatus occurs primarily in the Asian population and affects the premolars. **Evagination** of the layers of the tooth germ results in the formation of a tubercle that arises from the occlusal surface and consists of enamel, dentin, and pulp tissue. This tubercle tends to break when it occludes with the opposing dentition and may result in pulp exposure and subsequent pulp necrosis. Dens invaginatus occurs mainly in maxillary lateral incisors and ranges in severity from an accentuated lingual pit to what is known as a *dens in dente.* This phenomenon is caused by **invagination** of the layers of the tooth germ. Food becomes trapped in the pit, and caries begin early.

9. **What are the causes of generalized intrinsic discoloration of teeth?**

   - Amelogenesis imperfecta
   - Dentinogenesis imperfecta
   - Tetracycline staining

   - Fluorosis
   - Rh incompatibility

   - Congenital porphyria
   - Biliary atresia

10. **Why do teeth discolor from ingestion of tetracycline during odontogenesis?**
Tetracycline binds with the calcium component of bones and teeth and is deposited at sites of active mineralization, causing a yellow-brown endogenous pigmentation of the hard tissues. Because teeth do not turnover the way bone does, this stain becomes a permanent label that fluoresces under ultraviolet light.

11. **Which teeth are most commonly missing congenitally?**
Third molars, maxillary lateral incisors, and second premolars are the most common.

12. **What conditions are associated with multiple supernumerary teeth?**
Gardner syndrome and cleidocranial dysplasia are two important conditions.

13. **What are the most common sites for supernumerary teeth?**
Midline of the maxilla (mesiodens), posterior maxilla (fourth molar or paramolar), and mandibular bicuspid areas.

INTRABONY LESIONS

14. **A 40-year-old Black woman presents with multiple periapical radiolucencies and radiopacities. What is the diagnosis?**
The U.S. Black population is prone to developing benign fibro-osseous lesions of various types. They range from localized lesions, such as focal cemento-osseous dysplasia, usually involving the apex of a mandibular molar, to periapical cemento-osseous dysplasia, usually involving the mandibular anterior teeth, to florid (multifocal) cemento-osseous dysplasia, involving all four quadrants. The term *cemento-osseous* is preferred to *cemental* because a combination of cementum droplets and woven bone is usually present (Fig. 4-1).

15. **Are fibrous dysplasias of bone premalignant lesions?**
Fibrous dysplasia, a malformation of bone, is of unknown cause and is not premalignant, although a mutation of a gene (*GNAS*) has been identified for this condition. The monostotic form often affects the maxilla unilaterally. The polyostotic form is associated with various other abnormalities, such as skin pigmentations (café-au-lait macules) and endocrine dysfunction (McCune-Albright and Jaffe-Lichtenstein syndromes). Cherubism, which used to be termed *familial fibrous dysplasia,* is probably not a form of fibrous dysplasia and is associated with a different gene mutation (*SH3BP2*). In the past, fibrous dysplasia was treated with radiation, which sometimes caused the development of osteosarcoma. The best way to treat fibrous dysplasia and cherubism is by recontouring the bone after the pubertal growth spurt and when lesions become quiescent.

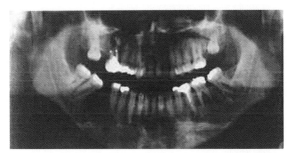

Fig. 4-1. Florid cemento-osseous dysplasia affecting at least three quadrants.

16. True or false: The globulomaxillary cyst is a fissural cyst.

False. Historically, the globulomaxillary cyst was classified as a nonodontogenic or fissural cyst thought to result from the entrapment of epithelial rests along the line of fusion between the lateral maxillary and nasomedial processes. Current thinking puts it into the category of odontogenic cysts of (a) developmental origin, and possibly related to the development of the lateral incisor or canine (if the teeth are vital), or of (b) inflammatory origin (radicular cyst) if the teeth are nonvital. The two embryonic processes mentioned do not fuse. The fold between them fills in and becomes erased by mesodermal invasion so that there is no opportunity for trapping of epithelial rests. This cyst occurs between the roots of the maxillary lateral incisor and cuspid.

17. True or false: The median palatal cyst is a true fissural cyst.

True. The epithelium of this intrabony cyst arises from proliferation of entrapped epithelium when the right and left palatal shelves fuse in the midline. This should be distinguished from a nasopalatine duct cyst, which arises from remnants of the duct in the area of the nasopalatine foramen. The soft tissue counterpart, which also occurs in the midline of the palate and is known as the palatal cyst of the newborn (Epstein pearl), is congenital and exteriorizes on its own.

18. A neonate presents with a few white nodules on the mandibular alveolar ridge. What are they?

They are most likely dental lamina cysts of the newborn (Bohn nodules). The epithelium of these cysts arises from remnants of dental lamina on the alveolar ridge after odontogenesis. Sometimes they appear at the junction of the hard and soft palate. Dental lamina cysts of the newborn tend to involute and do not require treatment.

19. A boy presents to the dental clinic with multiple jaw cysts and a history of jaw cysts in other family members. What syndrome does he most likely have?

The boy most likely has nevoid basal cell carcinoma (Gorlin-Goltz/Gorlin) syndrome, which is inherited as an autosomal dominant trait. The cysts are odontogenic keratocysts, which have a higher incidence of recurrence than other odontogenic cysts. It is now known that more than 90% of sporadic and syndromic keratocysts harbor mutations in *PTCH*.

Other findings in syndromic patients include palmar pitting, palmar and plantar keratosis, calcification of the falx cerebri, hypertelorism, ovarian tumors, and neurologic manifestations, such as intellectual disabilities and medulloblastomas.

20. Are all jaw cysts that produce keratin considered odontogenic keratocysts?

No. The odontogenic keratocyst/keratocystic odontogenic tumor is a specific histologic entity. There is some controversy as to whether this is a cyst or cystic tumor, with the new terminology favoring the former. The epithelial lining exhibits corrugated parakeratosis, uniform thinness (unless altered by inflammation), and palisading of the basal cell nuclei. The recurrence rate is high, and multiple childhood keratocysts are associated with nevoid basal cell carcinoma syndrome. Odontogenic cysts that produce orthokeratin do not show the basal cell nuclei changes, do not have the same tendency to recur, and are not associated with the syndrome. These cysts are referred to as orthokeratinized odontogenic cysts. The histologic distinctions are important because they have clinical and prognostic implications.

21. What neoplasms may arise in a dentigerous cyst?

Ameloblastoma, mucoepidermoid carcinoma and, least commonly, squamous cell carcinoma may arise in a dentigerous cyst. Odontogenic tumors that may arise in a dentigerous relationship, although not within a dentigerous cyst, include adenomatoid odontogenic tumor, calcifying cystic odontogenic tumor (Gorlin cyst), and calcifying epithelial odontogenic tumor (Pindborg tumor). The odontogenic keratocyst is often seen in a dentigerous relationship with an impacted tooth (Fig. 4-2).

22. What is the difference between a lateral radicular cyst and a lateral periodontal cyst?

A lateral radicular cyst is an **inflammatory** cyst in which the epithelium is derived from rests of Malassez (similar to a periapical or apical radicular cyst). It is in a lateral rather than an apical location because the inflammatory stimulus is emanating from a lateral accessory canal. The associated tooth is always nonvital. The lateral periodontal cyst is a **developmental** cyst in which the epithelium probably is derived from rests of dental lamina. It is usually located between the mandibular premolars, which are vital.

23. What is the incidence of cleft lip and/or cleft palate?

Cleft lip and cleft palate should be considered as two entities, (1) cleft palate alone and (2) cleft lip, with or without cleft palate. The former is more common in females and the latter in males. The incidence of cleft palate alone is 1 in 2000 births, whereas the incidence of cleft lip with or without cleft palate is 1 in 1500-3000 births (highest in Asians and Native Americans).

SOFT TISSUE CONDITIONS

24. Name some conditions in the mouth that may appear yellow.

Fibrinous material—ulcers
Sebaceous material—Fordyce granules
Fat—lipoma or other fatty tumors
Keratin—oral lymphoepithelial cyst (yellow nodules on the base of the tongue, floor of the mouth, or tonsils), epidermoid cyst, dermoid cyst

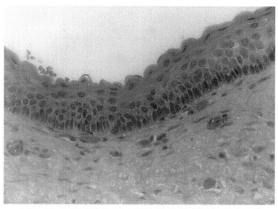

Fig. 4-2. Odontogenic keratocyst/keratocystic odontogenic tumor.

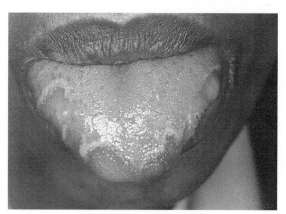

Fig. 4-3. Benign migratory glossitis.

25. Is benign migratory glossitis ("geographic tongue") associated with any systemic conditions?

Most cases of benign migratory glossitis are associated with atopy (history of hay fever, asthma, eczema, and food sensitivities) and some human leukocyte antigen (HLA) types.

Some cases have been associated with fissured tongue and patients with psoriasis, especially generalized pustular psoriasis, have a higher incidence of benign migratory glossitis (Fig. 4-3).

26. What predisposes to the formation of a coated or hairy tongue?

Hairy tongue is not a developmental lesion but a benign reactive condition. It is caused by reduced shedding and increased buildup of the keratin of the filiform papillae of the tongue. Factors that predispose to this include dehydration, smoking, and reduced intake of coarse foods such as fresh fruits and vegetables. Most patients have a history of a recent illness and have been on antibiotics, systemic steroids, and alcoholic mouth rinses. The papillae are colonized by chromogenic bacteria, so the tongue may appear black, brown, or even green from bacterial metabolic products, as well as from food coloring. It does not represent candidiasis.

This is different from oral hairy leukoplakia, which is caused by Epstein Barr virus and generally located on the lateral tongue.

INFECTIONS
FUNGAL INFECTIONS

27. Discuss the main clinical forms of candidiasis.
- Pseudomembranous candidiasis (the most common type, with curdy white patches, also known as *thrush,* tends to have an acute onset)
- Atrophic or erythematous candidiasis often seen under dentures (referred to as denture sore mouth or denture stomatitis); usually present for a long time because the denture often acts as a fomite; may be acute or chronic

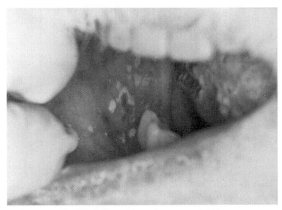

Fig. 4-4. Acute pseudomembranous candidiasis.

- Angular cheilitis presenting as cracked, weepy red areas at the corners of the mouth; tends to be chronic and recurrent
- Median rhomboid glossitis presenting as a red plaque in the midline of the posterior tongue, just anterior of the circumvallate papillae
- Chronic hyperplastic candidiasis presenting as white patches that do not wipe off easily
- Chronic mucocutaneous candidiasis (associated with skin candidiasis and an underlying systemic condition such as an endocrinopathy; Fig. 4-4)

28. **What are the common species of *Candida* that cause oral disease?**
The most common is *C. albicans*. However, some candida species such *C. tropicalis*, *C. glabrata*, and *C. dubliniensis* may be resistant to nystatin and fluconazole. *C. auris* may cause severe resistant infections and systemic infections may lead to mortality rate of 30%-60%.

29. **What factors predispose to candidal infection?**
Predisposing factors include the following: (1) alteration of the local oral milieu (such as from hyposalivation), (2) local immunosuppression (such as use of topical antibiotics or corticosteroids), (3) systemic use of antibiotics, (4) immunosuppression whether intrinsic or iatrogenic, and/or (5) other systemic conditions such as endocrinopathy or diabetes mellitus.

30. **A culture performed on an oral ulcer grows *Candida* spp. Does this mean that the patient has candidiasis?**
No. Approximately one-quarter to one-third of the adult population harbors *Candida* spp. in the mouth. Swabs from patients who are carriers for candida who do not have candidiasis, will grow candida.

31. **How do you make a diagnosis of candidiasis?**
   a. Good clinical judgment: Pseudomembranous plaques of candidiasis usually wipe off with difficulty, leaving a raw, bleeding surface.
   b. Cytology preparation: This is done in a similar manner to the Papanicolaou cytology preparation. The white plaques are scraped, and the scrapings are put on a glass slide, fixed with alcohol, and sent to be evaluated by a cytopathologist.
   c. Biopsy: This shows hyphae penetrating the tissues (too invasive for routine use).
   d. Cultures: Although cultures are not the ideal way to diagnose candidiasis, the quantity of candidal organisms that grow on culture correlates somewhat with clinical candidiasis. Cultures are particularly important for recalcitrant candidiasis to identify drug-resistant species.

32. **What are common antifungal agents for treating oral candidiasis?**
   - Polyenes: nystatin (topical), amphotericin (topical, systemic)
   - Imidazoles: clotrimazole, ketoconazole
   - Triazoles: fluconazole, itraconazole, voriconazole, posaconazole
   - Echinocandins

33. **True or false: Actinomycosis represents a fungal infection.**
False. *Actinomycetes* is a gram-positive filamentous bacteria. Do not be misled by the suffix *-mycosis*.

34. **What are sulfur granules?**
These yellowish granules (hence the name) are seen within the pus of lesions of actinomycosis. They represent aggregates of *Actinomycetes* (usually *A. israelii*), which are invariably surrounded by neutrophils.

35. **Name two opportunistic fungal diseases that often present in the orofacial region.**
Aspergillosis and mucormycosis tend to infect immunocompromised hosts; the latter causes rhinocerebral infections in patients with diabetes mellitus.

36. **Name the deep fungal infections that are endemic in North America.**
Histoplasmosis (caused by *Histoplasma capsulatum*) is endemic in the Ohio-Mississippi basin, coccidioidomycosis (caused by *Coccidioides immitis*) is endemic in the San Joaquin Valley in California, and blastomycosis (caused by *Blastomyces dermatitidis*) is endemic from the Great Lakes basin to the Mississippi valley.

VIRAL INFECTIONS

37. **Name the six most common viruses of the Herpesviridae family that often present in the orofacial area.**

Herpes simplex virus types 1 and 2 (HSV-1 and -2) (HHV-1 and 2)   Varicella-zoster virus (VZV) (HHV-3)
Epstein-Barr virus (EBV) (HHV-4)   Cytomegalovirus (HHV-5) (CMV)
Kaposi sarcoma herpesvirus (HHV-8)

*HHV—Human herpes virus

38. **True or false: Antibodies against HSV-1 protect against further outbreaks of the disease.**
False. The herpes viruses are unique in that they exhibit lifelong latency. Once a person has been infected by HSV-1, the virus remains latent within the sensory ganglia (e.g., trigeminal ganglion) for life. When conditions are favorable (for the virus, not the patient), HSV travels along nerve fibers and causes a mucocutaneous lesion at a peripheral site, such as a cold sore on the lip. A positive antibody titer (immunoglobulin G [IgG]) indicates that the patient has been previously exposed, and at the time of reactivation the titer may rise. Erythema multiforme is an ulcerative mucocutaneous condition that results from a hypersensitivity to recurrent HSV infections.

39. **How do you differentiate between recurrent aphthous ulcers and recurrent herpetic ulcers?**
Clinically, recurrent aphthous ulcers (minor) occur mostly on the nonkeratinized mucosae of the labial mucosa, buccal mucosa, sulci, ventral tongue, soft palate, and faucial pillars. Recurrent herpetic ulcers occur on the vermilion border of the lips (cold sores or fever blisters) and on the keratinized mucosae of the palate and attached gingiva in immunocompetent individuals. A polymerase chain reaction (PCR) test confirms the presence of the virus. In immunocompromised hosts, however, recurrent herpetic lesions may occur on the keratinized and nonkeratinized mucosae and may mimic aphthous ulcers (Fig. 4-5).

40. **An older patient with long-standing rheumatoid arthritis presents with a history of upper respiratory tract infection, ulcers of the right hard palate, right facial weakness, and vertigo. What does this patient have?**
The patient most likely has a reactivation of varicella-zoster virus that is equivalent to shingles of the skin, which typically presents as unilateral coalescent ulcers. The patient also has Ramsay-Hunt syndrome, which is caused by infection of cranial nerves VII and VIII with herpes zoster, leading to facial paralysis, tinnitus, deafness, and vertigo.

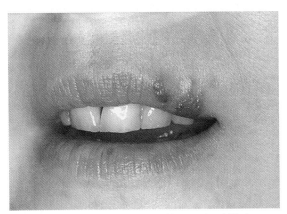

Fig. 4-5. Recurrent herpes labialis (cold sores or fever blisters).

41. What lesions associated with the Epstein-Barr virus may present in the orofacial region?

- Infectious mononucleosis
- Burkitt lymphoma
- Hodgkin lymphoma
- Nasopharyngeal carcinoma
- Oral hairy leukoplakia
- EBV mucocutaneous ulcers

42. How does infectious mononucleosis present in the mouth?

Infectious mononucleosis usually presents as multiple, painful, punctate ulcers of the posterior hard palate and soft palate in young adults or adolescents. It is often associated with regional lymphadenopathy and constitutional signs of a viral illness, such as fever and malaise.

43. What oral lesions have been associated with infection by human papillomavirus (HPV)?

- Squamous papilloma
- Verruca vulgaris
- Oral condyloma acuminatum
- Focal epithelial hyperplasia (Heck disease)
- Carcinoma of the oropharynx (tonsil)
- Oral carcinoma and HPV-associated dysplasia (less than 5% of oral carcinoma)

The benign conditions are usually associated with HPV-6 and -11; the malignant ones are usually associated with HPV-16, 18, 31, 33, 45, 52, and 58.

Gardasil™ is a nonavalent vaccine that is effective against these HPV types.
Heck disease is associated with HPV-13 and HPV-32.

44. What oral conditions does coxsackievirus cause?

Herpangina and hand-foot-and-mouth disease are caused by the type A coxsackievirus and generally affect children, who then develop oral ulcers associated with an upper respiratory tract viral prodrome. Lymphonodular pharyngitis is also caused by coxsackievirus.

45. What are Koplik spots?

Koplik spots are early manifestations of measles or rubeola (hence they are also called *herald spots*). They are 1- to 2-mm, yellow-white ulcers with surrounding erythema that occur on the buccal mucosa, usually a few days before the body rash of measles is seen. Koplik spots are not usually seen in German measles.

OTHER INFECTIONS

46. What are the organisms responsible for noma?

Noma, which is a gangrenous stomatitis resulting in severe destruction of the orofacial tissues, is usually encountered in areas in which malnutrition is rampant. The bacteria are similar to those associated with necrotizing ulcerative periodontitis, namely spirochetes, fusiform bacteria, and others. It is sometimes seen in patients with AIDS.

47. What are the oral findings in syphilis?

Primary: oral chancre
Secondary: mucous patches, condyloma lata
Tertiary: gumma (ulcerated nodules)
Congenital: enamel hypoplasia, mulberry molars, notched (Hutchinson) incisors

48. What is a granuloma?

Strictly speaking, a granuloma is a collection of epithelioid histiocytes that is often associated with multinucleated giant cells such as the Langhans-type giant cells seen in granulomas of tuberculosis (caused by *Mycobacterium tuberculosis*). Many infectious agents, including fungi (e.g., *Histoplasma* spp.) and those causing tertiary syphilis (*Treponema pallidum*) and cat scratch disease (*Bartonella henselae*), can produce granulomatous reactions. Foreign body reactions are often granulomatous. Orofacial granulomatosis may be related to hypersensitivity to foods, flavorings, and preservatives. Crohn disease and sarcoidosis are granulomatous diseases of unclear etiology (Fig. 4-6).

49. What are Langhans cells?

Langhans cells are multinucleated giant cells seen in granulomas, usually those caused by *M. tuberculosis*. Their nuclei have a characteristic horseshoe pattern. Do not confuse them with Langerhans cells, which are antigen-processing cells.

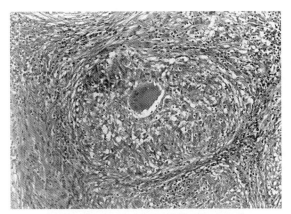

Fig. 4-6. Tuberculous granuloma with Langhans giant cell.

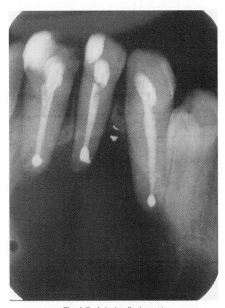

Fig. 4-7. Apical radicular cyst.

REACTIVE, HYPERSENSITIVITY, AND AUTOIMMUNE CONDITIONS
INTRABONY AND DENTAL TISSUES:

50. True or false: The periapical granuloma is composed of a collection of histiocytes, that is, a true granuloma.
    False. The periapical granuloma is a tumor-like (*-oma*) proliferation of granulation tissue found around the apex of a nonvital tooth. It is associated with chronic inflammation from pulp devitalization. The inflammation can stimulate proliferation of the epithelial rests of Malassez to form an apical radicular or periapical cyst (Fig. 4-7).

51. What is condensing osteitis?
    Condensing osteitis, a relatively common condition, manifests as an area of radiopacity in the bone, usually adjacent to a tooth that has a large restoration or endodontic therapy, although occasionally it may lie adjacent to what appears to be a sound tooth. It is asymptomatic. Histologically, condensing osteitis consists of dense bone, with little or no inflammation. It probably arises as a bony reaction to a low-grade inflammatory stimulus from the adjacent tooth. Idiopathic osteosclerosis, bone scar, and dense bone island are terms used for similar bone lesions unassociated with teeth.

52. What are the different causative factors between the wearing down of teeth caused by attrition, abrasion, erosion, and abfraction?
Attrition: tooth to tooth contact
Abrasion: a foreign object to tooth contact (e.g., toothbrush bristles, bobby pins, nails)
Erosion: a chemical agent to tooth contact (e.g., lemon juice, gastric juices)
Abfraction: occlusal stress leading to excessive tensile forces, which cause enamel at cervical areas of the teeth to shear off

SOFT TISSUE CONDITIONS

53. Name some systemic conditions associated with aphthous-like ulcers.

- Iron, folate, or vitamin B_{12} deficiency
- Inflammatory bowel disease
- Behçet disease
- Hypersensitivity to food or medications
- HIV (Human Immunodeficiency Virus) infection
- Conditions predisposing to neutropenia

54. True or false: An aphthous ulcer is the same as a traumatic ulcer.
False, but with reservations. A traumatic ulcer is the most common form of oral ulcer and, as its name suggests, occurs at the site of trauma, such as the buccal mucosa, lateral tongue, lower labial mucosa, or sulci. It follows a history of trauma, such as mastication or toothbrush injury. An aphthous ulcer may occur at the same sites, but often with no history of trauma. However, patients prone to developing aphthae tend to do so after episodes of minor trauma (Fig. 4-8).

55. A child returns after a visit to the dentist at which several amalgam restorations were placed. The child now has ulcers of the lateral tongue and buccal mucosa on the same side as the amalgams. What is your diagnosis?
This is a factitial injury. Children may inadvertently chew their tongue and buccal mucosae while tissues are numb from local anesthesia because the tissues feel strange to the child. Children and parents should be advised to be alert for such behavior.

56. Is the mucocele a true cyst?
No. The term *mucocele* refers loosely to a cyst-like lesion that contains mucus and usually occurs on the lower lip, ventral tongue, or floor of the mouth. However, it may occur wherever mucous glands are present. In most cases, it is not a true cyst because it is not lined by epithelium. It is caused by escape of mucus into the connective tissue when an excretory salivary duct is traumatized. Therefore, the mucocele is lined by fibrous and granulation tissue. When there is distention of the excretory duct because of a distal obstruction or the presence of a sialolith, the lesion is *salivary duct cyst.*

57. What is the cause of necrotizing sialometaplasia?
This painless ulcer usually develops on the hard palate but may occur wherever salivary glands are present. It represents vascular compromise and subsequent infarction of the salivary gland tissue, with reactive squamous metaplasia of the salivary duct epithelium that may mimic squamous cell carcinoma. The lesion resolves on its own.

58. Name the major denture-related findings in the oral cavity.
- Atrophic/erythematous candidiasis, especially of the palatal mucosa (denture sore mouth)
- Inflammatory papillary hyperplasia of the palatal mucosa
- Fibrous hyperplasia of the sulcus where the denture flange impinges (epulis fissuratum)
- Traumatic ulcers from overextension of flanges

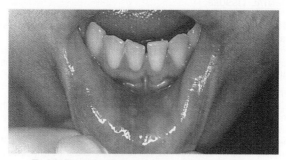

Fig. 4-8. Recurrent aphthous ulcer (minor) of lower labial mucosa.

- Angular cheilitis (candidiasis) from overclosure
- Denture base hypersensitivity reactions (uncommon; resembles atrophic candidiasis)

59. A patient is suspected of having an allergy to denture materials. What do you recommend?

The first thing is to rule out atrophic/erythematous candidiasis (denture stomatitis or denture sore mouth) because this is much more common. The patient should be treated with fluconazole (much more effective than nystatin or clotrimazole) or nystatin–triamcinolone cream applied directly to the denture to be worn by the patient; the denture must also be soaked in an antifungal agent overnight because it is a fomite. If these measures are taken and there is no response, the patient should be patch-tested by an allergist or dermatologist to a panel of denture base materials, which include metals and acrylic polymerization products. Usually, the lesions resolve with topical steroids.

60. What is a gum boil (parulis)?

A gum boil is an erythematous nodule usually located on the attached gingiva or even the alveolar mucosa. It may have a yellowish center that drains pus, and it may be asymptomatic. The nodule consists of granulation tissue and a sinus tract that usually can be traced to the root of the underlying tooth, with a thin gutta percha point. It indicates an infection of pulpal or periodontal origin (Fig. 4-9).

61. What is plasma cell gingivitis?

Plasma cell gingivitis presents as intensely erythematous gingivitis (desquamative gingivitis) and represents a contact hypersensitivity reaction to flavoring agents in toothpaste, mouthwash, chewing gum, and candies such as cinnamon or mint and other allergens including preservatives.

62. What is the differential diagnosis for desquamative gingivitis? What special handling procedures are necessary if you obtain a biopsy?

Desquamative gingivitis, which usually affects middle-aged women, is characterized by painful, red, eroded, and denuded areas of the gingiva. Most cases represent lichen planus and mucous membrane pemphigoid. Other causes include contact hypersensitivity reactions (such as plasma cell gingivitis), and less than 10% represent pemphigus vulgaris, or other autoimmune conditions, such as lupus erythematosus, linear IgA disease, and epidermolysis bullosa acquisita (Fig. 4-10). Definitive diagnosis requires direct immunofluorescence studies of the gingiva to look for autoantibodies. To preserve the integrity of immune reactants, the biopsy specimen should be split; half should be submitted in formalin for routine histopathology and the other half in Michel solution or fresh in saline. Alternately, two specimens can be harvested from different sites.

63. How does classic lichen planus present?

Classic lichen planus presents with white, reticular lesions (Wickham striae), often with erythema and sometimes ulcers, usually in a bilaterally symmetric fashion on the buccal mucosa, ventral tongue, and gingiva, although any site may be affected.

64. What medications can give a lichen planus-like (lichenoid) mucosal reaction (Fig. 4-11)?

- Drugs for treating hypertension, such as hydrochlorothiazide, angiotensin-converting enzyme (ACE) inhibitors, and beta blockers
- Levothyroxine
- Antigout agents, such as allopurinol
- Medications for treating inflammatory bowel disease, such as sulfasalazine
- Nonsteroidal anti-inflammatory drugs (NSAIDs)
- New biologic agents

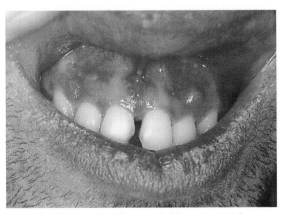

Fig. 4-9. Two parulides. The one on the left was about to drain.

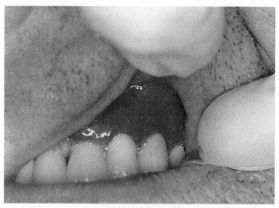

Fig. 4-10. Desquamative gingivitis.

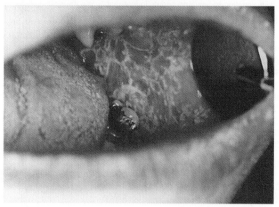

Fig. 4-11. Lichenoid stomatitis associated with hydrochlorothiazide.

65. **Name the medications that can be used to treat symptomatic lichen planus.**
    Most of the medications involved are immunomodulating agents. The most commonly used are corticosteroids (e.g., fluocinonide or clobetasol gels/creams) applied topically, injected intralesionally, or taken systemically or tacrolimus applied topically. Hydroxychloroquine, azathioprine, cyclosporine A, and retinoids have been used with some success.

66. **True or false: Dental restorations may cause lichen planus-like reactions.**
    True. In some people, amalgam and composite restorations have been shown to cause a lichenoid reaction in the mucosa in contact with the restoration. Replacement of the restoration may lead to resolution.

67. **What are the typical skin lesions of erythema multiforme called?**
    They are called *target, iris,* or *bull's-eye lesions*. Erythema multiforme is an acute mucocutaneous inflammatory process that may recur periodically in chronic form. It often leads to ulcers and erythema of the oral mucosa. It is no longer considered a variant of Stevens-Johnson syndrome.

68. **Name the most common factors responsible for recurrent erythema multiforme.**
    The most common etiology is hypersensitivity reaction to herpes simplex virus and, less frequently, hypersensitivity to some medications. Do not expect to be able to culture herpes simplex virus from the lesions of recurrent erythema multiforme, which is a hypersensitivity reaction to some component of the virus. Usually, the viral infection precedes the lesions of erythema multiforme.

69. **What is Stevens-Johnson syndrome?**
    Stevens-Johnson syndrome is a condition leading to blistering and necrolysis of the epidermis; the more severe form is called *toxic epidermal necrolysis*, a potentially fatal disorder. It is usually caused by hypersensitivity to medications. The condition is characterized by extensive involvement of the mucous membranes of the oral cavity,

eyes, genitalia, and occasionally the upper gastrointestinal and respiratory tracts. Desquamation and ulceration of the lips, with crusting, is usually dramatic. Atypical target lesions may be seen on the skin.

70. **What is the difference between pemphigus and pemphigoid?**
Both are autoimmune vesiculobullous diseases. In pemphigus (usually vulgaris when in the mouth), autoantibodies attack desmosomes of the epithelial cells, leading to acantholysis and formation of an intraepithelial bulla. In pemphigoid (usually mucous membrane), autoantibodies attack the junction between the epithelium and connective tissue, leading to the formation of a subepithelial bulla (Fig. 4-12).

71. **What two forms of pemphigoid involve the oral cavity?**
The two forms are mucous membrane pemphigoid and bullous pemphigoid. These autoimmune vesiculobullous diseases have antigens located in the lamina lucida of the basement membrane. Mucous membrane pemphigoid involves the oral mucosa, conjunctiva, esophageal, genital, and other mucosal sites, whereas bullous pemphigoid presents primarily with skin lesions and occasionally with mucosal lesions. IgG, IgA, and/or C3 localize at the basement membrane zone.

72. **Differentiate between a Tzanck test and Tzanck cell.**
The **Tzanck test** involves direct examination of cells that may indicate a herpes simplex virus infection. The test is done by scraping the lesion (which may be a vesicle, ulcer, or crust) and smearing the debris on a slide. The slide is then stained and examined with a microscope for virally infected cells, which show multinucleation and ground glass nuclei. **Tzanck cells** are acantholytic cells seen within the bulla of pemphigus vulgaris (Fig. 4-13).

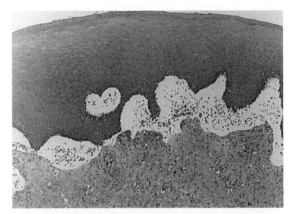

Fig. 4-12. Subepithelial bulla formation in mucous membrane pemphigoid.

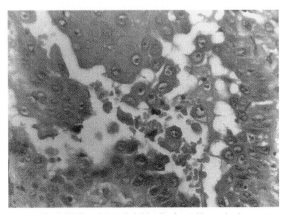

Fig. 4-13. Tzanck (acantholytic) cells of pemphigus vulgaris.

73. **What is the difference between systemic lupus erythematosus (SLE) and discoid lupus erythematosus (DLE)?**
SLE is the prototypical multisystem autoimmune disease characterized by circulating antinuclear antibodies; the principal sites of injury are skin, joints, and kidneys. The oral mucosa is often involved, and the lesions may appear lichenoid, with white reticulations, erythema, or ulcers. DLE is the limited form of the disease; most manifestations are localized to the skin and mucous membranes, with no systemic involvement. DLE does not usually progress to SLE, although certain phases of SLE are clinically indistinguishable from DLE. The oral findings are similar in both.
Patients with SLE demonstrate circulating antibodies, such as antinuclear antibody (ANA) and anti-Smith antibody.

74. **Define midline lethal granuloma.**
These terms describe a destructive ulcerative process, usually located in the midline of the hard palate, that may lead to palatal perforation. Conditions that may cause this clinical entity include deep fungal infections, syphilitic gummas, granulomatous polyangiitis, IgG4 disease, chronic cocaine use, and malignant neoplasms, such as sinonasal lymphomas, salivary gland malignancy, or squamous cell carcinoma.

CHEMOTHERAPY AND HUMAN IMMUNODEFICIENCY VIRUS INFECTION

75. **What are the common oral side-effects of chemotherapy?**
Chemotherapy is often directly toxic to the oral mucosa. The mucosa becomes atrophic and ulcerates. The chemotherapeutic agents also act on other rapidly dividing cells in the body, such as hematopoietic tissues. The results are neutropenia (low neutrophil count), anemia, and thrombocytopenia (low platelet count). Neutropenia may have an indirect stomatotoxic effect by allowing oral bacteria to colonize the ulcers. Usually, these ulcers develop during the period of profound neutropenia and resolve when neutrophils reappear in the blood circulation. In addition, patients are at increased risk for developing oral candidiasis, oral herpetic lesions, and deep fungal infections. Thrombocytopenia may cause oral petechiae, ecchymoses, and hematomas, especially at sites of trauma (Fig. 4-14).

76. **A patient who has undergone cancer chemotherapy now has recurrent intraoral herpetic lesions but no history of cold sores or fever blisters. Is this likely?**
Yes. Many people have been exposed to HSV without their knowledge and are completely asymptomatic. The virus becomes latent in the sensory ganglia and reactivates to give rise to recurrent or recrudescent herpetic lesions. The prevalence of those who have been exposed to HSV increases with age, immunosuppression, and immunosenescence.

77. **What are the complications of leukemia in the oral cavity, aside from those associated with chemotherapy?**
Leukemic infiltration of the bone marrow leads to reduced production of functional components of the marrow, although white blood cells and platelets may be increased in number but are cancerous and not functional. Neutropenia (quantitative or qualitative) results in more frequent and more aggressive odontogenic infections and soft tissue infections (including viral infections); thrombocytopenia results in petechiae, ecchymoses, and hematomas in the oral cavity, which is subject to trauma from functional activities. In addition, some leukemias, especially acute monocytic leukemia, have a propensity to infiltrate the gingiva, causing localized or diffuse gingival enlargement.

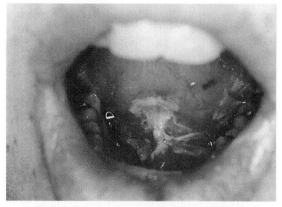

Fig. 4-14. Chemotherapy-associated oral ulcerative mucositis.

78. **A patient has undergone a matched allogeneic hematopoietic stem cell transplant for the treatment of leukemia. Three months later, he has erosive and lichenoid lesions in his mouth. What is your diagnosis?**

The likely diagnosis is chronic oral graft-versus-host disease. The allogeneic hematopoietic stem cell transplant or graft contains immunocompetent cells that recognize the host cells as foreign and attack them. The oral lesions of chronic graft-versus-host disease resemble the lesions of lichen planus (Fig. 4-15).

79. **What are the effects of radiation on the oral cavity?**

Short term: oral erythema and ulcers, candidiasis, dysgeusia, dysosmia, parotitis, acute sialadenitis, hyposalivation

Long term: hyposalivation, erythema and ulcers, candidiasis, dysgeusia, dysosmia, dental caries, osteoradionecrosis, epithelial atrophy, and fibrosis (leading to trismus)

80. **What factors predispose to osteoradionecrosis?**

This necrotic process affects bone that has been in the radiation field. Predisposing factors include a high total dose of radiation (especially if >6500 cGy), presence of odontogenic infection (e.g., periapical pathosis, periodontal disease), trauma (e.g., extractions), and site (the mandible is less vascular and more susceptible than the maxilla).

81. **What is the basic cause of osteoradionecrosis?**

The breakdown of hypocellular, hypovascular, and hypoxic tissue results in a chronic, nonhealing wound containing sequestra that can be secondarily infected.

82. **Other than radiation, what other situations may lead to osteonecrosis?**

- Medications: antiresorptive agents such as bisphosphonates and denosumab; antiangiogenic agents such as bevacizumab and sunitinib
- Trauma (especially of the lingual plate in the area of the molars)
- Odontogenic infection, osteomyelitis leading to sequestrum formation; aggravated by primary sclerotic bone disease (e.g., cemento-osseous dysplasia)
- Viral infection (e.g., oral shingles)

83. **True or false: A patient can only be said to have medication-related osteonecrosis of the jaws if she or he has exposed dead bone.**

False. Patients can have stage 0 (nonexposed) osteonecrosis if there are signs and symptoms that the clinician thinks are not related to odontogenic pathology if they are on medications that predispose to this. These include pain and sinus tracts not related to odontogenic infection, and poorly defined radiolucencies with sequestrum.

84. **What are the common oral manifestations of human immunodeficiency virus (HIV) infection?**

Soft tissue: candidiasis, recurrent herpetic infections, deep fungal infections, aphthous-like ulcers, oral hairy leukoplakia, viral warts

Periodontium: nonspecific gingivitis, necrotizing ulcerative periodontitis, severe and rapidly destructive periodontal disease, often with unusual pathogens

Tumors: Kaposi sarcoma, B-cell lymphoma, squamous cell carcinoma

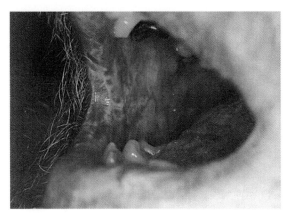

Fig. 4-15. Chronic oral graft-versus-host disease of buccal mucosa.

85. A patient who tested positive for HIV antibodies presents with a CD4 count of 150/μL but has never had an opportunistic infection or been symptomatic. Does he have AIDS?
Yes. By the Centers for Disease Control (CDC) definition, patients with CD4 counts below 200 cells/μL are considered to have Stage 3 AIDS. Stages 1 and 2 diseases are based on clinical findings such as generalized lymphadenopathy, opportunistic infections, and weight loss.

86. True or false: Like other leukoplakias, oral hairy leukoplakia has a tendency to progress to malignancy.
False. Oral hairy leukoplakia is associated with EBV infection and usually a superimposed candidiasis, with no malignant potential. However, patients infected with HIV are more susceptible to oral cancer in general. The word "leukoplakia" used in this context is misleading but historical.

87. Are HIV-associated aphthous ulcers similar to recurrent major aphthae?
Yes. They tend to be larger than 1 cm, persist for extended periods (weeks to months) and are difficult to treat. They may be associated with neutropenia caused by AIDS or medications or because of generalized immunosuppression (Fig. 4-16).

88. Should HIV-associated aphthous ulcers be evaluated for infection?
Yes. Often the culture/PCR or biopsy is positive for HSV, CMV, or even deep fungal infections, and the patient needs to be treated appropriately.

89. You have a patient with HIV-AIDS whom you have been treating with fluconazole. More recently, his candidiasis has been recalcitrant, even with double the dose of fluconazole. What should you do?
Culture the lesions of candidiasis and specifically ask the laboratory to check for resistance to fluconazole. Fluconazole resistance occurs not uncommonly in patients who have been treated for a long time with fluconazole. Other medications are voriconazole, itraconazole, and posaconazole.

BENIGN NEOPLASMS AND TUMORS
ODONTOGENIC TUMORS

90. Name the benign odontogenic tumors that are purely epithelial.
- Ameloblastoma
- Calcifying epithelial odontogenic tumor (Pindborg tumor)
- Adenomatoid odontogenic tumor
- Squamous odontogenic tumor

91. Which odontogenic tumor is associated with amyloid production? With ghost cells?
Calcifying epithelial odontogenic tumor (Pindborg tumor) is associated with amyloid production; calcifying odontogenic cyst (Gorlin cyst, calcifying cystic odontogenic tumor) is associated with ghost cells.

92. Which two lesions, one in the long bones and one in the cranium, resemble the ameloblastoma?
In the long bones, it is adamantinoma; in the cranium, it is craniopharyngioma.

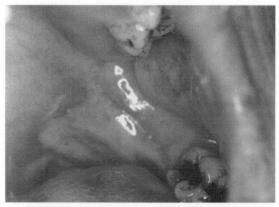

Fig. 4-16. HIV-associated aphthous ulcers of the soft palate and oropharynx.

93. True or false: All forms of ameloblastoma behave aggressively and tend to recur.
    False. One form of ameloblastoma, which occurs in adolescents and young adults, behaves less aggressively, and has a lower tendency to recur. It is called *unicystic ameloblastoma*. Peripheral (extraosseous) ameloblastomas also behave in a benign fashion and do not recur.

94. True or false: Because ameloblastoma is so aggressive, it can be considered a malignancy.
    False. Ameloblastoma is a locally destructive lesion that has no tendency to metastasize. However, it has two malignant counterparts, ameloblastic carcinoma and malignant ameloblastoma.

95. To which teeth are cementoblastomas usually attached?
    They are usually attached to the mandibular permanent molars.

96. Name the three most common odontogenic tumors that produce primarily mesenchymal tissues.
    These are central cemento-ossifying fibroma, odontogenic fibroma, and odontogenic myxoma.

97. An adolescent presents with a mandibular radiolucency with areas that histologically resemble ameloblastoma and dental papilla. What is your diagnosis?
    The diagnosis is ameloblastic fibroma, one of the rare odontogenic tumors that has both neoplastic epithelial and mesenchymal components.

FIBRO-OSSEOUS TUMORS

98. True or false: Central cemento-ossifying fibroma is a mesenchymal odontogenic neoplasm.
    True. While this used to be considered a primary bone neoplasm, it has been reclassified into a mesenchymal odontogenic neoplasm that likely arises from stem cells in the periodontal ligament, producing cementum-like droplets and bone (Fig. 4-17).

99. Is it possible to distinguish histologically between fibrous dysplasia and central cemento-ossifying fibroma?
    Sometimes yes, often no. The clinical and radiographic findings are the most important for differentiating between the two. Fibrous dysplasia tends to occur in the maxilla of younger individuals and presents as a poorly defined "ground-glass," homogenous, faint radio-opacity that blends with the normal adjacent bone. The central cemento-ossifying fibroma is a well-demarcated radiolucency, often with a distinct border, and may contain areas of radiopacity within the lesion. It is more common in the mandible.

SOFT TISSUE TUMORS

100. True or false: Fibroma of the oral cavity is a true neoplasm.
    False. As its name suggests, fibroma of the oral cavity is a tumor (*-oma*) composed of fibrous scar tissue. It tends to occur as a result of trauma and therefore usually presents on the buccal mucosa, lower labial mucosa, and lateral tongue. It is nonencapsulated and may enlarge with continued local trauma/irritation.
       Neoplasm has been defined as an uncontrolled proliferation of tissues generally driven by molecular changes such as mutations. Therefore, an oral fibroma is not a true neoplasm but just a tumor of fibrous scar tissue. Some pathologists prefer the term *fibrous hyperplasia* or *fibroepithelial polyp* instead of *fibroma* because it more accurately reflects its nature. The pathogenesis is similar to that of fibrous hyperplasia caused by poorly fitting dentures (epulis fissuratum) (Fig. 4-18).

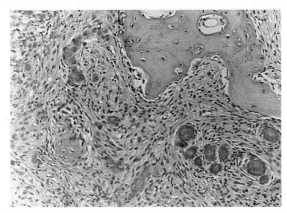

Fig. 4-17. Central cemento-ossifying fibroma with round globules of cementum and trabeculae of osteoid.

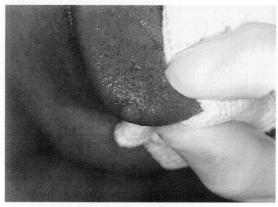

Fig. 4-18. Fibroma of the tongue.

101. **What are Verocay bodies?**
Verocay bodies consist of amorphous-looking, eosinophilic material and the adjacent palisaded nuclei which is a characteristic feature of schwannoma, a benign nerve sheath tumor of Schwann cells. The eosinophilic material represents duplicated basement membrane produced by Schwann cells and is an important component of Antoni A tissue.

102. **What is the most common tumor that contains neural structures?**
Traumatic neuroma is the most common. This is caused by trauma and severance of nerves. When the nerve branches try to regrow (Wallerian degeneration regeneration), they form a tangled mass of nerve fibers of varying sizes admixed with scar tissue. They are particularly common under denture flanges close to the mental foramen.

103. **What are venous lakes?**
Venous lakes or varices are purplish-blue nodules or papules, often present on the lips, tongue, and buccal mucosa of older people, that represent dilated venules.

104. **What is the most common benign salivary gland tumor?**
Pleomorphic adenoma is the most common.

105. **Why is pleomorphic adenoma sometimes called a benign mixed tumor?**
Pleomorphic adenoma is called a *mixed tumor* because histologically it has a mixture of epithelial and connective tissue components. The tumor arises from a progenitor cell that can produce ducts, myoepithelial cells, and stroma, which may contain cartilage and bone.

106. **What is a brown tumor?**
A brown tumor is histologically a central giant cell granuloma associated with hyperparathyroidism. It appears brown when excised because it is a highly vascular lesion. Most conventional central giant cell granulomas occur in children and young adults in the absence of hyperparathyroidism.

MALIGNANT NEOPLASMS

107. **What percentage of the population has leukoplakia? What percentage of leukoplakias have dysplasia or carcinoma when first biopsied as compared with erythroplakias?**
Leukoplakia occurs in 0.5%-1% of the population, and 15%-40% of leukoplakias have dysplasia or carcinoma at the time of biopsy, whereas 90% of erythroplakias show such changes at the time of biopsy (Fig. 4-19).

108. **What is leukoplakia and which forms of leukoplakia have a higher association with dysplasia?**
Leukoplakia is a white plaque, usually well-demarcated, that is the most common premalignant mucosal lesion. Those that have verrucous, nodular, or red components have a higher chance of harboring dysplasia.

109. **What is proliferative verrucous leukoplakia?**
It is a clinically progressive and multifocal form of leukoplakia with a high rate of malignant transformation (up to 70%) compared to localized leukoplakias. The term proliferative leukoplakia is more appropriate because all lesions are not verrucous and some may be homogenous or even erythroleukoplakia.

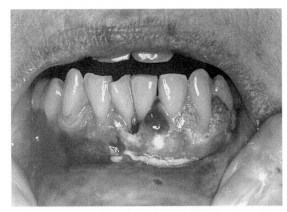

Fig. 4-19. Squamous cell carcinoma presenting as leukoplakia with erythematous and verrucous areas.

110. What is the prevalence of oral cancer in the United States? Which country has the highest prevalence of oral cancer?
Oral cancer accounts for 3% of all cancers in the United States if oropharyngeal lesions are included. India has the highest prevalence of oral cancer; it is the most common cancer there and is related to the use of areca nut and tobacco products.

111. What are the risk factors for oral cancer?
- Tobacco products
- Alcohol (especially in conjunction with smoking)
- Areca nut products also cause oral submucous fibrosis (especially in East Indians and some Southeast Asian cultures)
- Sunlight (especially for cancer of the lip in men)
- Immunosuppression and autoimmune disease
- Personal history of oral cancer or other cancer
- Family history of cancer
- Age
- Plummer-Vinson syndrome
- Familial cancer syndromes such as dyskeratosis congenita and Li Fraumeni syndrome

112. True or false: Patients with HPV-associated tonsillar carcinoma have a better prognosis than those with tobacco-associated tonsillar carcinoma.
True.

113. What is the difference in prognosis between a squamous cell carcinoma and verrucous carcinoma?
Approximately 50% of squamous cell carcinomas have metastasized at the time of diagnosis. The larger they are, the more likely that metastases will develop. Verrucous carcinomas do not tend to metastasize despite the rather large size of some lesions; they are locally aggressive lesions.

114. What is a so-called rodent ulcer?
A "rodent ulcer" refers to a basal cell carcinoma of the skin that, despite its low tendency to metastasize, erodes through adjacent tissues like the gnawing of a rodent; it may cause destruction of the facial structures.

115. What are the three most common intraoral malignant salivary gland tumors?
These are mucoepidermoid carcinoma, polymorphous adenocarcinoma, and adenoid cystic carcinoma.

116. Which two salivary gland tumors often show perineural invasion (neurotropism)?
These are adenoid cystic carcinoma and polymorphous adenocarcinoma. However, any malignancy (particularly carcinomas) can show perineural invasion.

117. True or false: Lymphoepithelial sialadenitis (formerly known as myoepithelial sialadenitis and benign lymphoepithelial lesion) of Sjögren syndrome is an innocuous autoimmune sialadenitis.
False. The "benign" lymphoepithelial lesion is not so benign. Patients with this condition have a higher incidence of lymphoma (up to 16 times more) than the general population.

118. A patient with Sjögren syndrome is referred for a labial salivary gland biopsy to identify a lymphoepithelial sialadenitis. Does this sound right?

No. The lymphoepithelial sialadenitis of Sjögren syndrome is found in the major glands, mainly the parotid, especially if parotid enlargement is present. A labial salivary gland biopsy will show an autoimmune sialadenitis characterized by lymphocytic infiltrates that form "foci" which are collections of at least 50 lymphocytes around a duct. The more "foci," the more likely the diagnosis of an autoimmune sialadenitis.

119. Do lymphomas of the oral cavity occur outside Waldeyer ring?

Yes. Oral lymphomas are most common in Waldeyer ring, but they may occur in the palatal mucosa, buccal mucosa, tongue, floor of the mouth, and retromolar areas. Primary bone lymphomas also occur in the jawbones.

120. What does monoclonal plasma cell proliferation mean?

Plasma cells produce immunoglobulin that contains heavy and light chains. Each plasma cell and its progeny produce either kappa or lambda light chains and never both. A group of plasma cells that produces only kappa or lambda light chains is most likely caused by proliferation of a single malignant clone of plasma cells, such as a plasmacytoma or multiple myeloma. The presence of both light chains in a plasma cell proliferation is more likely to be polyclonal proliferation, which characterizes inflammatory lesions.

121. Name the different epidemiologic forms of Kaposi sarcoma.

1. Classic or European form: usually Eastern European men (often Jewish); multiple red papules on the lower extremities, with rare visceral involvement and a more indolent course
2. Endemic or African form: young men or children in equatorial Africa; frequent visceral involvement that may be fulminant
3. Epidemic form: HIV-associated; may be widely disseminated to mucocutaneous and visceral sites; variable course
4. Organ transplantation-associated form: patients who have undergone organ (especially renal) transplantation, with immunosuppressive therapy
5. Kaposi sarcoma in HIV-negative men who have sex with men which is clinically similar to classic type except in a younger age group

122. A patient has a suspected metastatic tumor to the mandible. What are the likely primary tumors?

- Lung
- Breast
- Prostate
- Kidney
- Gastrointestinal tract
- Thyroid
- Skin

123. True or false: Osteosarcoma of the jaws occurs in younger patients more often than osteosarcoma of the long bones.

False. Patients with osteosarcoma of the jaws are 1 to 2 decades older than patients with osteosarcoma of the long bones.

124. Which conditions predispose to osteosarcoma?

Many cases of osteosarcoma in young adults occur *de novo*. However, there are well-documented cases of osteosarcoma in association with Paget disease, chronic osteomyelitis, history of retinoblastoma, and prior radiation to the bone for fibrous dysplasia.

NONVASCULAR PIGMENTED LESIONS

125. What medications can cause mucosal melanosis?

- Oral contraceptives
- Antimalarial agents
- (e.g., hydroxychloroquine)
- Tetracycline and minocycline
- Imatinib

126. Why does heavy metal poisoning primarily cause staining of the gingiva?

Heavy metals such as lead, bismuth, and silver may cause a grayish-black line to appear on the gingival margins, especially in patients with poor oral hygiene. Plaque bacteria can produce hydrogen sulfide; this combines with the heavy metals to form heavy metal sulfides, which are usually black.

127. What can cause mucosal melanosis?

Benign: physiologic pigmentation, post-inflammatory hyperpigmentation (especially in dark-skinned people), oral melanotic macule, smoking (may be post-inflammatory), mucosal melanocytic nevus, melanoacanthosis

Malignant: melanoma

Systemic conditions: Peutz-Jegher syndrome, McCune Albright syndrome, Addison disease, neurofibromatosis

128. What are the different forms of oral melanocytic nevi?
Intramucosal nevus: tends to be elevated, papular, or nodular
Junctional nevus: tends to be macular
Compound nevus: tends to be papular or nodular
Blue nevus: tends to be macular

129. What is the most common site for oral melanoma?
It is the hard palatal mucosa.

130. What is the difference between a melanocyte and melanophage?
A melanocyte is a neuroectodermally derived cell that contains the intracellular apparatus to manufacture melanin. A melanophage is a macrophage (scavenger cell) that has phagocytosed melanin pigment and therefore can resemble a melanocyte because it contains melanin. However, it lacks the enzymes to produce melanin.

METABOLIC LESIONS ASSOCIATED WITH SYSTEMIC DISEASE

131. What are the various presentations of Langerhans cell histiocytosis?
Single system disease with unifocal or multifocal involvement: single or multiple lesions in one or multiple bones. In the jaw bones, this presents as a radiolucency often with teeth floating in it.
Multisystem disease with or without risk organ involvement, with risk organs being liver, spleen, and bone marrow. Involvement of risk organs is associated with a poorer prognosis.

132. What are Birbeck granules?
Birbeck granules are racket-shaped cytoplasmic inclusions seen in Langerhans cells of Langerhans cell histiocytosis (Fig. 4-20).

133. What are two common oral changes associated with pregnancy?
These are gingivitis and pyogenic granuloma (epulis gravidarum).

134. An older man complains that his jaw seems to be getting too big for his dentures and that his hat does not fit him anymore. What do you suspect?
This could be Paget disease of bone (osteitis deformans), a metabolic bone disease in which initial bone resorption is followed by haphazard bone repair, with resulting marked sclerosis. This condition may lead to narrowing of the skull base foramina and neurologic deficits.
The maxilla is often affected, and a cotton wool appearance has been described on radiographs.

135. What oral lesions are associated with gastrointestinal disease?
The most common gastrointestinal disease associated with oral signs is inflammatory bowel disease, especially Crohn disease. Patients may manifest with swelling of the lips, cobblestoning of the mucosa, papillary growths, and linear aphthous-like ulcers. Biopsy shows non-necrotizing granulomas. Patients may also develop glossitis associated with vitamin B_{12} deficiency if part of the ileum has been resected for the disease. Those with gluten-sensitive enteropathies such as celiac disease may also present with aphthous-like ulcers. Patients with ulcerative colitis may also develop pyostomatitis vegetans.

136. What are primary and secondary Sjögren syndrome?
Primary Sjögren syndrome consists of dry eyes (keratoconjunctivitis sicca) and dry mouth (hyposalivation) in the absence of other systemic conditions. Secondary Sjögren syndrome consists of primary Sjögren syndrome plus

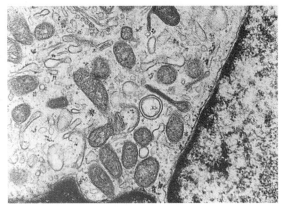

Fig. 4-20. Racket-shaped Birbeck granule of Langerhans cell histiocytosis.

a connective tissue disorder such as rheumatoid arthritis, systemic lupus erythematosus, or progressive systemic sclerosis. Most patients with Sjögren's syndrome have circulating autoantibodies (antinuclear antibodies).

137. **What is the dental significance of the Sturge-Weber syndrome?**
This syndrome is characterized by vascular malformations of the leptomeninges, facial skin innervated by the fifth nerve (nevus flammeus), and corresponding ipsilateral areas in the oral mucosa and bone. Bleeding is therefore an important consideration in dental treatment. Patients may also exhibit intellectual disabilities and seizure disorders. Treatment may include phenytoin which can cause gingival hyperplasia.

DIFFERENTIAL DIAGNOSES AND GENERAL CONSIDERATIONS
INTRABONY LESIONS

138. **Name two pseudocysts of the jaw bones.**
    • Traumatic (simple) bone cyst: radiolucency scallops between tooth roots; empty at surgery.
    • Static bone cyst (Stafne bone cavity): salivary gland depression beneath the inferior alveolar canal.
    While aneurysmal bone cyst used to be considered a pseudocyst, it is now considered a neoplasm because it has been found to harbor mutations. It consists of giant cells lining blood-filled spaces.

139. **What is the differential diagnosis for a multiloculated radiolucency?**
    Odontogenic cysts or tumors
    • Dentigerous cyst
    • Odontogenic keratocyst (also known as a keratocystic odontogenic tumor)
    • Ameloblastoma
    • Odontogenic myxoma
    Lesions that contain giant cells
    • Central giant cell granuloma
    • Aneurysmal bone cyst
    • Cherubism
    Vascular malformations
    Intraosseous salivary gland tumors

SOFT TISSUE LESIONS

140. **What is the differential diagnosis for a solitary upper lip nodule?**
    Salivary gland pathology: sialolith, benign salivary gland tumor (especially pleomorphic adenoma and canalicular adenoma), malignant salivary gland tumor

    Vascular tumor: pyogenic granuloma
    Neural tumor: neurofibroma, schwannoma, neuroma
    Nasolabial cyst
    Skin appendage tumors

141. **What may cause diffuse swelling of the lips?**
    • Vascular malformations
    • Angioedema
    • Hypersensitivity reactions
    • Cheilitis glandularis
    • Orofacial granulomatosis (e.g., Melkersson-Rosenthal syndrome)
    • Crohn disease

142. **What is the differential diagnosis for a solitary gingival nodule?**
    The most common diagnoses are fibroma or fibrous hyperplasia, pyogenic granuloma (especially in a pregnant patient), peripheral giant cell granuloma, peripheral ossifying fibroma (essentially a fibrous hyperplasia with metaplastic bone formation), and parulis. Other less common conditions include gingival cyst of the adult, benign extraosseous odontogenic tumors, and malignant tumors, including metastatic tumors.

143. **What may cause generalized overgrowth of gingival tissues?**
    Common causes include plaque accumulation, medications such as phenytoin, cyclosporine, valproic acid, diltiazem, and nifedipine (the last two are calcium channel blockers), hormonal factors (puberty and pregnancy), granulomatosis with polyangiitis, orofacial granulomatosis, fibromatosis gingivae, and leukemic infiltrate.

144. **A labial salivary gland biopsy is useful for diagnosis of certain systemic conditions. What are they?**
    • Sjögren syndrome
    • Amyloidosis

- Sarcoidosis
- IgG4 disease

145. What may cause chronic hyposalivation?

Common causes include ingestion of anticholinergic medications, aging (although many experts believe this to be drug-related), insufficient oral intake of fluids, excessive consumption of caffeinated products, and chronic anxiety. Less common conditions include autoimmune sialadenitis (such as Sjögren syndrome and graft-versus-host disease) and radiation to the gland.

146. Name possible causes of bilateral parotid swelling.

Mumps
Sjögren syndrome
Radiation-induced acute parotitis
Diabetes mellitus
Malnutrition
Alcoholism
Bulimia
Warthin tumor
Lymphoepithelial cysts in HIV infection

147. What may cause depapillation of the tongue?

Vitamin B, iron, and/or folate deficiency
Median rhomboid glossitis (focally)
Benign migratory glossitis (focally)
Syphilis
Plummer-Vinson syndrome
Lichen planus
Chronic hyposalivation

148. What may cause diffuse enlargement of the tongue?

Congenital macroglossia	Angioedema
Lymphatic malformation (with vesicles)	Acromegaly
Vascular malformation	Trisomy 21
Neurofibromatosis	Amyloidosis
Hyperpituitarism	Hypothyroidism

149. What is the differential diagnosis of midline swellings of the floor of the mouth?

Ranula (mucocele, usually to one side)
Dermoid cyst
Epidermoid cyst

150. What may cause diffuse white plaques in the buccal mucosa?

Cannon white sponge nevus
Pachyonychia congenita
Candidiasis
Proliferative leukoplakia
Hereditary benign intraepithelial dyskeratosis
Chronic bite keratosis (Morsicatio mucosae oris)
Contact hypersensitivity
Contact desquamation from strong dentifrices

151. Name the conditions that may give rise to papillary lesions of the oral cavity.

These are squamous papilloma, verruca vulgaris, condyloma, inflammatory papillary hyperplasia of the palatal mucosa (denture injury), localized spongiotic gingival hyperplasia, verrucous carcinoma, papillary squamous cell carcinoma, and verruciform xanthoma.

152. What lesions may occur in the oral cavity of neonates?

Lesions in the oral cavity of neonates include congenital granular cell tumor of the newborn, gingival cyst of the newborn, palatal cyst of the newborn (Bohn nodules, Epstein pearls), lymphangiomas of the alveolar ridge, natal teeth, and neuroectodermal tumor of infancy.

153. What may cause burning symptoms of the tongue?

Patients may report burning symptoms of the tongue secondary to mucosal disease such as atrophic glossitis, candidiasis, lichen planus, and migratory glossitis. However, this syndrome may also occur in the absence of any organic mucosal disease. In these cases, it is referred to as primary burning mouth (oral dysesthesia) syndrome, a neuropathic pain disorder with a strong association with anxiety, depression, and other somatoform disorders.

154. **What may cause oral paresthesia?**
Oral paresthesia may be caused by manipulation or inflammation of a nerve or tissues around a nerve, direct damage to a nerve or tissues around a nerve, tumor impinging on or invading a nerve, primary neural tumor, and central nervous system disorder or tumor.

155. **Why do lesions appear white in the oral cavity?**
Lesions appear white because of the following:
• Thickened keratin or keratin where none was present before
• Edema of the epithelium cells
• Thickened epithelium
• Altered epithelium from dyskeratotic syndromes (often genetic) or from dysplasia (leukoplakia)
• Scarring of the connective tissue

156. **Why do lesions appear red in the oral cavity?**
• Loss of the usual keratin layer
• Erosion or atrophy of the epithelium
• Increased or dilated vasculature (e.g., in inflammation)
• Change in the intrinsic nature of the epithelial cell, such as epithelial dysplasia (erythroplakia)

157. **Distinguish among macules, papules, and plaque.**
A macule is a localized lesion that is flush with the adjacent mucosa and is better seen than felt. The term is often used to describe localized pigmented lesions, such as amalgam tattoos and melanotic macules. Papules and plaque are broad-based, raised lesions; the papule is smaller than 5 mm, and the plaque is larger than 5 mm.

158. **What is the difference between a bulla and a vesicle?**
Both are fluid-filled. A bulla is usually larger than 5 mm; a vesicle is smaller than 5 mm.

159. **Differentiate between a hamartoma and a choristoma.**
A **hamartoma** is a tumor-like growth consisting of an overgrowth of tissues that histologically appears mature and is native to the area. A hamartoma of the skin and mucosa is sometimes called a *nevus* (e.g., vascular, epidermal, or melanocytic nevus). A **choristoma** is a tumor-like growth consisting of an overgrowth of tissues that histologically appears mature but is not native to the area (e.g., cartilaginous choristoma, bony choristoma of the tongue).

160. **What are oncocytes?**
Oncocytes are eosinophilic swollen cells found in many salivary gland tumors, such as oncocytomas and Warthin tumor, and in oncocytic metaplasia of salivary ducts. They are swollen because they contain many mitochondria.

161. **What are Russell bodies?**
Russell bodies are round eosinophilic bodies found in reactive lesions; they represent globules of immunoglobulin in plasma cells.

BIBLIOGRAPHY

Developmental Conditions

Bilodeau EA, Collins BM. Odontogenic cysts and neoplasms. *Surg Pathol Clin.* 2017;10(1):177–222.
Davidova LA, Bhattacharyya I, Islam MN, Cohen DM, Fitzpatrick SG. An analysis of clinical and histopathologic features of fibrous dysplasia of the jaws: A series of 40 cases and review of literature. *Head Neck Pathol.* 2020;14(2):353–361.
Lo Muzio L, Mascitti M, Santarelli A, et al. Cystic lesions of the jaws: a retrospective clinicopathologic study of 2030 cases. *Oral Surg Oral Med Oral Pathol Oral Radiol.* 2017;124(2):128–138.
Mainville GN, Turgeon DP, Kauzman A. Diagnosis and management of benign fibro-osseous lesions of the jaws: a current review for the dental clinician. *Oral Dis.* 2017;23(4):440–450.
Nelson BL, Phillips BJ. Benign fibro-osseous lesions of the head and neck. *Head Neck Pathol.* 2019;13(3):466–475.
Tabareau-Delalande F, Collin C, Gomez-Brouchet A, et al. Diagnostic value of investigating GNAS mutations in fibro-osseous lesions: a retrospective study of 91 cases of fibrous dysplasia and 40 other fibro-osseous lesions. *Mod Pathol.* 2013;26(7):911–921.

Infections

Betz SJ. HPV-related papillary lesions of the oral mucosa: a review. *Head Neck Pathol.* 2019;13(1):80–90.
Fitzpatrick SG, Cohen DM, Clark AN. Ulcerated lesions of the oral mucosa: clinical and histologic review. *Head Neck Pathol.* 2019;13(1):91–102.
Guarner J, Brandt ME. Histopathologic diagnosis of fungal infections in the 21st century. *Clin Microbiol Rev.* 2011;24(2):247–280.
Hellstein JW, Marek CL. Candidiasis: red and white manifestations in the oral cavity. *Head Neck Pathol.* 2019;13(1):25–32.
Stojanov IJ, Woo SB. Human papillomavirus and Epstein-Barr virus associated conditions of the oral mucosa. *Semin Diagn Pathol.* 2015;32(1):3–11.
Woo SB, Challacombe SJ. Management of recurrent oral herpes simplex infections. *Oral Surg Oral Med Oral Pathol Oral Radiol Endod.* 2007;103(Suppl):S12 e1–e8.

Reactive, Hypersensitivity, and Autoimmune Conditions

Akintoye SO, Greenberg MS. Recurrent aphthous stomatitis. *Dent Clin North Am.* 2014;58(2):281–297.

Benli M, Batool F, Stutz C, Petit C, Jung S, Huck O. Orofacial manifestations and dental management of systemic lupus erythematosus: a review. *Oral Dis.* 2021;27(2):151–167.

Carey B, Setterfield J. Mucous membrane pemphigoid and oral blistering diseases. *Clin Exp Dermatol.* 2019;44(7):732–739.

Celentano A, Tovaru S, Yap T, Adamo D, Aria M, Mignogna MD. Oral erythema multiforme: trends and clinical findings of a large retrospective European case series. *Oral Surg Oral Med Oral Pathol Oral Radiol.* 2015;120(6):707–716.

Fortuna G, Calabria E, Ruoppo E, et al. The use of rituximab as an adjuvant in the treatment of oral pemphigus vulgaris. *J Oral Pathol Med.* 2020;49(1):91–95.

Idrees M, Farah CS, Khurram SA, Firth N, Soluk-Tekkesin M, Kujan O. Observer agreement in the diagnosis of oral lichen planus using the proposed criteria of the American Academy of Oral and Maxillofacial Pathology. *J Oral Pathol Med.* 2021;50(5):520–527.

Jham BC, Nikitakis NG, Scheper MA, Papadimitriou JC, Levy BA, Rivera H. Granulomatous foreign-body reaction involving oral and perioral tissues after injection of biomaterials: a series of 7 cases and review of the literature. *J Oral Maxillofac Surg.* 2009;67(2):280–285.

Kuten-Shorrer M, Menon RS, Lerman MA. Mucocutaneous diseases. *Dent Clin North Am.* 2020;64(1):139–162.

Lo Russo L, Fierro G, Guiglia R, et al. Epidemiology of desquamative gingivitis: evaluation of 125 patients and review of the literature. *Int J Dermatol.* 2009;48(10):1049–1052.

Lucchese A. From HSV infection to erythema multiforme through autoimmune crossreactivity. *Autoimmun Rev.* 2018;17(6):576–581.

Muller S. Oral lichenoid lesions: distinguishing the benign from the deadly. *Mod Pathol.* 2017;30(s1):S54–S67.

Shen WR, Chang JY, Wu YC, Cheng SJ, Chen HM, Wang YP. Oral traumatic ulcerative granuloma with stromal eosinophilia: a clinicopathological study of 34 cases. *J Formos Med Assoc.* 2015;114(9):881–885.

Shulman JD, Carpenter WM. Prevalence and risk factors associated with geographic tongue among US adults. *Oral Dis.* 2006;12(4):381–386.

Sultan AS, Villa A, Saavedra AP, Treister NS, Woo SB. Oral mucous membrane pemphigoid and pemphigus vulgaris—a retrospective two-center cohort study. *Oral Dis.* 2017;23(4):498–504.

Wang D, Woo SB. Histopathologic spectrum of intraoral irritant and contact hypersensitivity reactions: a series of 12 cases. *Head Neck Pathol.* 2021;15(4):1172–1184.

Zoghaib S, Kechichian E, Souaid K, Soutou B, Helou J, Tomb R. Triggers, clinical manifestations, and management of pediatric erythema multiforme: a systematic review. *J Am Acad Dermatol.* 2019;81(3):813–822.

Chemotherapy and HIV Disease

Kuten-Shorrer M, Woo SB, Treister NS. Oral graft-versus-host disease. *Dental Clin North Am.* 2014;58(2):351–368.

Otto S, Pautke C, Van den Wyngaert T, Niepel D, Schiodt M. Medication-related osteonecrosis of the jaw: prevention, diagnosis and management in patients with cancer and bone metastases. *Cancer Treat Rev.* 2018;69:177–187.

Patton LL, Ramirez-Amador V, Anaya-Saavedra G, Nittayananta W, Carrozzo M, Ranganathan K. Urban legends series: oral manifestations of HIV infection. *Oral Dis.* 2013;19(6):533–550.

Woo SB, Treister NS. *Management of the Oncologic Patient.* Philadelphia, PA: WB Saunders Company; 2008.

Benign Neoplasms and Tumors

Mainville GN. Non-HPV papillary lesions of the oral mucosa: clinical and histopathologic features of reactive and neoplastic conditions. *Head Neck Pathol.* 2019;13(1):71–79.

Malignant Neoplasms

Seethala RR, Stenman G. Update from the 4th Edition of the World Health Organization Classification of Head and Neck Tumours: Tumors of the Salivary Gland. *Head Neck Pathol.* 2017;11(1):55–67.

Villa A, Menon RS, Kerr AR, et al. Proliferative leukoplakia: proposed new clinical diagnostic criteria. *Oral Dis.* 2018;24(5):749–760.

Villa A, Woo SB. Leukoplakia—a diagnostic and management algorithm. *J Oral Maxillofac Surg.* 2017;75(4):723–734.

Westra WH, Lewis Jr JS. Update from the 4th Edition of the World Health Organization Classification of Head and Neck Tumours: Oropharynx. *Head Neck Pathol.* 2017;11(1):41–47.

Nonvascular Pigmented Lesions

Buchner A, Merrell PW, Carpenter WM. Relative frequency of solitary melanocytic lesions of the oral mucosa. *J Oral Pathol Med.* 2004;33(9):550–557.

Donnell CC, Walton RL, Carrozzo M. The blue palate—a case series of imatinib-related oral pigmentation and literature review. *Oral Surg Oral Med Oral Pathol Oral Radiol.* 2021;131(1):49–61.

Koppang HS, Roushan A, Srafilzadeh A, Stolen SO, Koppang R. Foreign body gingival lesions: distribution, morphology, identification by X-ray energy dispersive analysis and possible origin of foreign material. *J Oral Pathol Med.* 2007;36(3):161–172.

Natarajan E. Black and brown oro-facial mucocutaneous neoplasms. *Head Neck Pathol.* 2019;13(1):56–70.

Metabolic Lesions Associated With Systemic Disease

Al Johani KA, Moles DR, Hodgson TA, Porter SR, Fedele S. Orofacial granulomatosis: clinical features and long-term outcome of therapy. *J Am Acad Dermatol.* 2010;62(4):611–620.

Little JW, Miller CS, Rhodus NL. *Little and Falace's Dental Management of the Medically Compromised Patient.* 9th ed. St. Louis, MO: Elsevier Health Sciences; 2018.

Mawardi H, Alsubhi A, Salem N, et al. Management of medication-induced gingival hyperplasia: a systematic review. *Oral Surg Oral Med Oral Pathol Oral Radiol.* 2021;131(1):62–72.

Monsereenusorn C, Rodriguez-Galindo C. Clinical characteristics and treatment of Langerhans cell histiocytosis. *Hematol Oncol Clin North Am.* 2015;29(5):853–873.

Differential Diagnoses and General Considerations

Neville BW, Damm DD, Allen C, Chi AC. *Oral and Maxillofacial Pathology.* 4th ed. Philadelphia, PA: Elsevier Health Sciences; 2015.

Woo SB. *Oral Pathology: A Comprehensive Atlas and Text.* 2nd ed. Philadelphia, PA: Elsevier; 2016.

CHAPTER 5

ORAL RADIOLOGY

Bernard Friedland, Gustavo Machado Santaella

RADIATION PHYSICS AND BIOLOGY

1. **How are x-rays produced?**
   X-rays are produced by "boiling off" electrons from a filament (the cathode) and accelerating the electrons to the target at the anode. The accelerated x-rays are decelerated by the target material, resulting in bremsstrahlung (German for "braking radiation"). Characteristic x-rays are produced when the incoming electrons knock out an inner K- or L-shell electron in the target and an electron from the L- or M-shell falls in to fill the void.

2. **At the energies typically used in dental radiography, what interactions do the x-rays undergo with tissues?**
   X-rays undergo three interactions with tissue—elastic (or coherent) scatter, Compton scatter (also known as inelastic or incoherent scatter), and photoelectric absorption. Pair production occurs at much higher energy values (1.02 megaelectron volts [MeV]) than those used in dentistry.

3. **What is the effect on a patient and on the image as a result of these interactions?**
   - In elastic scattering, a low-energy x-ray photon interacts with an atom and causes it to be momentarily excited. The atom then returns to ground state and emits an x-ray photon with the same energy as that of the incoming photon. The resulting photon can be emitted in any direction, causing scattering of the incoming/primary photon. There is no transfer of energy from the photon to the atom (Fig. 5-1).
   - In Compton scatter, an incoming x-ray photon interacts with an electron in the outer orbital shell, removing that electron and causing ionization of the atom. The incoming photon can be scattered in any direction. Depending on the degree of scatter, the scattered photon may "hit" and interact with the sensor or miss it. Both the scattered photon and the ejected electron can undergo additional interactions as they travel through the patient (Fig. 5-2).
   - In photoelectric absorption, the incoming x-ray photon interacts with an electron in the inner shell of an atom, transfers all its energy to the electron which then gets ejected from its orbital shell and travels with the remaining kinetic energy. When photoelectric absorption occurs, the incoming photon disappears and thus does not interact with the sensor.

4. **Which of the different interactions of x-rays with a patient is primarily responsible for patient dose?**
   In the photoelectric process, the incoming x-ray transfers all its energy to the tissue. Photoelectric absorption, therefore, contributes the most to patient dose.

5. **Which interaction of x-rays with a patient is primarily responsible for image quality degradation due to the scattering of the x-rays?**
   Compton scatter. In this interaction, the incoming x-ray photon is scattered in direction. As the trajectory of photons is changed, they cause image degradation when they reach the image receptor, as the density interpreted by the sensor does not correspond anymore to the known origin of the image projection. The sensor "sees" the photon as

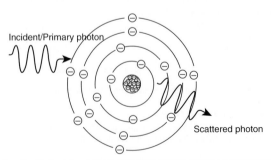

Incident/Primary photon

Scattered photon

Fig. 5-1. Elastic (coherent) scatter. The incoming photon is scattered in direction, but there is no net transfer of energy to the atom.

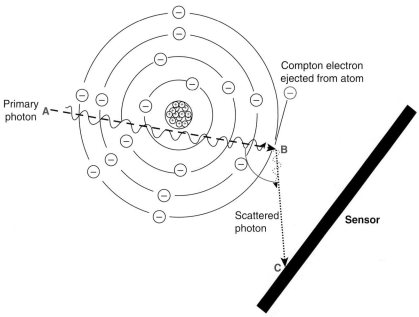

Fig. 5-2. Compton scatter. The sensor "sees" the photon as having come from direction B-C, when in fact it originally came from direction A-B. Thus, Compton scatter results in the sensor getting incorrect information, which degrades the image.

having originated from a particular direction and as having passed through certain tissues, when in fact the photon originated from a different direction and passed through different tissues. See Fig. 5-2.

6. **What is resolution and how is it measured?**
   Resolution, more accurately termed spatial resolution, is a measure of how well a radiographic system can distinguish fine line detail. Stated differently, resolution quantifies how close lines can be to each other and still be seen as separate. In analog systems, such as film-based radiography, resolution is measured using a line-pair resolution phantom and is expressed in line pairs per millimeter (lp/mm). An example of how resolution applies to clinical practice is the ability to see the lamina dura and periodontal ligament space, both small structures that are adjacent to one another. A system with good resolution (a periapical image) allows one to distinguish between the lamina dura and periodontal ligament space, whereas a system with poorer resolution (a panoramic image) may not allow this to be done.

   If a line-pair resolution phantom is used to evaluate a digital system, the resulting resolution can also be expressed in lp/mm. With digital systems, however, spatial resolution is more complicated. For example, it may be different in the horizontal (rows) and vertical (columns) directions. In digital systems, spatial resolution in effect refers to the number of independent pixel values per unit length and is limited by the minimum pixel size. Resolution of digital systems is measured by the modulation transfer function (MTF), which incorporates a number of variables. A full discussion of MTF is beyond the scope of this text (Fig. 5-3).

7. **How do each of the digital systems, CCD, CMOS, and CdTe detectors,* and storage phosphor plates work to produce an image?**
   Each pixel of a charge-coupled device (CCD), complementary metal–oxide–semiconductor (CMOS), and cadmium telluride (CdTe) sensor acts as an analog device. When x-rays strike the pixel, the energy deposited is stored as a small electrical charge. The charges are converted to a voltage one pixel at a time as they are read from the chip. Further circuitry then converts the voltage into digital information that can be displayed on a monitor. The difference between these three is that CCD and CMOS sensors have a scintillator layer that converts x-rays to light, that gets captured by the sensor, while CdTe does not need a scintillator, as it works by doing a direct conversion of the x-ray photons to an electrical charge.

   With storage phosphor plates, the energy deposited by x-ray photons is stored within the phosphor. This energy is released when the phosphor is stimulated with a visible wavelength laser light.

---

*The words detector and sensor are used interchangeably in this text. CCD, CMOS, and CdTe detectors are hereinafter collectively referred to as solid-state or rigid detectors.

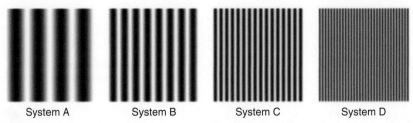

| System A | System B | System C | System D |

Fig. 5-3. Line pairs/mm (lp/mm) is how spatial resolution is measured in analog systems. In the systems shown, system A has the lowest and system D has the highest resolution.

8. **Which radiosensitive organs are in the field of typical dental x-ray examinations?**
   The thyroid is an extremely radiosensitive organ, along with lymphoid tissue and bone marrow in the exposed areas. The salivary glands are of importance too, as they often lie within the primary beam in intraoral and extraoral projections.

9. **What evidence suggests a risk of carcinogenesis from exposures to low levels of ionizing radiation such as those in dentistry?**
   No single study has proven the association between carcinogenesis and exposure to x-rays at the low dose levels used in dentistry. Studies that followed patients who were exposed to higher levels, however, provide evidence of a link. The current understanding of the mechanism for radiation-induced cancer comes from extrapolating from the results of studies on human populations who were exposed to large doses of radiation (e.g., in Nagasaki, Hiroshima, Chernobyl, and in radium watch dial painters, and patients exposed to multiple fluoroscopies for tuberculosis).

10. **What units are used to describe radiation exposure and dose? What do they measure?**
    a. The roentgen (R) is the basic unit of radiation exposure for x-rays and gamma radiation. It is defined in terms of the number of ionizations produced in air. It is a measure of the amount of radiation to which a person has been exposed but does not measure how much radiation was absorbed.
    b. The rad (roentgen-absorbed dose) is a measure of the amount of energy absorbed by an organ or tissue. Different organs or tissues absorb a different amount of energy when exposed to the same amount of radiation or roentgens.
    c. The rem (roentgen equivalent man or roentgen equivalent mammal) is a measure of the degree of damage caused to different organs or tissues. Different organs or tissues show differing amounts of damage even when they have absorbed the same amounts of rads.
       The International System of Units (SIs) are the coulomb/kilogram (C/kg), gray (Gy), and sievert (Sv) for the roentgen, rad, and rem, respectively.

11. **What is the difference between density and contrast?**
    Density refers to the overall degree of blackening of a radiograph. Contrast refers to the differences in densities between adjacent areas of a radiograph (Fig. 5-4).
       Adjusting the contrast will also affect the density to some extent.

12. **Which technique factors control radiographic density?**
    The longer a sensor is exposed, the darker the image will be; hence, time of exposure controls density. The number of amps flowing through the filament determines how hot it gets and thus how many electrons are boiled off. The higher the filament current, the hotter the filament and the more electrons are boiled off to reach the anode and produce x-rays; hence, mA also controls density. As a result of the kilovolt peak (kVp), which is the potential voltage difference between the cathode (filament) and anode, electrons that are boiled off are accelerated to the anode. The greater the potential difference between the cathode and anode, the greater the acceleration of the electrons toward the anode. Electrons that hit the anode at higher speed result in x-rays with higher energies. X-rays with higher energies are more likely to reach the sensor and darken it. Thus, kVp also controls sensor density. The distance from the source to the sensor also has a great effect on sensor density (see question 18).

13. **Which technique factors control film contrast? How do they affect contrast?**
    Contrast is controlled only by the kVp. The higher the kVp, the lower the contrast, and vice versa. kVp also affects density; the higher the kVp, the greater the density, and vice versa. Time, mA, and distance affect only density and not contrast.

14. **What is cone beam CT (CBCT), and how does it differ from medical or conventional CT in acquiring the images?**
    CBCT is a relatively new (c. 2000) computed tomographic imaging modality that provides three-dimensional images of anatomic structures. Unlike medical CT, in which the data are acquired axially by a thin, fan-shaped

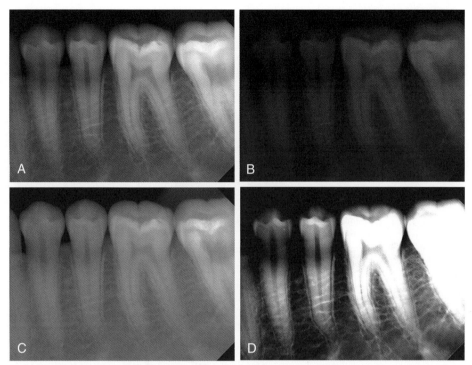

Fig. 5-4. (A) Ideal density and contrast; (B) high-density image. The contrast is the same as in (A), but the density is too high for the eye to appreciate it; (C) low-contrast image. Note that the density is satisfactory; (D) high-contrast image.

beam, the beam in CBCT is shaped like a cone. The medical CT scanner acquires individual image slices, which are then stacked to obtain the field of view (FOV). CBCT, with its large cone-shaped beam, acquires all the data in a single rotation. Thus, whereas in medical CT the x-rays are parallel to one another, in CBCT the x-rays are divergent.

15. **How is magnification defined?**
    Magnification is the ratio of the image size to the object size. It is, for example, the ratio of the length of the tooth as measured on the monitor compared to the actual tooth length. In real life, it is rarely possible to measure the size—for example, the length—of an object because the object is in the patient and may not be visible at all (e.g., an impacted tooth, osseous landmarks on a lateral cephalogram) or is only partly visible (e.g., an erupted tooth). Thus, we use a formula to calculate magnification.

    Magnification = target–detector distance/target–object distance (Fig. 5-5).

16. **How do the target-detector and object-detector distances affect magnification?**
    Fig. 5-6 shows how to calculate magnification and how the target-detector and object-detector distances affect magnification. When the target in the anode in the x-ray tube is in position A, the target-detector distance is 6 cm, and the target-object distance is 4 cm. Thus, the magnification is 6/4 or 1.5. If we move the target to position B, the target-detector distance is now 3 cm and the target-object distance is 1 cm, resulting in a magnification of 3/1 or 3.0. Thus, it is evident that, all other factors remaining unchanged, the longer the target-detector distance, the less the magnification. This is the rationale behind using the long cone technique for intraoral imaging and the long distance in cephalometric radiography. Using the formula and Fig. 5-6 as an example, you should now be able to determine how the object-detector distance affects magnification.

17. **What is the ideal geometric setup to get the most accurate image in intraoral radiography?**
    It is the paralleling technique, in which the central x-ray is perpendicular to the long axis of the object (e.g., tooth, head) and to the long axis of the detector. To accomplish this, the long axis of the detector must be parallel to the long axis of the object.
    • Large target-detector distance: The longer this distance, the less the magnification (see question 16).
    • Small object-detector distance: The smaller this distance, the less the magnification (see question 16).

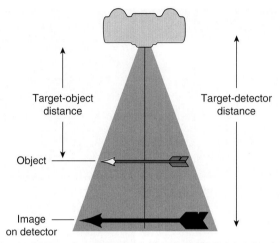

Fig. 5-5. Magnification is the ratio of the image size to the object size. (From Bushong SC: Radiologic Science for Technologists, ed 10, St. Louis, 2013, Mosby.)

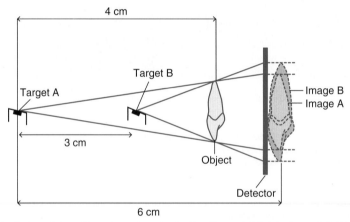

Fig. 5-6. Changing the target-detector distance changes magnification. (From Frommer HH, Stabulas-Savage JJ: Radiology for the Dental Professional, ed 9, St. Louis, 2011, Mosby.)

18. **What is the inverse square law?**
The intensity or exposure rate of radiation at a given distance from the source is inversely proportional to the square of the distance. For example, if we double the distance from the source, the intensity of the radiation is reduced fourfold. This is why the tube should be close to the patient and to the sensor to ensure that the image is not underexposed. The inverse square law can also be used to our advantage. By standing further away from the x-ray source, the intensity of the x-ray beam is reduced. Although the exact distance may vary from state to state, generally if one stands 6 feet away from the dental x-ray source, no additional radiation protection is needed for the operator.

19. **How do you trouble-shoot a radiographic image that is too dark (overexposed) or too light (underexposed)?**
For both film-based and digital systems, check the exposure factors (kVp, mA, time) to ensure that they are appropriate for the patient. For digital systems, one of these will almost always be the cause of the problem. With film, changes in radiographic quality usually result from errors in processing. For film-based systems, check the chemicals to ensure that they are at the correct temperature, have been stirred, and are fresh. If all these factors are satisfactory, evaluation of the x-ray unit, digital sensor, or batch of film may be necessary. It is important to remember to adjust the preset exposure parameters (kVp, mA, time) of the x-ray unit when using different types of receptors, as storage phosphor plates may require slightly higher exposure time than sensors, and films require a significantly higher exposure time compared to digital systems.

Another error that may cause an underexposed image is failure to depress the x-ray exposure button for the duration of the exposure. It is not possible to overexpose an image by holding the exposure button too long because there is a fail-safe mechanism that will automatically stop the exposure after the time that was set. Placing the tube too far from the sensor will also result in an underexposed image because of the effect of the inverse square law (see question 18).

20. What is the difference between internal and external scatter?
When x-rays interact with material, including body tissues, a number of interactions may take place, including scatter (see question 2). Scatter may result from x-rays interacting with material outside the patient's body and undergoing a change in direction so that the scattered photons hit the patient and thus increase the dose. This type of scatter is called external scatter. An example is an x-ray photon that hits the wall and is scattered in the direction of the patient. The second type of scatter is called internal scatter. This type of scatter occurs when x-ray photons interact with tissues in the patient and are directed to other parts of the patient's body. Because these photons arise from interactions that occur in the patient's body, they are known as internal scatter. An example is x-rays that interact with an object in the mouth (e.g., tooth restoration) and are scattered toward the thyroid gland. Neither a lead apron nor thyroid collar will help to reduce internal scatter.

21. What is meant by the quality of an x-ray beam, and how it is measured?
The quality of the beam refers to the penetrating power of the beam. The penetrating power is greater the higher the energy levels of the photons. A higher kVp results in higher photon energies and thus a more penetrating beam. The word quality is a term of art and refers only to the energy level of the beam. The number of x-rays in a beam is described by the beam intensity. Although kVp affects both beam quality and intensity (quantity), the two parameters are distinct and separable.
 Beam quality is measured by the half-value layer (HVL). The HVL is defined as the thickness of a given substance which, when introduced in the path of a given beam of rays, will reduce its intensity by half. Different materials (e.g., lead, aluminum, barium plaster) have different half-value layers. The half-value layer also differs for different energy (kVp) beams.

22. What is meant by the terms sensitivity, specificity, and predictive value when applied to the efficacy of radiographic examinations?
Sensitivity refers to the ability of a test, in our case a radiograph, to detect disease in patients who have the disease. Thus, sensitivity is a measure of the frequency of the true-positive and false-negative rate of test results in patients with disease. Stated differently, a test's sensitivity is its ability to correctly identify those with the disease (the true positives) while minimizing the number of false negative results.
 Specificity refers to the ability of a test to screen out patients who do not in fact have the disease. Thus, specificity is a measure of the frequency of true-negative and false-positive test results in patients without disease. Stated differently, a test's specificity is its ability to correctly identify those without the disease (the true negatives) while minimizing false positive results.
 The predictive value of a radiograph is the probability that a patient with a positive test result actually has the disease (positive predictive value) or the probability that a patient with a negative test result actually does not have the disease (negative predictive value).

23. What is the basic technology behind magnetic resonance imaging (MRI)? What are the indications for MRI in dentistry?
Nuclei of atoms that have an unpaired proton or neutron in the body act like bar magnets. In an MRI procedure, the area to be examined is subjected to an external magnetic field. The long axes of the nuclei line up with the magnetic field. Once the nuclei are aligned, they are subjected to a radiofrequency (RF) pulse. The nuclei absorb some of the radio wave's energy and lean over or tilt (the technical term is precess) to a transverse magnetization. When the RF pulse is turned off, the nuclei begin to return to their original low-energy state (relax) and emit the energy that they absorbed. This variation in the transverse magnetization can be picked up by appropriate receivers and converted into an image.
 Currently, the most significant use of MRI in dentistry is for TMJ evaluation, especially to localize the disk. MRI can also be used to determine soft-tissue extent, lymph node involvement, perineural invasion of neoplasms, and of salivary gland and vascular lesions. Other potential applications of MRI for dental indications include caries detection, pulpal/periapical disease characterization, and some efforts at inferior alveolar nerve identification, but these have been limited largely to research/experimental reports.

24. How does an MRI image produce tissue contrast so that one can distinguish between various types of tissue?
The operator selects the technical parameters of an MRI scan. The most important of these is the RF pulse sequence. The most basic characteristics of a pulse sequence are the repetition time (length of time between successive RF pulses) and echo time (how long after the RF pulse is applied when the magnetic resonance signal is read). The contrast is determined by the repetition time (TR) and echo delay time (TE), as well as by the T1 (time to return to the original low-energy state and restore the longitudinal magnetization) and T2 (time to dissipate the transverse magnetization) times. The latter are fixed by the intrinsic characteristics of the tissue under examination.

- T1-weighted images: Tissues with fast T1 times appear bright (e.g., fat, subacute hemorrhage, gadolinium-enhanced brain tumor). The high signal from short T1 substances is enhanced on short TR–short TE images.
- T2-weighted images: Tissues with long T1 times appear bright (e.g., cerebrospinal fluid [water], mucus, late subacute hemorrhage). The high signal from long T2 substances is enhanced on long TR–long TE images.
    Contrast agents may be administered to enhance image contrast. These agents, which are administered orally or intravenously, work by altering the relaxation times of atoms.

25. **What is the difference between stochastic and deterministic effects as the terms are used in radiation biology?**
Stochastic effects result from sublethal damage inflicted on the DNA of individual cells exposed to radiation. The greatest concern of a stochastic effect is carcinogenesis. Although mutations inherited by the offspring of the exposed individual are possible, they are much less likely.
    Deterministic effects are concerned with changes to the macromolecules of intracellular structures. These changes may result in cell death.
    Other differences between stochastic and determinative effects include the following:
- Deterministic effects require a threshold dose; for stochastic effects, even a single x-ray photon could cause cancer or lead to an inheritable mutation
- With deterministic effects, once the threshold dose is attained, all individuals display the effect; with stochastic effects, the higher the dose, the greater the chance of having the effect
- With deterministic effects, the severity of the clinical outcome is proportional to the dose; with stochastic effects, the results are an all-or-nothing proposition—one either experiences the effect or does not

RADIOGRAPHIC TECHNIQUES

26. **From the standpoint of the detector, what types of intraoral digital radiographic systems are available today? How do they differ from one another? What are the advantages and disadvantages of each system?**
There are four types of detectors—CCD, CMOS, CdTe, and storage phosphor plates (PSP). CMOS detectors have largely replaced CCDs, and CdTe is a technology more recently used in sensor that does not require a scintillator layer to convert x-rays to light. The most basic clinical differences among the systems lie in the physical nature of the detector and the manner in which images are transferred to the computer. CCD, CMOS, and CdTe detectors are rigid or solid, whereas PSP detectors are flexible. In the solid-state detector systems, the detector is connected directly (hard-wired) to a computer, whereas with PSP systems, the latent image must first be processed by putting the detector into a laser-scanning device. The latter is connected to the computer.

Advantages of a Storage Phosphor Plate
- Detectors are thin and flexible, more comfortable for the patient, and easier for the operator to use.
- It is less expensive, especially when multiple operatories and operators are involved.

Advantages of Solid-State Detectors
- Image appears on the monitor almost instantaneously.
- Infection control is easier and quicker. The detector is merely enclosed in a protective sleeve.

Disadvantages of Storage Phosphor
- When a full-mouth series is done, multiple plates must be used, just as with film; each plate must be wrapped before use and then unwrapped after use before placement in the scanner.
- The images appear only after the sensors have been placed in a laser reader.
- The position of the images in the digital mount on the monitor depends on the position of each plate in the laser scanner. This means that the images are jumbled when they first appear and must be digitally mounted in the correct position.
- The sensors are easily scratched, giving rise to artifacts.
- Information begins to be lost within a few minutes of exposure, so it is important to place the sensors in the laser reader as soon as possible.
- Exposure to light affects the image, so the sensors should be stored away from even ambient light until they are needed.

Disadvantages of Rigid Detector Systems
- Rigid detectors are more uncomfortable for the patient than storage phosphor plates.
- Because of their total inflexibility, obtaining images of certain regions is difficult. The most typical example is where the arch has its greatest curvature, and the sensor cannot be adapted to fit the curvature. This is seen especially in the canine area. Thus, capturing the distal aspect of the canine on a bitewing is difficult.
- The cable connecting the sensor to the computer makes it impossible for the teeth to be fully in occlusion. This results in a small open bite, which, on a bitewing, may make it difficult to assess periodontal bone height, especially if there is bone loss.
- Biting or pressure on the cable may introduce artifacts or noise into an image.
- The presence of a cable limits the distance that the computer may be from the chair.
- These are expensive compared with storage phosphor systems.

27. **What are the major advantages of digital radiography over conventional film-based systems?**
    - With a solid-state (CdTe, CCD, or CMOS) detector, images are visible almost instantaneously.
    - The need for a film processor and/or darkroom is eliminated.
    - Archiving of images is easier, and so is retrieval.
    - Digital images can be optimized—density and contrast can be changed; images can be magnified.
    - Built-in digital rulers enable one to perform measurements on the image.
    - Patient dose is reduced. Importantly, however, it is unclear whether the reduction in dose has any biologic benefits (e.g., reduced number of cancers, cataracts). There is much controversy in the radiation biology and radiation physics literature over this issue.

28. **What are the differences between a long cone and short cone? When is each one used? What is a recessed or built-in long cone, and what are its advantages?**
    Until approximately the 1970s, two types of x-ray cones were available, long and short cones. The short cone was used with the bisecting angle technique. With this technique, there is no aiming device, so that one has to "eyeball" the position of the tube in all dimensions. Obtaining the precise vertical angulation is difficult for most operators. Because it is easier to eyeball something over a shorter rather than a longer distance, a short cone was used.
    When using beam-indicating devices, and eyeballing is not necessary, the lead-lined long cone is preferred. The long cone technique has two primary benefits. It reduces patient dose by reducing the field size and increases the target-film distance, thereby reducing magnification. Because of the advantages of the long cone, it is always desirable to use it, even for the bisecting angle technique. This became feasible when Dr. Albert Richards invented the recessed or built-in long cone in the mid-1960s. The recessed cone has the advantage of a short-appearing cone, thus making it easier for the operator to execute the bisecting angle technique successfully, but with the benefits of the long cone. The recessed long cone takes up less space, which may be important in cramped quarters. The principle of the recessed cone is schematically illustrated in Fig. 5-7.

29. **How has the use of occlusal radiography changed in recent years?**
    Occlusal images are used, among other reasons, to determine the buccolingual position of an impacted tooth, demonstrate the buccolingual dimensions of a lesion and the buccal and lingual cortices in the mandible, visualize the intermaxillary suture, demonstrate arch form, and replace periapical films in young children. An occlusal image also may be used when one wishes to visualize on one film a lesion that is too large to fit on a single periapical film, such as a large nasopalatine duct cyst.
    The use of occlusal imaging has declined markedly in recent years for two reasons. The first is related to digital radiography. With the introduction of digital radiography, occlusal-size sensors are not as readily available. Because of their prohibitive cost, no rigid detectors come in an occlusal size. Very few manufacturers of storage phosphor plates make occlusal-size plates, so unless one uses storage phosphor plates from a manufacturer that makes them, one is not likely to use them. The second reason for the drop in occlusal radiography is the advent of CBCT. The dose from CBCT is relatively low compared to medical CT (but higher than from a single occlusal exposure), so CBCT has become widely used to provide information that would otherwise have been acquired from an occlusal image.

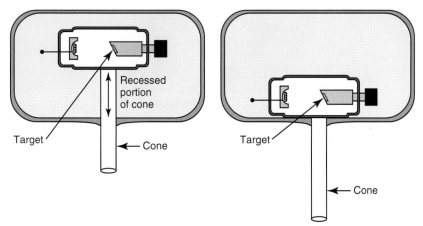

Fig. 5-7. The recessed long cone compared to the traditional long cone. By moving the anode and target deeper into the x-ray unit, it became possible to build part of the cone into the machine. From the outside, the recessed long cone has the appearance of a short cone.

30. **What operator error results in a foreshortened image?**

Foreshortening results when the vertical angulation of the tube is too great; that is, the tube is angled too steeply. Elongation, by contrast, results from a vertical angle that is too shallow. A good way to remember cause and effect is to think of the sun and your shadow. Your shadow is shortest at noon when the sun is highest in the sky (a steep vertical angle) and longest in the late afternoon when the sun is low in the sky (a shallow vertical angle).

31. **On a panoramic image, some structures may be clearly visible while others are not or appear blurry or out of focus. Why is this?**

For structures to be visible on a panoramic image, they must be in what is termed the focal trough. The focal trough determines the distance between the nearest and farthest objects that appear acceptably sharp in the image. The width of the focal trough in different machines varies in different parts of the jaw. It is widest in the posterior region and narrowest in the anterior. For structures to appear clearly on a panoramic image, the structures must be in the focal trough. Structures that are perfectly positioned in the focal trough will show up sharpest. As structures move farther away from the focal trough, they become blurrier, until they are no longer visible. Think of the focal trough as akin to the depth of field in photography. The manner in which the focal trough and depth of field are determined is wholly different, but conceptually they are similar (Fig. 5-8).

32. **Why is the focal through in panoramic radiography narrower anteriorly and larger posteriorly?**

In panoramic radiography, there is a trade-off between the width of the focal trough and the sharpness of the image. The narrower the focal trough, the sharper the image. Because the posterior segment is larger than the anterior segment, the former requires a wider focal trough compared to the narrower anterior segment.

33. **Which radiographic view is considered the primary view for evaluating the alveolar bone for periodontal disease?**

The bitewing view is the primary view for evaluating radiographic changes consistent with periodontal disease, which include loss of crestal cortication, changes in the contour of the interdental bone, horizontal and angular bone loss, and furcation involvement. The bitewing film is superior to a periapical film because distortion, including elongation or foreshortening, is slight. The reason is that in the case of a bitewing, the vertical angle is small (approximately plus 5 to 10 degrees), and the central ray is directed at right angles to the sensor.

34. **Is there a generally accepted protocol for the frequency of radiographic evaluation in adult dental patients?**

Yes. The U.S. Food and Drug Administration (FDA), in cooperation with the American Dental Association and other major organizations, has developed and disseminated protocols for exposing dental patients to x-ray examinations. These protocols require a history and clinical examination before prescribing an individualized radiographic examination. For more information, go to http://www.fda.gov/Radiation-EmittingProducts/Radiation-EmittingProductsandProcedures/MedicalImaging/MedicalX-Rays/ucm116504.html. One not infrequently hears that a patient should get a full-mouth series every 5 years. This adage arises from the fact that dental insurance will cover a full-mouth series every 5 years. The fact that insurance will or will not cover an x-ray does not imply that one should or should not be taken.

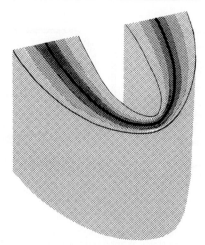

Fig. 5-8. Focal trough. Structures positioned on the black line will be in the sharpest focus. As one moves farther away from this line, the structures are less sharp, until they eventually become almost invisible. (From White SC, Pharoah MJ: Oral Radiology: Principles and Interpretation, ed 6. St. Louis, 2009, Mosby.)

35. How should radiographic protocols be altered for pregnant dental patients?

With the use of standard radiation protection, there is no additional risk to the fetus from x-ray exposures commonly used in dentistry and pregnant women can be treated, for radiographic purposes, like all other female patients. However, because of the concerns many women still have about receiving radiation during pregnancy, it is probably still advisable to limit x-ray exposures to the minimum necessary.

36. Describe the use of CBCT in dentistry with regard to implants, endodontics, orthodontics, and impacted teeth, especially third molars.

Implants. The use of CBCT in implant planning is well accepted and widely practiced. If there is any disagreement, it is whether CBCT should be used in *all* cases. This is still an open question.

Endodontics. Today CBCT is widely used in endodontic therapy. This is especially true for teeth that are being retreated after failing or failed endodontic therapy. It is also used for cases in which additional canals are suspected but cannot be found clinically, for teeth that have unusual anatomy that complicates diagnosis and/or treatment, as well as for suspected fractures. CBCT should not be used routinely in all endodontic cases. There are guidelines on the use of CBCT in endodontics (https://www.aae.org/specialty/clini cal-resources/cone-beam-computed-tomography/).

Orthodontics. The use of CBCT in the discipline of orthodontics remains one of the most unsettled and contentious issues concerning this modality. Although CBCT is used by some private practitioners and some educational institutions in all orthodontic cases, many—probably most—dentists are opposed to its routine use or at least have serious reservations about it. This is based on the young age of most orthodontic patients with the greater susceptibility of their tissues to the adverse effects of radiation and the lack of evidence showing that the routine use of CBCT affects the outcome. There are some situations in which there is almost complete unanimity and in which the use of CBCT is appropriate. These include localizing impacted, unerupted, or supernumerary teeth, in patients with cleft palate, and patients for whom orthognathic surgery is a consideration.

Impacted teeth. CBCT is also used to locate impacted teeth, most commonly mandibular third molars, to assess their proximity to the mandibular canal, as well as impacted maxillary canines to better localize them. CBCT should not be routinely used in all third molar impactions. Although there are as yet no guidelines for when CBCT should be used in these circumstances, certain signs seen on the panoramic image should serve as a starting point. See question 98.

37. What is the buccal object rule? What do you need to apply it? How is it applied?

The buccal object rule, also known as the tube shift rule and the SLOB rule ("same lingual, opposite buccal"), is a method for determining the relative location of objects that cannot be directly visualized. Examples include the location of an impacted tooth or an additional root or canal. To apply the rule, one needs a reference object and two images taken at different angles.

The rule is applied as follows. In tube position 1, the images of the three objects are as depicted in Fig. 5-9. Assume that one wants to determine the relative position of the circular and black objects. The horizontal position of the tube is changed, in this case by moving the tube distally to position 2. Another way of looking at it is to say that the tube is directed anteriorly in position 2, but most people find it easier to think simply in terms of the mesiodistal position of the tube.

Assume that the red circle represents an erupted tooth. With the tube in position 2, the images of all three objects are projected more mesially. However, their absolute position on the detector is not important. In applying the buccal object rule, we are interested only in their relative positions to one another. From Fig. 5-9, it is evident with the tube in position 2 that the black square has moved mesially with respect to the red circle, an erupted tooth that is serving as the reference object. Now apply the SLOB rule. As the tube was moved distally, the black object moved mesially with respect to the erupted tooth; that is, the black object moved in the *opposite* direction to the tube. Thus, the black object is buccal (opposite buccal) to the reference tooth.

Using the two periapical images below in Fig. 5-10, determine whether the crown of the impacted bicuspid is buccal or lingual to the first molar.

The image on the right was taken distally compared to the image on the left. As the tube was moved more distal from the left to the right image, the crown of the bicuspid moved distal relative to the mesial root of the first molar. Thus, the impacted tooth moved distally—relative to the first molar—as the tube was moved distally, i.e., it moved in the same direction as the tube. Based on the SLOB rule (same lingual), the impacted tooth's crown is thus lingual to the first molar.

38. When performing CBCT, which technical parameters should be taken into account? How can they be adjusted?

kVp, mA, and time. These are important technical parameters. Different manufacturers allow a varying amount of control over these parameters. In some machines, it may not be possible to adjust these technical factors at all, which are preset and must be used for all studies. In others, the factors come preset for specific studies. For example, machines allow one to select a patient by size, such as child, small adult, or adult. Selecting a child patient will result in certain default settings, whereas selecting an adult for the same study will cause the machine to apply different default settings. Some machines allow one to set the default settings in each group (e.g., adult or child), as opposed to the manufacturer setting them. Some manufacturers allow one to alter these default

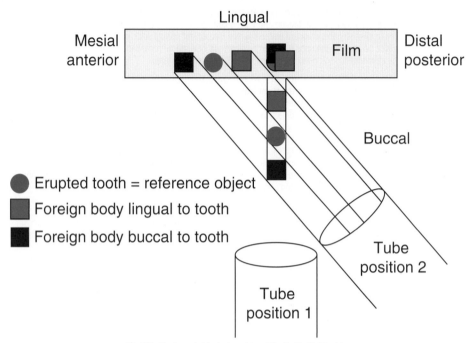

Fig. 5-9. The buccal object rule or tube shift rule (the SLOB rule).

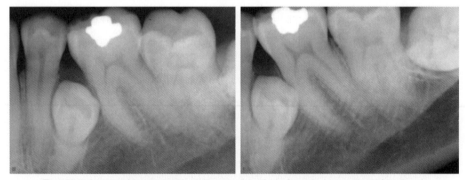

Fig. 5-10. Is the crown of the impacted bicuspid buccal or lingual to the first molar (see question 37)? It is lingual.

settings for a specific patient—for example, a particularly obese or small-framed patient. In this situation, if one chooses "adult" and the default kVp is 90, one should change the kVp for this one patient only. It is important for the operator to understand what each machine permits and how to alter the settings in order to minimize patient dose and obtain the best-quality image.

Resolution. Not every study requires the highest resolution. For example, an implant CT is commonly done at a resolution of 0.3 voxel, although some may do it at 0.2 voxel. Rarely is any higher resolution required for an implant study or for the evaluation of pathology. On the other hand, for endodontic studies, where one is looking for individual canals, one would generally choose the highest resolution of which the machine is capable. Remember that the smaller the number, the higher the resolution. Thus, a resolution of 0.2 voxel is greater than one of 0.4 voxel.

Field of view. This refers to the physical size of the x-ray field. CBCT machines come in three FOV categories—small, medium, and large. One wants to select the smallest FOV that is compatible with the desired clinical information. The ability to adjust the FOV varies by manufacturer and model of machine. In some of the large FOV machines, one can adjust the height of the field, but not the anteroposterior FOV. Thus, one can image one arch (small vertical FOV), both arches (larger FOV), or the whole head (largest vertical FOV), but one cannot

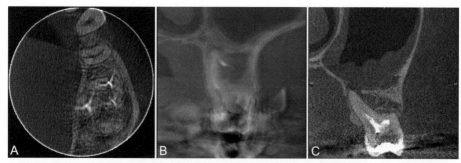

Fig. 5-11. (A) Axial view of a CBCT scan demonstrating artifacts—the white streaks—caused by the gutta-percha fill. (B) Sagittal view demonstrating the blurred edges and double contours caused by motion. (C) Example of a sagittal view demonstrating significant image noise.

image just part of one jaw—for example, only the right posterior mandible. Some machines have a number of preset FOVs. In this case, the operator selects the most appropriate FOV but cannot customize it further. It is up to the operator to understand the limitations and capabilities of each machine.

39. **Cone beam CT presents some problems inherent to its acquisition that can show up in the volume as artifacts. Describe the most common types of artifacts and how they occur.**

    Artifacts caused by high-density objects, such as metal, gutta-percha, post, and cores, can result in white and dark striped being projected on the areas around these objects, which may mask or mimic areas of interest, affecting the diagnostic abilities of the scan (Fig. 5-11A).

    Motion artifacts are caused by misregistration of data due to the patient moving during the scan. It may appear as blurred or double contours in the reconstructed image and severely affect the image quality. Motion artifacts can be minimized by restraining the patient's head and using a shorter scan time (Fig. 5-11B).

    Scattering of the x-ray photons can happen when diffracted from their original path after interacting with matter and may cause an overall image degradation ("salt and pepper aspect") (Fig. 5-11C).

40. **What are some limitations of CBCT for different types of diagnosis?**
    - CBCT demonstrates various types of image artifacts, mainly those produced by high-density restorations such as crowns and composites. These materials produce streak artifacts. Streak artifacts are worse in the axial (horizontal) plane than in the vertical plane and compromise the evaluation of caries lesions and alveolar bone loss.
    - It is not able to accurately represent the different densities of an internal structure of soft tissues and soft-tissue lesions, which limits the ability of detecting alterations in soft tissues. Stated differently, CBCT has poor soft tissue contrast.
    - It is not possible to correlate with Hounsfield Units for standardized quantification of bone density in implant assessment sites.

41. **Do panoramic images portray objects with sufficient accuracy to permit reliable measurements to be made on the image?**

    Although magnification (or minification) is generally undesirable, it is not a major impediment to obtaining accurate measurements if one knows the amount of magnification. All one needs to do is to apply a correction factor. In panoramic images, however, magnification varies from one part of the image to another. Varying magnification of different parts of the same image is termed distortion. If one wants to do measurements on a panoramic image, one should place an opaque object of known dimensions (ball bearings are commonly used) in the area of interest. By then measuring the size of that object's image, one can calculate a conversion factor. That measurement will be accurate only for that specific location. There is less variation in vertical magnification than in horizontal magnification on panoramic images.

42. **In panoramic radiography, what are ghost and double images? How are they formed, and how can one tell them apart?**

    Panoramic radiography produces two broad categories of images, real images and ghost images. Real images can be divided into true real images and double images. True real and double images are formed by objects that are between the center of rotation and the sensor in both projections (Fig. 5-12). Ghost images occur when structures are located between the x-ray source and the rotation center (Fig. 5-13).

    One can tell them apart by the following characteristics:

    A double image:
    - is reversed with respect to the true real image—that is, it is a mirror image of the true real image.
    - has the same proportions as the true real image.

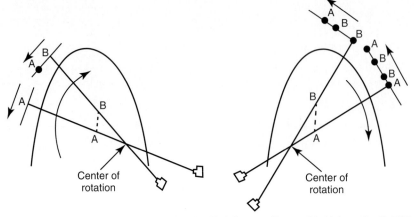

Fig. 5-12. Formation of a double image. Note that for the formation of both the true real image and double image, the object AB is located between the center of rotation and the detector.

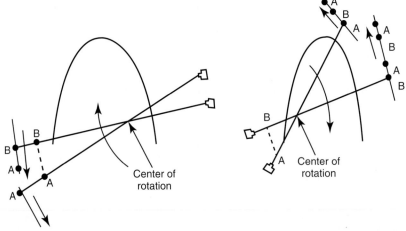

Fig. 5-13. Formation of a ghost image. Note that for the formation of the true real image, AB is located between the center of rotation and the detector, but in the formation of the second (ghost) image, object AB is located between the x-ray tube and center of rotation.

- has the same location, including vertical position, on the opposite side.
    A ghost image:
- is more blurred compared to the true real image.
- is more blurred in the vertical than the horizontal.
- is magnified especially in the vertical runs in the same direction as the real image—that is, it is not a mirror image of the true real image.

43. **What are the names of the major salivary glands? How are they studied radiographically?**
    The three major salivary glands are the parotid, submandibular, and sublingual glands. Because the salivary glands consist of soft tissue, they cannot be seen on radiographs unless special steps are taken to make them visible. In a technique called sialography, a radiopaque dye or contrast is injected through the duct openings into the gland. Iodine is the agent normally used to provide contrast. If patients are allergic to iodine, a different contrast agent must be used. Calcifications of the duct may be seen on intraoral radiographs, especially calcifications of Wharton's duct, the submandibular gland duct. The stones or sialoliths may be seen on periapical radiographs, but an occlusal radiograph or CBCT is needed for localizing. If a stone is detected, it is obviously present. However, if none is detected, it does not mean that there is not a stone. Up to 40% of parotid sialoliths and 20% of submandibular sialoliths are not radiopaque. MRI is increasingly replacing sialography as the modality of choice for studying the salivary glands.

44. **What are the indications for the use of MRI versus CT?**
There is no simple answer to this question. In general, MRI is better for imaging soft tissue—for example, a tumor in the tongue. CT, on the other hand, provides better images of bone; thus, for an intraosseous tumor, CT is the technique of choice. Not uncommonly, one may want to use both MRI and CT. For example, when a patient has a tumor in the floor of the mouth, one may use MRI to determine its extent in the soft tissue and CT to determine whether there is any bone involvement. For temporomandibular joint (TMJ) imaging, MRI is better at depicting the soft tissue of the disk, but CT is better for almost all other TMJ studies. For most dental purposes, where the primary interest is bone and soft tissue discrimination is not a factor (e.g., implant or endodontic studies), CBCT is the modality of choice.

45. **What is tomosynthesis and why is it a promising imaging modality for dentistry in the future?**
Tomosynthesis, also known as limited-angle tomography, is a quasi-3D modality using reduced angular coverage, fewer projection images, and a lower dose than CT.
Tomosynthesis works by taking a number of views from different angles. Unlike CT and cone-beam CT, the source is stationary when exposing an image. The concept is illustrated in Fig. 5-14.
While tomosynthesis has been used for some in other disciplines such as mammography, owing to technical issues, it was not available for dental use until very recently. A dental tomosynthesis unit was approved by the FDA in 2021 (https://portrayxray.com; https://surroundmedical.com).
The advantage of tomosynthesis over other 3D modalities, such as CT or cone-beam CT scans, include a lower dose reduction of artifacts and simpler hardware.
Its advantage over periapical and bitewing images is that tomosynthesis allows one to see the anatomy slice by slice. (For a short video on a demonstration of tomosynthesis, (https://www.wral.com/unc-researchers-develop-3d-dental-x-ray-method/14923174/.)

BASIC RADIOLOGIC INTERPRETIVE CONCEPTS

46. **What are the radiographic features of a lesion or area of interest that should be described and recorded?**
    1. Location of the lesion as exactly as possible. This is an important feature, as many lesions have a propensity to occur in certain locations.
    2. Shape. As a result of their being fluid filled, resulting in hydraulic pressure, most cysts tend to be round). Two exceptions are the odontogenic keratocyst (OKC), which has a tendency to grow along the internal aspect of the jaw (in the length of the bone), thus causing minimal expansion and the simple bone cyst, a pseudocyst, that tends to scallop between the teeth.
    3. Appearance of borders. This is a critical feature that may help distinguish between benign (usually well-defined borders) and malignant lesions (usually poorly defined borders). A corticated lesion is by definition well defined, but a non-corticated lesion may still be well defined.

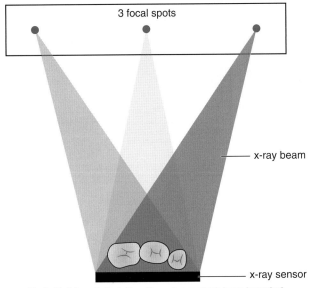

Fig. 5-14. Schematic illustration of how a tomosynthesis image is acquired.

4. Internal structure. The internal structure may have septations, resulting in a multilocular lesion. Pay particular attention to whether the lesion is radiolucent, radiopaque, or mixed, and note the nature of the opacity, if any is present. For example, is the opacity homogeneous and is it the density of bone or tooth?

5. Effects of the lesion on adjacent structures. Has the lesion displaced structures (e.g., moved teeth, the canal, sinus floor)? Has it caused resorption of teeth or destroyed the bone around them, leaving the teeth themselves untouched? Is there any reactive response—for example, a periosteal response or sclerosis of the bone?

6. Localized versus generalized. When lesions are generalized, one has to consider a different differential diagnosis than if just a single lesion is present.

7. Size. Although many people describe size before any of the other features, size by itself is generally not helpful. A snapshot of a lesion does not indicate how long it has been present. Even a benign lesion will grow to a large size if left untreated. Size may be helpful if one has two or more images taken at different times and one knows the time frame between them.

47. **Once you have described the features of a lesion (see question 46), you need to arrive at a differential diagnosis. Describe a method or algorithm for doing this.**
Although there is no one correct way to do this, the initial step should be to determine whether the area in question is normal or abnormal. If normal, you should be able to identify the structure. If you decide that the area in question is abnormal, Fig. 5-15 illustrates one way to proceed.
    One reason for following at least the initial steps outlined here is that patients typically want to know whether something is normal and, if it is not, whether the abnormality is benign or malignant, so it is desirable to reach that conclusion as soon as possible. After that, there is more leeway. Some clinicians, for example, may prefer to decide on the odontogenic versus nonodontogenic nature of a lesion before deciding whether it is a cyst or tumor, whereas others may reverse that step.

48. **What is the most likely interpretation of a bilaterally symmetric radiographic appearance in the jaws?**
A bilateral symmetric appearance, with extremely few exceptions, is indicative of normality (Fig. 5-16). Among the few exceptions to this are cherubism and infantile cortical hyperostosis (Caffey's disease).

49. **The location of a lesion may be a clue about its origin. What single anatomic structure in the mandible is most useful for differentiating between a lesion of possible odontogenic versus nonodontogenic origin?**
The mandibular or inferior alveolar canal is extremely useful in distinguishing between a lesion of odontogenic or nonodontogenic origin. Because one does not expect to find odontogenic tissues inferior to the canal, it is most unlikely that lesions situated below the canal are odontogenic in origin. Lesions of odontogenic origin rarely, if ever, begin below the canal. However, any lesion, including one of odontogenic origin, may begin above the canal and extend below it.

50. **If you wish to view pathology in soft tissue, would you order a CBCT? Explain your answer.**
Although CBCT has a number of advantages over medical CT, it also has disadvantages. One of the greatest is that relative to medical CT, CBCT lacks soft tissue contrast. This means that CBCT does not discriminate well between different soft tissues, such as fat and muscle. Thus, CBCT is not the modality of choice if the primary purpose is to examine the soft tissues. Usually, an MRI is the modality of choice for viewing soft tissue, but a medical CT

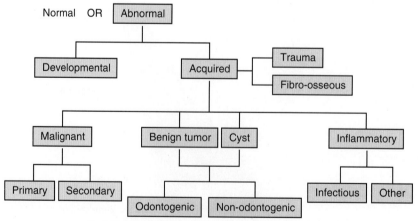

Fig. 5-15. Algorithm for arriving at a radiographic differential diagnosis.

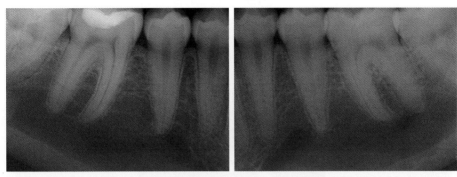

Fig. 5-16. Patient with a bilaterally symmetrical radiolucency in each posterior quadrant of the mandible, indicative of normal anatomy (submandibular gland fossa). If one saw only the image on the right or only the one on the left, one may think it is a simple bone cyst as it appears to scallop between the teeth.

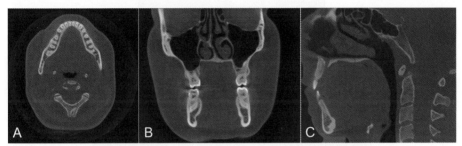

Fig. 5-17. Axial (A), coronal (frontal; B), and sagittal (C) views of a CBCT scan.

might be a reasonable choice, depending on the situation. If one has an intraosseous lesion and simply wants to determine whether it has broken through into the surrounding soft tissue, CBCT is useful.

51. **What general radiographic features are indicative that the findings may be due to a systemic cause?**
When a systemic cause underlies a problem, both the mandible and maxilla are affected. Furthermore, the jaws are typically affected bilaterally, often symmetrically. If the condition affects the teeth, one would expect them also to be affected in a bilaterally symmetric fashion.

52. **What do we call the three different perspectives from which one can view images on a cone beam CT, medical CT scan, or an MRI?**
The axial view is considered as viewing the patient from below, the coronal or frontal view is considered as viewing the patient from the front, and the sagittal view is considered as viewing the patient from the side (Fig. 5-17).
    In dentistry, the coronal view through the alveolus, as depicted in Fig. 5-18, is also referred to as a cross section or cross-sectional view. Also, in dentistry, a panoramic reconstruction is frequently obtained (Fig. 5-19).

53. **What are the usual radiographic signs of inflammatory disease involving the paranasal sinuses observed in radiographs or CBCT?**
    • Mucous membrane thickening
    • Air-fluid levels
    • Partial or complete opacification of a sinus cavity
    • Presence of a soft tissue mass
    • Changes in the cortical margins of a sinus

54. **What common radiographic signs help one distinguish between a cyst, benign neoplasm, and malignant neoplasm?**
With a few exceptions, cysts tend to be radiolucent and round or oval in shape, with intact cortical margins. Benign neoplasms are more variable than cysts in density and shape. Malignant neoplasms of the jaws classically have ragged, ill-defined margins. Malignant lesions often grow rapidly, destroying the less highly mineralized bone and leaving roots of teeth unaffected, giving the appearance of teeth floating in space. Cysts and benign neoplasms are more likely than malignant neoplasms to resorb tooth roots.

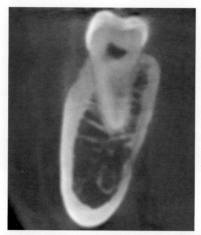

Fig. 5-18. Coronal view, also known as a cross-sectional view, through the posterior mandible.

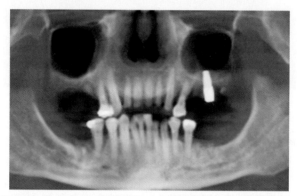

Fig. 5-19. Panoramic reconstruction from a CT scan. Note that there is a difference between a panoramic reconstruction from a CT scan and a panoramic image.

55. **Which modality, CBCT, panoramic imaging, or intraoral radiography, is best for interpreting and diagnosing conditions radiographically?**
    Contrary to what is commonly thought, and what purveyors of the latest products might lead one to believe, the latest and/or most expensive imaging technology is not always best for interpretation and diagnosis. What is best depends on what information is being sought. For example, CBCT is of little to no use in diagnosing caries. The scatter from metals such as amalgams, posts and cores, crowns, and, to a lesser extent, other less dense materials such as gutta-percha results in so much scatter as to render CBCT scans almost useless for caries detection., as well as for assessing the status of periodontal bone Panoramic images provide a useful overview of the jaws, but may lack sufficient detail to visualize small structures. For example, in some cases, the lamina dura may not be visible on a panoramic image because this modality lacks sufficient resolution. The panoramic image does not show the buccolingual dimension, so it is not useful when this information is being sought. Intraoral images, with their high resolution, provide exquisite images of small structures, but the views are limited in size. Before ordering a particular image, the dentist should think about what information is being sought and select the appropriate imaging modality accordingly (Fig. 5-20).

56. **Is it possible for a patient to have an asymmetry, yet for it not to be clinically evident?**
    Yes, both the osseous structures and soft tissues contribute to a person's appearance. It is possible to have an osseous hypoplasia or hyperplasia, which is compensated for by soft tissue. In such a case, the asymmetry will only be noticeable with radiography. In these cases, treatment may not be necessary for aesthetic purposes. The reverse is also true; one may have a soft tissue asymmetry, but not an osseous one.

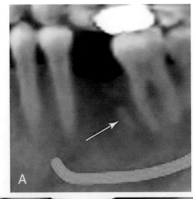

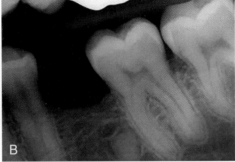

Fig. 5-20. (A) A cropped, full-thickness panoramic reconstruction of a large field of view CBCT scan taken at a resolution of 0.4 mm. An opacity (*arrow*) is visible mesial to the apical third of the root of the second molar. Based on this and other perspectives (not shown) on the CBCT scan, the differential diagnosis includes dense bone (enostosis), condensing osteitis, and a tooth root. (B), A periapical image of the area clarifies the nature of the opacity, which can be clearly seen to be surrounded by a uniform lucency (the periodontal ligament space), which is in turn surrounded by a cortical border (the lamina dura). One is therefore looking at a tooth root.

57. **How do primary teeth differ from permanent teeth? How does the difference affect the radiographic evidence of caries in primary teeth?**
    Primary teeth are smaller and have relatively larger pulp chambers, with pulp horns in closer proximity to the external surface of the crown. The roots of primary molars are more splayed (wider apart) than those of permanent molars. The enamel layer is thinner in dimension. Primary teeth are slightly less opaque on film because of a higher inorganic content. As a result, caries in primary teeth tends to progress more rapidly from initial surface demineralization to involvement of the dentin. Thus, careful interpretation is especially important when evaluating the primary dentition (Fig 5.21).

58. **What is the differential diagnosis for a short root on a radiograph?**
    - Variation of normal
    - Tooth that hasn't completed formation (Fig 5-22A)
    - A tooth that has undergone apical external resorption (Fig 5-22B)
    - Foreshortening of the image (Figs 5-22C and D)

59. **Which CBCT view, axial, coronal, sagittal, or panoramic, is best for viewing pathology?**
    There is no single view that is always best. It is always important to look at all three views because each one conveys different information. It is only by viewing all three perspectives that one obtains the complete picture (Figs. 5-23 and 5-24).

60. **What is the rule of 3s for radiographic assessment of the development of permanent teeth?**
    It takes approximately 3 years for a permanent tooth bud to calcify after matrix formation is complete, approximately 3 more years for the tooth to erupt after calcification is complete, and about 3 more years after initial eruption for root formation to be complete.

61. **In pathology of the maxilla, which feature seen on a periapical image is most useful in determining whether the pathology arose inside or outside the sinus?**
    The floor of the sinus is the most useful feature. If the pathology arose inside the sinus, the floor is intact and in its normal position or perhaps depressed inferiorly. Additionally, the superior aspect of the lesion will not be

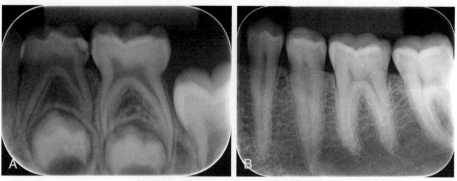

Fig. 5.21. (A) Periapical image of the left mandible in a child. (B) Periapical image of the left mandible in an adult.

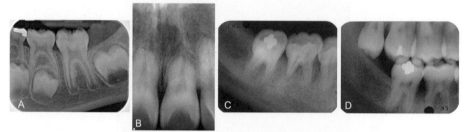

Fig. 5-22. (A) Note that the first molar has an open apex and a blunderbuss appearance. The latter indicates that the tooth has not yet completed formation. (B) Apical external resorption of the maxillary central incisors. Note that, as in (A), the apices of the central incisors are open; however, the walls of the canal are convergent, indicating that these teeth had completed formation and then underwent external resorption. (C) Periapical image of the mandibular right molars demonstrating short-appearing roots. (D) Bitewing radiograph of the same area as (C), showing normal length roots, thus confirming that the short roots were a result of foreshortening.

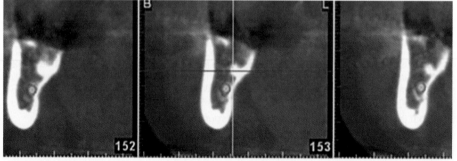

Fig. 5-23. Cross-sectional views of the posterior mandible show a rounded opacity toward the lingual aspect of the alveolus. The differential diagnosis includes bone (enostosis, condensing osteitis) and tooth material. It is not possible to determine definitively which it is.

corticated. If the pathology arose outside the sinus and the floor of the sinus is intact, it may be in its normal position or be displaced superiorly. If the sinus floor has been destroyed, it may not be possible to determine whether the pathology arose from without or within the sinus (Fig. 5-25).

62. Foramina may be superimposed over the apices of teeth, mimicking the presence of periapical disease. Which radiographic features are most useful in distinguishing between normal structures and apical pathology?
   If the lucency is caused by the superimposition of a foramen, the periodontal ligament space and the lamina aura around the tooth are intact. The exposure of a second radiograph, with the tube in a different position from the first exposure, also is frequently useful. If the lucency moves relative to the apex of the tooth, the lucency is not associated with the tooth and is not caused by periapical pathology. This exercise, however,

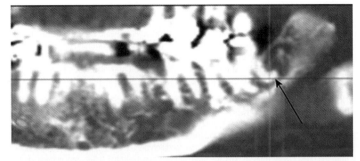

Fig. 5-24. A view through a thin section of a panoramic reconstruction shows a dilacerated distal root (*arrow*) of the third molar. It is this dilaceration that is seen in the cross section. One can now say with certainty that the opacity noted in the cross section is a root.

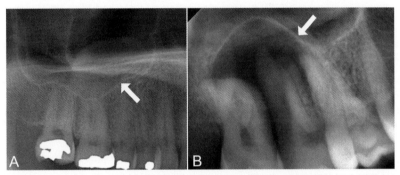

Fig. 5-25. (A) Cropped panoramic radiograph demonstrating intact floor of the maxillary sinus (*arrow*) in a normal position in a case of a mucous retention cyst. (B) Periapical radiograph demonstrating the floor of the maxillary sinus pushed superiorly (*arrow*) in a case of a radicular cyst.

does not rule out the possibility that the lesion is abnormal; it merely means that the lesion is not related to the tooth.

63. **What is the differential diagnosis of a radiopacity in the soft tissues in and around the jaws?**
It is easiest to answer this question if the radiopacities are classified into groups—tooth, bone, foreign body, and calcification. Foreign bodies are mostly metallic but need not be. Gutta-percha, endodontic sealer, some composites, and contrast media are opaque but not metallic. Although bone is a form of calcification or mineralization, it is distinctive enough to warrant a separate category. In a given case it may be difficult to distinguish even among these categories, but the classification is nevertheless useful. In most cases, one can easily rule out a tooth in soft tissue, although in cases of trauma, fragments of a tooth or even a whole tooth may be found in the lips, tongue, or cheeks. Ossification of the stylohyoid ligament is common, but bone in soft tissue is otherwise rare. Examples of the latter are choristomas and ossifying hematomas. A number of entities involve calcification. These include sialoliths, lymph node calcification (e.g., in granulomatous diseases such as tuberculosis), tonsilloliths, calcification of the cartilage found in the neck, for example, the thyroid cartilage and calcified atheromatous plaques. Less common examples include phleboliths, calcified acne lesions, and parasitic larvae (e.g., cysticercosis). Antroliths and rhinoliths are calcifications (stones) that occur in a sinus or the nasal cavity, respectively. When an opacity is seen in a cavity such as the sinus, fluids and soft tissue should be considered in the differential diagnosis. They are not as dense as the other opacities.

64. **Is it possible for a patient to be in acute pain as a result of a periapical abscess, yet have a completely normal periapical radiograph?**
Yes. This finding is not unusual because sufficient mineralization must occur before bone destruction is radiographically evident. In an acute situation, there frequently has not been sufficient time for this amount of bone destruction to occur. Thus, the radiographic picture may lag behind the clinical picture. The same may be true in the healing phase—a patient may be improving clinically but still show radiographic signs of pathology.

65. **Is a widened periodontal ligament space at the apex of a tooth always indicative of pathology?**
No. When a radiolucency such as the mental foramen or mandibular canal is superimposed over the periodontal ligament (PDL) space, the ligament space appears to be widened. Such a widening is purely artifactual. The PDL space also may appear wider, usually at the neck of a tooth, as a normal variation, or may be widened around the entire tooth as a result of orthodontic treatment. Traumatic occlusion may also result in widening of the PDL space. Generalized widening of the PDL space may be caused by disease, such as scleroderma.

66. **Some serious conditions may mimic periodontal disease. Name two such conditions and indicate how bone loss from these conditions can be differentiated from periodontal bone loss..**
The two conditions that usually mimic periodontal bone loss are Langerhans cell histiocytosis (LCH) and squamous cell carcinoma. One can usually determine LCH because this condition begins *in* the bone, whereas periodontal disease progresses from the crest down. Thus, in LCH, the alveolar crest may be intact. If the crest is destroyed, then this feature is less useful in differentiating the two conditions. Another feature that may be useful is that in periodontal disease, once the bone loss extends to the apex, it usually does not progress further or very little so, whereas in LCH, one may see bone loss well beyond the apices of the teeth. Patients with LCH may also manifest a periosteal reaction.

Squamous cell carcinoma (SCCA) most frequently begins in the overlying soft tissue, extending into the bone. When SCCA invades the bone in this fashion, it destroys the alveolar crest, so this feature is not useful to distinguish between SCCA and periodontal disease. Periodontal disease, especially when there is significant bone loss, is usually generalized, so what looks like periodontal disease in only a localized area should heighten one's degree of suspicion that something more sinister is occurring.

A lucency caused by SCCA is unlikely to be surrounded by a sclerotic border, whereas in periodontal disease there may be a sclerotic border. As in the case of LCH, one may see bone loss well beyond the apices of the teeth in SCCA.

67. **What are the radiographic manifestations in the jaws of patients infected with the human immunodeficiency virus (HIV)?**
There are no unique oral or maxillofacial radiographic manifestations of HIV infection, although infected patients are at a higher risk for severe periodontal disease.

68. **What is the efficacy of dental radiographs?**
Studies of standard dental radiography (bitewing, periapical, and panoramic views) show considerable variation in the ability to detect common dental diseases such as caries, periodontal disease, and apical periodontitis. Radiographs should not be considered to be perfect; they are most valuable when combined with a thorough history and clinical examination.

RADIOGRAPHIC INTERPRETATION

69. **What is the earliest radiographic sign of periapical disease of pulpal origin?**
In permanent teeth, widening of the periodontal ligament space is seen around the apex of the tooth. In primary teeth, by contrast, the infection presents as widening of the periodontal ligament space or an area of lucency, usually in the furcation area, although it may on occasion occur at the apex of a primary tooth.

70. **What is the next radiographic sign of periapical disease of pulpal origin?**
The next radiographic sign is loss of the lamina dura around the apex of the tooth or, in the case of primary teeth, in the furcation.

71. **Describe the radiographic differences that allow periapical abscesses, granulomas, radicular (periapical) cysts, and apical surgical scars to be distinguished.**
One cannot distinguish among periapical abscesses, granulomas, or radicular (periapical) cysts on radiographic grounds alone. All these lesions are radiolucent, usually with well-defined borders. Whereas an abscess may be expected to be less well corticated than a radicular cyst, this feature is not marked or constant enough to be useful.

72. **Radiographically, what are the features of a benign neoplasm in bone that help differentiate it from a malignant neoplasm?**
1. Margins are irregular and fade imperceptibly into surrounding bone.
2. The cortex tends to remain intact but may be thinned, and the part involved may be expanded.
3. Margins are usually defined and demarcated from surrounding bone.
4. There often is a perforation of the periosteum.
5. Some structures (e.g., teeth, the mandibular canal, sinus floor) are displaced.
   a. 1 and 2 only
   b. 1, 2, and 4 only
   c. 2, 3, and 5
   d. 2, 3, and 4 only
   Answer: c

73. At times, it may be difficult to distinguish between hypercementosis and a buccal or palatal dilaceration at the apex of a tooth. What radiographic feature permits a definitive diagnosis when this occurs?

    For both conditions, the periodontal ligament space is visible around the opacity; that is, the excess cementum or root is contained within the PDL space. In the case of a dilaceration, the PDL space surrounds the entire opacity, running across the root. In hypercementosis, by contrast, the PDL space does not cross the root (Fig. 5-26).

74. What is the earliest radiographic sign of periodontal disease?

    The earliest radiographic sign of periodontal disease is loss of density of the crestal cortex, which is best seen in the posterior regions. In the anterior region, the alveolar crests lose their pointed appearance and become blunted. In the posterior areas, the alveolar crests usually meet the lamina aura at right angles. In the presence of periodontal disease, these angles become rounded.

75. What is the earliest radiographic sign of furcation involvement caused by periodontal disease?

    In periodontal disease, one may see the loss of a cortical plate—the buccal or lingual cortical plate—on an intraoral radiograph. The plate may be lost to such a degree that the crest now occupies a position apical to the furcation. However, this appearance by itself, does not permit a diagnosis of furcation involvement. Widening of the periodontal ligament space in the furcation area is the earliest radiographic sign of furcation involvement.

76. What is the radiographic differential diagnosis of a radiolucency on the root of a periodontally healthy tooth?

    Internal resorption, external resorption, and superimposition are the most common causes. Note that the question refers to a periodontally healthy tooth. If bone loss has resulted in exposure of the root, caries, and abrasion, among other possibilities, enter the picture.

77. How can you distinguish among the above radiolucencies on the root of a tooth?

    In internal resorption, the canal is widened, whereas it is unaffected in external resorption. If the resorption began below the bone level, it has to be internal resorption because, without adjacent bone, there are no osteoclasts in the area to cause external resorption. If internal or external resorption involves both the canal and other tooth structure, it is not possible to distinguish between the two conditions. A superimposed radiolucency moves relative to the root if another view is obtained with the tube in a different position. The most common of these lucencies are normal

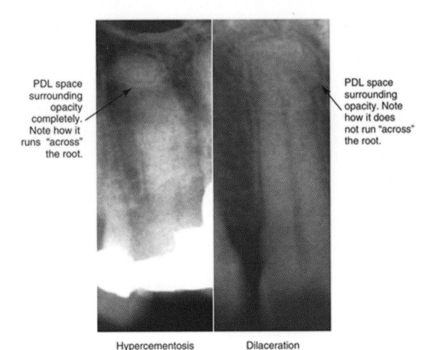

PDL space surrounding opacity completely. Note how it runs "across" the root.

PDL space surrounding opacity. Note how it does not run "across" the root.

Hypercementosis   Dilaceration

Fig. 5-26. Periapical images showing an example of a dilacerated root (buccal or palatal) and of hypercementosis. Note how, in hypercementosis, the PDL space runs across the tooth.

anatomy, such as foramina, the sinus, mandibular canal, and accessory or nutrient foramina or canals. Artifacts such as cervical burnout may also produce a lucency on the root at the junction of the enamel and cementum.

78. **What is the radiographic differential diagnosis of a radiolucency on the crown of an erupted tooth?**
Carious lesions, internal resorption, restorations, abrasions, erosions, and enamel hypoplasia are among the more common possibilities. Carious lesions typically have irregular margins; they may also have typical shapes, such as the triangular appearance of interproximal carious lesions. Internal resorption has smooth, well-defined margins. The same is true of radiolucent restorations, which frequently can be recognized by their shape and sometimes by the presence of an opaque base, such as calcium hydroxide, lining the floor of the preparation. Abrasions, particularly at the cervical margins, often have a V-shaped appearance. Other abrasions, such as those caused by a clasp on a denture, typically have well-defined borders and straight lines, unlike most naturally occurring phenomena. Erosions also have well-defined borders, and their shape is typically round or oval. Hypoplasia usually is not a single lucency on a tooth but rather many small lucencies.

79. **One can determine a tooth that has not completed formation compared to a tooth that has external resorption by which of the following?**
With a tooth that has not completed formation, the apex is open and the walls of the canal are divergent, whereas in a tooth that has completed formation and is resorbed, the apex is closed and the walls of the canal are convergent (Fig 5-27).

What is the differential diagnosis for an apical lucency?

The answer to this question is best begun by differentiating between vital and nonvital teeth. For nonvital teeth, the differential diagnosis includes:
- A periapical abscess
- A periapical cyst
- A periapical granuloma
- A periapical scar

For vital teeth, the differential diagnosis most commonly includes:
- The papilla of a still-developing tooth.
- Cemento-osseous lesions (COD) (a.k.a. periapical osseous dysplasia [POD], periapical cemental dysplasia [PCD], florid cemento-osseous dysplasia). COD may occur around the apex of a non-vital tooth, but it would be an unrelated finding, not associated to the non-vitality.

The differential diagnosis above includes the vast majority of lesions or conditions that occur at the apex of a tooth. It should be kept in mind that many other less common conditions may occur at the apex of a tooth. Leukemia and multiple myeloma are two such examples.

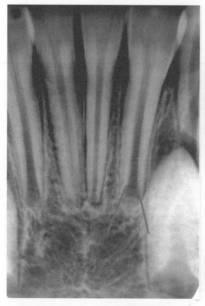

Still developing vs. External resorption

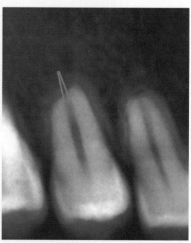

Fig. 5-27. In the image on the left, the apex is open, and the walls of the canal are divergent. The divergent walls indicate that the tooth has not completed formation. In the image on the right, the apex is open, but the walls of the canal are convergent. This indicates that the tooth had completed formation and that it was subsequently resorbed.

80. **If endodontic therapy on a maxillary molar is failing, what is the most likely cause?**
Maxillary molars were classically described as having three canals, one in the mesiobuccal (MB) root, one in the distobuccal (DB) root, and one in the palatal root. The majority of maxillary molars have an additional canal, which is a second canal in the MB root. The first canal in the MB root is called MB1 and is located buccal to the second canal, which is called MB2. With the use of microscopes in endodontics, it became evident that more maxillary molars have an MB2 than was originally thought. If MB2 cannot be located clinically, a high-resolution CBCT scan can frequently identify it (Fig 5-28).

81. **Name two serious and even potentially fatal conditions that may be detected by dental radiographs before clinical signs or symptoms develop. What are the dental signs and symptoms of these diseases?**
Gardner's syndrome and Gorlin-Goltz syndrome have radiographic signs that should alert a vigilant dental practitioner to the possibility of their presence. The oral or dental findings in Gardner's syndrome are classically characterized by multiple osteomas, dense bone islands and impacted teeth. Odontomas and supernumerary teeth may also be present. The non-dental finding of greatest concern is the presence of polyps in both large and small intestines. These polyps have a high propensity to become malignant. Other non-dental findings include the presence of desmoid tumors and epidermoid cysts. The oral or dental finding in Gorlin-Goltz syndrome (multiple basal cell nevoid carcinoma syndrome; basal cells nevus syndrome; bifid rib syndrome) is the presence of odontogenic keratocysts. The non-dental finding of greatest concern is the presence of basal cell carcinomas on the skin. While rarely fatal and not as serious as squamous cell carcinomas, if left untreated or treated too late, basal cell carcinomas may invade the deeper tissues, complicating their removal. Also, the later they are treated, the higher is the likelihood of recurrence. There are a host of other non-dental anomalies in in Gorlin-Goltz syndrome. These include bifid ribs, polydactyly, ocular and neurologic abnormalities, such as calcification of the falx cerebri.

82. **Can one diagnose osteomyelitis radiographically? What are other radiographic signs of osteomyelitis?**
Osteomyelitis may be present in the total absence of radiographic signs. To make a diagnosis of osteomyelitis *radiographically*, a sequestrum must be noted. A sequestrum is an area of bone that has been separated from the body of the bone. A radiographic sign that may be suggestive but is not pathognomonic of osteomyelitis is a periosteal reaction.

83. **In radiology, what do we mean when we say that something is a central lesion?**
Lesions can be central or peripheral. A central lesion is one that starts in the bone. A peripheral lesion is one that begins on the surface of the bone or in the overlying soft tissue. Most lesions are of one type or another, but some may be of either type. For example, odontogenic fibromas, the vast majority of which are of the central variety, also have a peripheral form. Peripheral lesions are less likely to be visualized in a radiograph because they are less likely to cause sufficient changes to mineralized tissues.

84. **How may periosteal reactions present radiographically?**
Onion skin: this is most commonly seen in the presence of infections.
Sunray or sunburst: this is most commonly seen with malignant lesions, for example, in osteosarcoma and chondrosarcoma.
Hair-on-end: this is most commonly seen in conditions such as thalassemia and sickle cell disease.
It should be borne in mind, however, none of the above periosteal reactions are pathognomonic. For example, one may on occasion see an onion-skin appearance in an osteosarcoma or a hair-on-end appearance in a metastatic lesion.

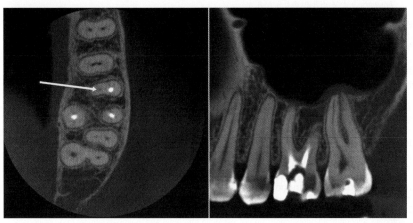

Fig. 5-28. The *yellow arrow* in the left image (axial slice) is pointing to an MB2 canal in tooth #14. Gutta-percha is visible in the other three canals. The red line in the right image (sagittal slice) indicates the level of the axial slice.

85. Simple bone cysts (traumatic bone cysts) occur in two distinct age groups. What are these age groups? How are the simple bone cysts in these age groups similar or different?
Simple bone cysts usually occur in the first two decades of life, with a mean age of occurrence of 17 years. In this age group, there is a male-to-female predominance of 2:1. Simple bone cysts in this age group are solitary. They are treated by curettage, which causes bleeding into the lesion which then heals.

The second group in whom simple bone cysts occur are middle-aged black women. It is in this group that cemento-osseous dysplasia is found. Simple bone cysts may be found in patients with cemento-osseous dysplasia, especially the florid variety, and there may be multiple simple bone cysts. One or more cysts form and heal, and then others may form.

As opposed to solitary simple bone cysts, which occur in the younger age group, cysts that occur in the presence of cemento-osseous dysplasia are not usually treated.

86. Explain how the lamina dura may fail to be visible on a periapical image..
The most common cause of loss of the lamina dura is infection; the vast majority are the result of infections of endodontic origin. Once infection has been ruled out, cemento-osseous dysplasia and less commonly malignancy should be considered. With infections and malignancy, the lamina is actually destroyed. With cemento-osseous dysplasia, the lamina dura may be present or absent.

There is, however, a third condition that may render the lamina dura invisible, but it is not destroyed, as in the aforementioned conditions. In fibrous dysplasia, the lamina dura may be converted to fibrous dysplastic bone, so that the contrast between the normal lamina dura and bone is lost. In osteoporosis and osteopetrosis, a similar process may result in loss of the lamina dura. If there is generalized destruction of the lamina dura, systemic conditions such as hyperparathyroidism should be considered. Finally, the lamina dura may not be visible because of radiographic technique and/or technical factors. A panoramic image, with its relatively poor resolution compared with intraoral radiographs, may not show the lamina dura. Even an intraoral image that is underexposed, overexposed, or very poor in contrast may render the lamina dura difficult or impossible to see.

87. What are the radiographic signs of a fracture?
The radiographic signs of a fracture include a demonstrable radiolucent fracture line, displacement of a bony fragment, disruption in the continuity of the normal bony contour, and increased density (caused by overlap of the adjacent fragments).

88. Match the lesion with the most common location for each one:.
1. Dentigerous cyst
2. Lateral periodontal cyst
3. Buccal-bifurcation cyst
4. Ameloblastoma
5. Adenomatoid odontogenic tumor
6. Periapical cemento-osseous dysplasia
   a. Mandibular incisors around the apices
   b. The mandibular first molars
   c. Third molars
   d. Mandible from the lateral incisor to the first premolar
   e. Canine area in maxilla
   f. Mandibular molar–ramus area
      Answers: 1, c; 2, d; 3, b; 4, f; 5, e; 6, a

89. What is the differential diagnosis for a large tooth, and how would you differentiate between the conditions?
The differential diagnosis includes a macrodont or megadont, a geminated tooth, and fused teeth.

A macrodont is simply a larger version of one of the normal complements of teeth. Aside from the fact that the tooth is larger, it is otherwise normal. For example, the root will be in proportion to the size of the crown. The pulp chamber and canal will be in proportion to the size of the crown and root, respectively.

As a practical matter, geminated or fused teeth have an altered shape—that is, they never completely resemble a normal tooth. On clinical examination, there may be a "cleft" running down part or all of the crown. On radiographic examination, the roots often do not appear normal.

Gemination and fusion are most easily distinguished by counting the teeth. If there is a normal complement (including the altered tooth), one is dealing with gemination. If there is one tooth less than in a normal dentition, one is dealing with fusion. Sometimes fusion can occur with a supernumerary tooth, such as a mesiodens, which will not alter the number of teeth.

90. To what extent do the amount and degree of calcification in a tumor indicate its benign or malignant nature?
Calcification has no significance in predicting the benign or malignant nature of a tumor. Benign tumors (e.g., odontomas, adenomatoid odontogenic tumors, ossifying fibromas) and malignant tumors (e.g., osteogenic

sarcoma) produce bone or calcifications. To determine the benign or malignant nature of a tumor, other features must be sought.

91. **Which lesions may present with a soap bubble or honeycomb appearance?**
Ameloblastoma
Giant cell lesions
Odontogenic keratocyst
Hemangioma
Primordial cyst
Calcifying epithelial odontogenic tumor
Aneurysmal bone cyst
Cherubism

92. **Assume that a bone (e.g., the mandible) is enlarged or expanded. Which feature would be most helpful when making an initially broad differential diagnosis?**
The most useful feature would be whether the disease process began inside or on the surface of the bone. If the original cortical boundary is intact and in its normal position, and the new bone has been laid down outside that bone, the new bone is of periosteal origin. With this appearance, the differential diagnosis would include conditions that result in a periosteal reaction. An infectious process would be most common. If the original cortex is on the outer surface of the expanded bone, the condition began in the bone. In that case, the differential would include diseases such as fibrous dysplasia, Paget's disease, cemento-osseous dysplasia, and central (benign) cysts and tumors (Fig. 5-29).

93. **At times, it is very difficult to differentiate dense bone from tooth. What features should be sought to identify opacities of this nature?**
Features to look for are the following:
- The shape of the opacity—teeth typically have a certain distinctive shape. Remember though that at times one may be looking at a cross section of a tooth or part of it.

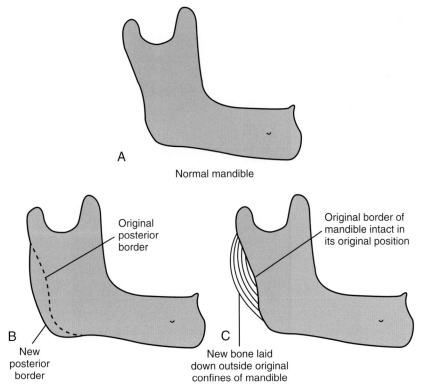

A
Normal mandible

B
Original posterior border
New posterior border

C
Original border of mandible intact in its original position
New bone laid down outside original confines of mandible

Fig. 5-29. (A) A normal mandible. (B) Depiction of an expanded mandible in which the expansion is a result of pathology within the body of the bone. (C) Representation of an expanded mandible in which the expansion is a result of new bone being laid down outside the confines of the original bone.

- Note the heterogeneity of the opacity. A tooth is not homogeneous, but has a denser outer surface (enamel) and a less dense bulkier portion (dentin) with a lucency, representing the chamber and/or canal in the center. If the opacity is a root only and not a whole tooth, there will be no enamel.
- A tooth is surrounded by a uniform radiolucency that represents the periodontal ligament space.
- In the case of a tooth, outside the periodontal ligament space will be a cortical border, the lamina dura.

94. What is the most common malignancy in bones, not just the jawbones?
Metastatic disease is the most common malignancy in bone. Interestingly, most metastatic lesions to the jaws arise from primary lesions below the level of the clavicle.

95. What is the differential diagnosis for an opacity in or about the coronal aspect (crown) of a tooth?
The most common finding is calculus (Fig. 5-30A). A pulp stone and enamel pearl should be included in the differential diagnosis (see Fig. 5-30B and C1-3). Calculus can be ruled in or out on clinical examination. It is

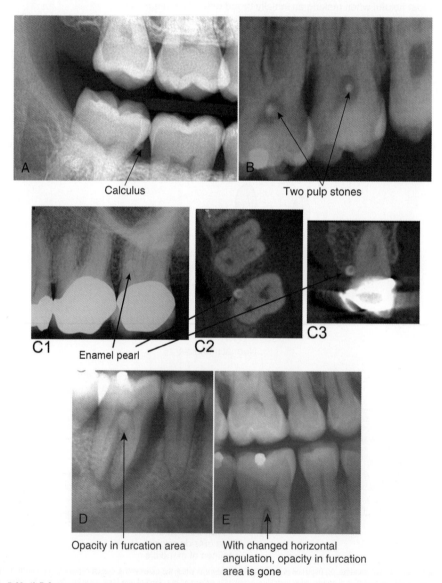

Fig. 5-30. (A-E) Some common coronal opacities—calculus. These can usually be easily distinguished by their radiographic location and a clinical examination.

easiest to differentiate between a pulp stone and enamel pearl by increasing the vertical angulation of the tube. If it is an enamel pearl, the opacity will move away from the pulp chamber. Finally, what appears to be an opacity may actually be an artifact. This occurs when x-rays pass obliquely through a molar, resulting in part of one root in the furcation area to be superimposed over another, causing an opacity. Another view taken at a different horizontal angle usually causes the opacity to disappear, revealing its true nature (see Fig. 5-30D and E).

96. **Certain teeth and locations are more prone to anomalies than others. List the teeth and locations in which anomalies are common and describe those anomalies..**
    - Third molars—congenital absence; malformation, for example, poorly formed roots
    - Mandibular second bicuspids—congenital absence of the tooth; supernumeraries (which may be multiple)
    - Maxillary lateral incisors—congenital absence; peg lateral; dens invaginatus
    - Maxillary midline—mesiodens

97. **On a panoramic image, what are some of the signs that suggest a close association between an impacted mandibular third molar and the mandibular canal?**
    Root darkening, narrowing of the tooth root, loss of the cortical boundaries of the canal, and diversion of the canal are some of the more common signs that suggest a close association between an impacted mandibular third molar and the mandibular canal. There is no agreement about which of these signs is the best predictor that exposure of the nerve or a clinical complication involving the nerve will occur as a result of surgery to remove the tooth. There does, however, appear to be general consensus that the absence of positive radiographic signs on the panoramic film is more useful than the presence of such signs. Without positive signs, the risk of injury to the nerve is considered miniscule, whereas the presence of one or more positive signs is not a good predictor of injury to the nerve.

98. **What lesion is highly suggestive of mandibular first molar roots that are displaced into the lingual cortex in a child?**
    It likely indicates a buccal bifurcation cyst. The finding of first molar roots that have been displaced into the lingual cortex, together with the lesion being centered over the furcation, is considered to be pathognomonic; no other lesion displays these features.

BIBLIOGRAPHY

American Association of Endodontists. American Academy of Oral and Maxillofacial Radiology: Use of cone-beam computed tomography in endodontics Joint Position Statement of the American Association of Endodontists and the American Academy of Oral and Maxillofacial Radiology. *Oral Surg Oral Med Oral Pathol Oral Radiol Endod*. 2011;111:234–237.

Christensen EE. *Christensen's Introduction to the Physics of Diagnostic Radiology*. 4th ed. Philadelphia: Lippincott Williams & Wilkins; 1990.

Farman AG. *Panoramic Radiology: Seminars on Maxillofacial Imaging and Interpretation*. Berlin: Springer-Verlag; 2010.

Fiorica JV. Breast cancer screening, mammography, and other modalities. *Clin Obstet Gynecol*. 2016;59(4):688–709.

Friedland B, Donoff RB, Chenin D. Virtual technologies in dentoalveolar evaluation and surgery. *Atlas Oral Maxillofacial Surg Clin North Am*. 2012;20:37–52.

Friedland B, Donoff RB, Dodson TB. The use of 3D reconstructions to evaluate the anatomical relationship of the mandibular canal and impacted mandibular third molars. *J Oral Maxillofac Surg*. 2008;66:1678–1685.

Inscoe CR, Platin E, Mauriello SM, et al. Characterization and preliminary imaging evaluation of a clinical prototype stationary intraoral tomosynthesis system. *Med Phys*. 2018;45(11):5172–5185.

Kapila S, Conley RS, Harrell Jr WE. The current status of cone beam computed tomography imaging in orthodontics. *Dentomaxillofac Radiol*. 2011;40:24–34.

Kocasarac HD, Geha H, Gaalaas LR, Nixdorf DR. MRI for dental applications. *Dental Clin Nor Am*. 2018;62(3):467–480.

Koenig L. *Diagnostic Imaging: Oral and Maxillofacial*, Salt Lake City, UT, 2011. In: Amirsys. Langlais RP. *Exercises in Oral Radiology and Interpretation*. 4th ed. Philadelphia: Saunders; 2003.

Langland OE, Langlais RP, Preece J. *Principles of Dental Imaging*. 2nd ed. Philadelphia: Lippincott Williams & Wilkins; 2002.

Larheim TA, Westesson PA. *Maxillofacial Imaging*. Berlin: Springer-Verlag; 2008.

Lee L, Wong Y. Pathogenesis and diverse histologic findings of sialoliths in minor salivary glands. *J Oral Maxillofac Surg*. 2010;68:465–470.

Mallya S, Lam E. *White and Pharoah's Oral Radiology*. 8th ed. St. Louis: Elsevier; 2019.

Miles D. *Color Atlas of Cone Beam Volumetric Imaging for Dental Applications*. Hanover Park, IL: Quintessence; 2008.

Tyndall DA, Price JB, Tetradis S, et al. Position statement of the American Academy of Oral and Maxillofacial Radiology on selection criteria for the use of radiology in dental implantology with emphasis on cone beam computed tomography. *Oral Surg Oral Med Oral Pathol Oral Radiol*. 2012;113:817–826.

CHAPTER 6

PERIODONTOLOGY

David M. Kim, Paul A. Levi Jr., Chia-Yu Chen

FUNDAMENTALS OF THE PERIODONTIUM

1. Anatomically, what makes up the components of periodontium?
   Gingiva, periodontal ligament, cementum, and alveolar bone.

2. Sharpey's fibers are mainly composed of what type of collagen?
   Type I collagen.

3. What connective tissue fibers are normally found in the gingiva?
   Histologically, the fibers that described are the dentogingival, dentoperiosteal, circular, and transseptal.

4. What portion of the root is covered by acellular cementum? What portion of the root is covered by cellular cementum?
   Acellular cementum is located in the coronal and middle portion of the root. Cellular cementum is located in the apical third of the root.

5. What blood vessels supply the gingiva?
   Supraperiosteal blood vessels from sublingual artery, mental artery, buccal artery, facial artery, greater palatine artery, infraorbital artery, and posterior superior dental artery.

6. What are the components of the organic matrix of alveolar bone?
   Mainly type I collagen (90%) with small amounts of non-collagenous proteins.

7. How is the width of attached gingiva determined?
   It is determined by subtracting the probing depth from the coronoapical width of gingiva.

8. What type of mucosal tissue is the gingiva?
   Masticatory mucosa. It is keratinized on the oral surface and non-keratinized on the sulcular surface.

9. What is the principal cell type of the gingival epithelium?
   Keratinocyte.

10. What are the different cell types present in the connective tissue of gingiva?
    Fibroblasts, mast cells, macrophages, and inflammatory cells.

11. What are the four layers of oral epithelium?
    Stratum basale, stratum spinosum, stratum granulosum, and stratum corneum.

12. Define gingival phenotype.
    Gingival thickness (buccolingually) (GT) and gingival width apico-occlusally (GW).

13. What is periodontal phenotype?
    Gingival phenotype and thickness of the facial and/or buccal bone plate (bone morphotype).

14. Can we modify the periodontal phenotype?
    Yes, it can be modified by environmental factors and clinical interventions.

15. Can we modify the gingival biotype?
    No, the biotype is genetically predetermined.

16. What are the common methods to measure the gingival phenotype?
    Direct visual inspection, dental probe transparency, transgingival probing, ultrasonic transducer, parallel profile periapical radiography, and cone-beam computed tomography.

17. Which method is non-invasive and highly reproducible to measure the gingival phenotype?
    Dental probe transparency is non-invasive and highly reproducible, with 85% agreement between duplicate recordings.

CLASSIFICATION AND ETIOLOGY OF PERIODONTAL DISEASES

18. **What is the primary etiologic agent in periodontal disease?**
The primary cause of gingivitis and periodontitis is bacterial plaque (biofilm), specifically gram-negative bacteria.

19. **How does the presence of gram-negative bacteria predispose the patient to periodontal disease?**
The toxins from bacteria may directly cause tissue destruction or may stimulate and modulate the host response.

20. **Name the predominant bacterial species associated with periodontal disease.**
Porphyromonas gingivalis, Aggregatibacter actinomycetemcomitans, Tannerella forsythia, Treponema denticola, Fusobacterium nucleatum, Prevotella intermedia, Campylobacter rectus, Peptostreptococcus micros, and *Eikenella corrodens.*

21. **Which bacteria are associated with periodontal health?**
Gram-positive facultative species and some members of *Streptococcus* and *Actinomyces* (e.g., *S. sanguis, S. mitis, A. viscosus, A. naeslundii).*

22. **What is the primary composition of plaque?**
Bacteria in a matrix of salivary glycoproteins and extracellular polysaccharides emanating as waste products from bacterial metabolism.

23. **What is the major difference between materia alba and plaque?**
Materia alba does not have the same organized structure as plaque, and thus can be easily displaced.

24. **Why is the tooth likely place for plaque accumulation?**
The tooth surface is nonshedding.

25. **What are the basic types of plaque? How do they differ in composition?**
The basic types of plaque are supragingival and subgingival. Supragingival plaque consists mostly of aerobes and facultative bacteria (mostly gram-positive), whereas subgingival plaque consists mostly of anaerobic bacteria (frequently gram-negative).

26. **What type of plaque is associated with caries?**
Supragingival plaque is associated with caries—predominantly the gram-positive cocci and rods (e.g., *Streptococcus mutans, lactobacilli).*

27. **What role does the salivary pellicle play in plaque retention?**
Salivary pellicle attaches to the tooth and allows for bacterial adhesion by a glycocalyx on the bacterial cell surface.

28. **Where is subgingival plaque located?**
On hard tissue (enamel, cementum, dentin), soft tissue (adheres to the epithelial cells), and loose in the sulcus.

29. **What are the two major factors determining the difference in composition between supra- and subgingival plaque?**
Presence/absence of oxygen and availability of blood products.

30. **What are the primary nutrient sources for bacterial metabolism?**
For supragingival bacteria, saliva is the primary nutrient source, and for the subgingival microbes, the gingival crevicular fluid (GCF) is the primary nutrient source. Dr. Socransky called these sources bulk fluid.

31. **Do gram-positive cariogenic bacteria promote colonization by periodontal pathogens?**
No, the cariogenic bacteria tend to inhibit the gram-negative rods associated with periodontal disease by producing bacteriocins and other substances that inhibit gram-negative bacterial growth.

32. **Why is subgingival calculus generally darker than supragingival calculus?**
Inflammation leads to ulceration of epithelium, which then leads to subgingival bleeding, and blood pigment permeates the calculus (Figs. 6-1 and 6-2).

33. **What terms are used to describe healthy gingiva?**
Healthy gingiva has scalloped, knife-like margins and a firm, stippled texture. In Caucasians, its color is uniform and is varying shades of pink.

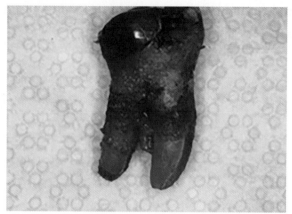

Fig. 6-1. Extracted mandibular molar due to severe periodontal destruction. Note the dark subgingival calculus located at the level of the furcation entrance and also on the roots. Due to the instrument limitation, it would be difficult to remove the calculus nonsurgically.

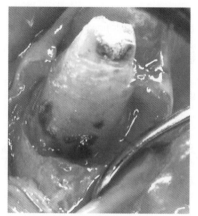

Fig. 6-2. Dark subgingival calculus was noted on the root surface, which led to an infrabony defect. Without the gingival flap elevation, it would not be easy to detect this clinically.

34. **What terms are used to describe inflamed gingiva?**
The key word is inflammation, and the cardinal signs of inflammation are calor, rubor, tumor, and dolor. All may apply to inflamed gingiva. The signs of inflammation in the gingiva may be marginal (within the free marginal gingiva) or diffuse (extending to or beyond the mucogingival junction), depending on the location of the inflammation. The margins are described as rolled, and interproximally it is often bulbous. The gingiva will be erythematous and edematous. The gingiva is frequently described as boggy or spongy due to edema, and stippling is lost in those areas (Fig. 6-3).

35. **Anatomically, what are the two parts of gingiva?**
Free gingiva (marginal gingiva) and attached gingiva.

36. **What is gingivitis?**
Gingivitis is inflammation of the gingiva that is not causing attachment loss.

37. **What bacterial groups are generally associated with gingivitis?**
Spriochetes, *Actinomyces* spp. (gram-positive filament), and *Eikenella* spp. (gram-negative rod).

38. **What other terms are used in the clinical description of gingival inflammation?**
Other terms describe severity (mild, moderate, severe), location (marginal or diffuse, and the presence or absence of ulceration, suppuration, and bleeding of probing. Other terms describing the architecture also may apply, such as blunting papilla and clefting.

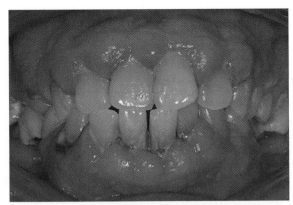

Fig. 6-3. Drug-induced gingival enlargement in a patient with poor oral hygiene and heavy supragingival calculus deposition. Gingival inflammation is evident in the presence of marginal erythema, and bulbous interdental papilla.

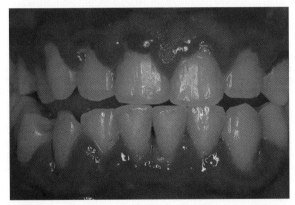

Fig. 6-4. The gingiva on this diabetic patient shows severe marginal erythema, evidence of edema, bulbousness, rolling margin, and an absence of marginal stippling.

39. How should the gingiva be described in this diabetic patient?
    Severe marginal erythema, evidence of edema/bulbousness/rolling margin, and absence of marginal stippling (Fig. 6-4).

40. What viral infection is associated with linear gingival erythema?
    Linear gingival erythema (LGE) is frequently seen in HIV gingivitis. The gingival margin shows significant erythema and hemorrhages easily.

41. Does all gingivitis become periodontitis?
    No, gingivitis may persist for long periods without advancing to periodontitis.

42. Does attachment loss occur without gingivitis?
    Yes, attachment loss can be induced by trauma (e.g., physical such as toothbrush trauma or factitious) rather than bacteria.

43. What causes gingivitis to become periodontitis?
    Microbial shift from gram-positive to gram-negative, from cocci to rods, from nonmotile to motile, from facultative anaerobe to obligate anaerobes. Additionally, the host resistance (immune system) plays a role.

44. What are the histologic characteristics of the initial lesion?
    Basically, vasculitis of the vessels is accompanied by an increase of gingival exudate from the sulcus. Polymorphonuclear neutrophils (PMNs) migrate into the sulcus and junctional epithelium. The most coronal portion of the junctional epithelium is altered, and some perivascular collagen is lost.

45. What are the histologic characteristics of the early lesion?
    Many of the changes are a continuation of the initial lesion. PMNs continue to migrate into the epithelium, and other lymphocytes follow. The collagen network continues to break down, and the junctional epithelial cells proliferate. Ulceration of the gingival sulcus is also noted.

46. **What are the histologic characteristics of the established lesion?**
A key component of the established lesion is the predominance of plasma cells in the connective tissue with the production of antibodies, continued loss of connective tissue substance, and proliferation of junctional epithelium with or without apical migration.

47. **What are the histologic characteristics of the advanced lesion?**
Many of the features are similar to the established lesion. The advanced lesion extends to the periodontal ligament and alveolar bone with pocket formation and goes through periods of exacerbations and remission. There are more extensive cellular changes due to inflammation.

48. **A patient presents with heavy plaque, calculus, and bleeding on probing without attachment loss. What is the periodontal diagnosis?**
Generalized (>30%), severe marginal gingivitis (Fig. 6-5).

49. **What are the clinical signs of necrotizing ulcerative gingivitis (NUG)?**
NUG is an acute, recurring infection of the gingiva characterized by necrosis of the papilla (leading to blunting), spontaneous bleeding, pain, and fetor oris (Fig. 6-6).

50. **What bacteria are associated with NUG?**
The bacteria associated with NUG are a fusospirochetal complex—fusiform bacteria and spirochetes.

51. **How is necrotizing ulcerative periodontitis (NUP) different from NUG?**
NUP exhibits a loss of clinical attachment and alveolar bone, whereas NUG shows no apical migration of the attachment apparatus (supracrestal attachment) and no loss of alveolar bone.

52. **What bacteria are associated with gingivitis during pregnancy? Why?**
Bacteria associated with gingivitis during pregnancy are the black-pigmenting *Bacteroides* spp., which utilize steroid hormones for their own metabolism. Therefore, pregnancy essentially selects for these bacteria. Patients who use birth control pills or receive steroid therapy (chronic autoimmune diseases) are also at risk.

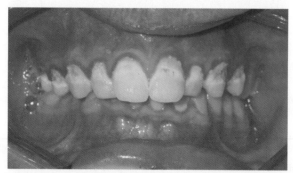

Fig. 6-5. Patient with plaque-induced gingival disease. Note the heavy plaque and calculus. No attachment loss was present.

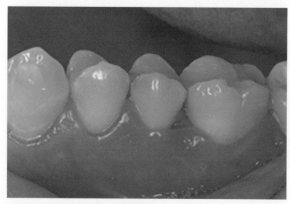

Fig. 6-6. The clinical signs of NUG included blunting of the papilla (between the first molar and second premolar), spontaneous bleeding, pain, and fetor oris.

53. A pregnant patient presents with gingival swelling on the palatal aspect of #12/13 area. The patient presents with minimal plaque build-up without radiographic evidence of bone loss. What is the ideal initial periodontal treatment?

The patient is diagnosed with pregnancy-associated gingivitis. The treatment will instruct with plaque control techniques and scaling if needed. Following the initial treatment, gingival swelling has been reduced (Figs. 6-7 and 6-8)

54. What is the American Dental Association's periodontal disease classification?

Type I: Gingivitis

Type II: Mild periodontitis

Type III: Moderate periodontitis

Type IV: Severe or advanced periodontitis

These categories are based on clinical and radiographic criteria such as the amount of bone loss, pocket depth, and mobility.

55. What is the American Academy of Periodontology's periodontitis classification?

The 2017 AAP/EFP Classification System for periodontitis is based on staging (disease severity and complexity) and grading (disease progression).

Stage I: Radiographic Bone Loss Coronal (RBL) third (<15%), No tooth loss due to periodontitis, greatest clinical attachment loss (CAL) 1 to 2 mm, maximum probing depth (MPD) $\leq$ 4 mm, mostly horizontal bone loss (HBL)

Stage II: RBL Coronal third (15%-33%), No tooth loss to periodontitis, greatest CAL 3 to 4 mm, MPD $\leq$ 5 mm, mostly HBL

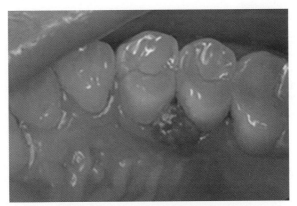

Fig. 6-7. Patient with pregnancy-associated gingivitis.

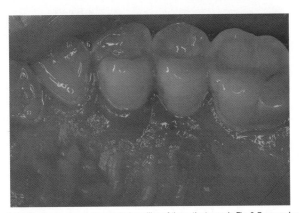

Fig. 6-8. After the treatment, the gingival swelling of the patient seen in Fig. 6-7 was reduced.

Stage III: Stage II complexity and RBL extends to mid-third of root, ≤4 teeth lost to periodontitis, CAL ≥ 5 mm, MPD > 6 mm, vertical bone loss (VBL) ≥ 3 mm, Furcation involvement (FI) Class II or III, moderate ridge defects

Stage IV: Stage III complexity and tooth loss to periodontitis ≤ 5 teeth, need for complex rehabilitation, secondary occlusal trauma, bite collapse, severe ridge defects, <20 remaining teeth (10 opposing pairs)

Grade A: Direct evidence of progression: RBL or CAL no loss over past 5 years, indirect evidence of progression % RBL ÷ age = <0.25, heavy biofilm deposits, nonsmoker, normoglycemic, no diagnosis of diabetes

Grade B: Direct evidence of progression: RBL or CAL, <2 mm over 5 years, indirect evidence of progression: % RBL ÷ age = 0.25-1.0, RBL and CAL commensurate with biofilm deposits, smokers: <10 cigarettes per day, diabetics: HbA1c ≤ 7.0%

Grade C: Formerly "aggressive" Direct evidence of progression: RBL or CAL ≥ 2 mm over 5 years, indirect evidence of progression: % RBL ÷ age = ≥1.0, RBL and CAL exceed expectations of given biofilm deposits, can be generalized or molar/incisor pattern, smokers: ≥ 10 cigarettes per day, diabetics: HbA1c ≥ 7.0 (Tables 6-1 and 6.2).

Table 6-1. Periodontitis: Staging

Staging intends to classify the severity and extent of a patient's disease based on the measurable amount of destroyed and/or damaged tissue as a result of periodontitis and to assess the specific factors that may attribute to the complexity of long-term case management.

Initial stage should be determined using clinical attachment loss (CAL). If CAL is not available, radiographic bone loss (RBL) should be used. Tooth loss due to periodontitis may modify stage definition. One or more complexity factors may shift the stage to a higher level. See perio.org/2017wwdc for additional information.

	PERIODONTITIS	STAGE I	STAGE II	STAGE III	STAGE IV
Severity	Interdental CAL *(at site of greatest loss)*	1-2 mm	3-4 mm	≥5 mm	≥5 mm
	RBL	Coronal third (<15%)	Coronal third (15%-33%)	Extending to middle third of root and beyond	Extending to middle third of root and beyond
	Tooth loss *(due to periodontitis)*	No tooth loss		≤4 teeth	≥5 teeth
Complexity	Local	• Max. probing depth ≤4 mm • Mostly horizontal bone loss	• Max. probing depth ≤5 mm • Mostly horizontal bone loss	In addition to Stage II complexity: • Probing depths ≥6 mm • Vertical bone loss ≥3 mm • Furcation involvement Class II or III • Moderate ridge defects	In addition to Stage III complexity: • Need for complex rehabilitation due to: • Masticatory dysfunction • Secondary occlusal trauma (tooth mobility degree ≥2) • Severe ridge defects • Bite collapse, drifting, flaring • <20 remaining teeth (10 opposing pairs)
Extent and distribution	Add to stage as descriptor	For each stage, describe extent as: • Localized (<30% of teeth involved); • Generalized; or • Molar/incisor pattern			

Table 6-2. Periodontitis: Grading

Grading aims to indicate the rate of periodontitis progression, responsiveness to standard therapy, and potential impact on systemic health.

Clinicians should initially assume grade B disease and seek specific evidence to shift to grade A or C.

See perio.org/2017wwdc for additional information.

	PROGRESSION		GRADE A: SLOW RATE	GRADE B: MODERATE RATE	GRADE C: RAPID RATE
Primary criteria	Direct evidence of progression	Radiographic bone loss or CAL	No loss over 5 years	<2 mm over 5 years	≥2 mm over 5 years
Whenever available, direct evidence should be used.	Indirect evidence of progression	% bone loss/age	<0.25	0.25 to 1.0	>1.0
		Case phenotype	Heavy biofilm deposits with low levels of destruction	Destruction commensurate with biofilm deposits	Destruction exceeds expectations given biofilm deposits; specific clinical patterns suggestive of periods of rapid progression and/or early onset disease
Grade modifiers	Risk factors	Smoking	Nonsmoker	<10 cigarettes/day	≥10 cigarettes/day
		Diabetes	Normoglycemic/no diagnosis of diabetes	HbA1c < 7.0% in patients with diabetes	HbA1c ≥ 7.0% in patients with diabetes

56. How is chronic periodontitis further subclassified and characterized?
    - Localized form: <30% of sites involved
    - Generalized form: ≥30% of sites involved
    - Location: generalized, molar/incisor pattern

57. Initial radiograph shows no bone loss on #13, however, radiographs that are taken 3 years and 6 years later showed an extensive progressive bone loss. What is the most appropriate periodontal diagnosis for this patient?
    Localized Stage III, Grade C periodontitis (Fig. 6-9).

58. What are the clinical features of generalized Grade C periodontitis?
    - Often affecting persons under 30 years of age (however, may be older).
    - Generalized proximal attachment loss affecting at least three teeth other than first molars and incisors.
    - Pronounced episodic nature of periodontal destruction.
    - Poor serum antibody response to infecting agents.
    - Often, they show chemotactic defects of their neutrophils.

59. This patient presented with significant bone and clinical attachment loss, but minimal local factors. What is the most likely classification of this patient's periodontal disease?
    Generalized Stage III, Grade C periodontitis (Fig. 6-10).

60. What bacteria is commonly associated with Grade C periodontitis?
    A. Actinomycetemcomitans.

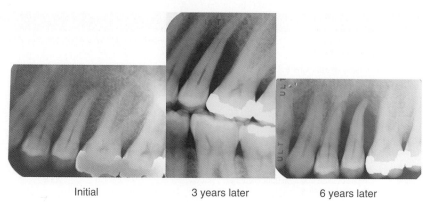

Initial   3 years later   6 years later

Fig. 6-9. Initial radiograph (*left*) and radiographs taken at 3 (*middle*) and 6 years (*right*) for a patient with localized aggressive periodontitis. Extensive progressive bone loss is shown.

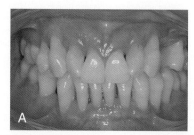

Fig. 6-10. (A) Clinical view of a patient with generalized Stage III, Grade c periodontitis. Significant bone loss and clinical attachment loss are present.

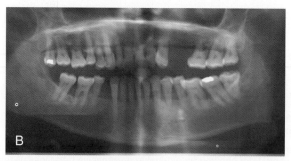

Fig. 6-10. (B) Panoramic view of a patient with generalized Stage III, Grade c periodontitis. Significant bone loss and clinical attachment loss are present.

61. What is the first cellular line of defense of the body against the periopathogens?
Other than the epithelial cell barrier, the first line of defense is the PMN.

62. What is meant by a "burn-out lesion" in a patient with Stage III, Grade C incisor/molar pattern periodontitis?
At one point, the patient with Stage III, Grade C incisor/molar pattern periodontitis had an infection with periodontal lesions in which the chief etiologic agent was *A. actinomycetemcomitans*. The body responds with an immunologic response and controls the infection, but the bony defect remains. The deep pocketing now becomes inhabited with bacterial flora, which is more characteristic of chronic periodontal lesions (Fig. 6-11).

63. Patients with deep periodontal pockets and heavy deposits of plaque and calculus may develop an acute periodontal abscess after scaling. Why?
This is due to incomplete removal of etiologic agents.

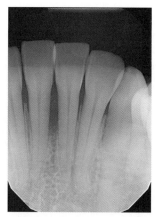

Fig. 6-11. Severe bone loss down to the middle-apical third of the mandibular incisors.

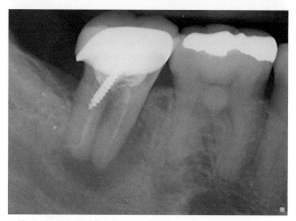

Fig. 6-12. Gingival swelling with sinus tract noted on the mesial-buccal of tooth #31 associated with a perio-endo lesion.

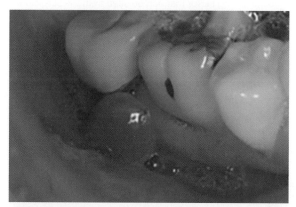

Fig. 6-13. Peri-apical film showing J-shaped radiolucency around tooth #31.

64. **What is a perio-endo abscess?**
    A perio-endo abscess is a combined lesion in which periodontal and endodontic problems occur simultaneously. The lesion can be initiated by extensive periodontitis, which creates pulpal pathology (Figs. 6-12 and 6-13).

65. **What treatment is frequently used for a periodontal abscess?**
    Initial treatment may consist of the establishment of drainage and the removal of the etiologic agents (incision and drainage through the sulcus along with scaling, root planing, and irrigation), followed first by a course of antibiotic therapy and then by surgical treatment when needed.

66. **When is it safe to treat a pregnant woman's nonacute periodontal problem?**
    In general, the second trimester is the window of treatment for most dental procedures. If antibiotics or other medications are indicated, consult with the obstetrician and *Physicians' Desk Reference*.

67. **Which periodontal pathogen most nearly fulfills Koch's postulates?**
    Koch's postulates state that a pathogenic bacterium causes disease, that the disease is transmissible through the bacteria, and that if you eliminate or control the bacteria, you eliminate the infection. *A. actinomycetemcomitans* (molar-incisor Stage III, Grade C) and *P. gingivalis* most nearly fulfill Koch's postulates.

68. **What bacterial group is associated with root caries?**
    Root caries may be a problem for patients with gingival recession and xerostomia (whether induced by drugs, radiation, or some other agent). The bacteria associated with root caries are gram-positive rods and filaments, particularly *Actinomyces viscosus* (Fig. 6-14).

69. **This patient presented with deep pocket depth and severe bone loss on #30. What is the most noticeable contributing factor that can be seen from the surgical exposure of the site?**
    Class 3 cervical enamel projection (Fig. 6-15).

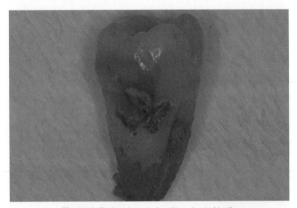

Fig. 6-14. Root caries noted on the extracted tooth.

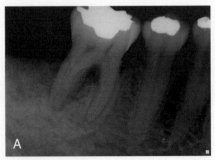

Fig. 6-15. (A) Radiographic view of severe bone loss and deep pocket depth on tooth #30.

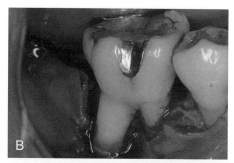

Fig. 6-15. (B) Clinical view of severe bone loss and deep pocket depth on tooth #30. Note the significant enamel projection.

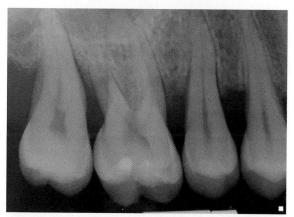

Fig. 6-16. Radiographic evidence of periodontitis as the crestal bone levels are more than 2 mm below CEJ.

CONCEPT OF DISEASE ACTIVITY

70. What is meant by active periodontitis?
    It refers to periodontal inflammation that causes an apical migration of epithelial attachment.

71. How is progressive periodontal disease activity measured?
    Classically, disease activity is measured as clinical attachment loss (CAL) by using a periodontal probe and a fixed reference point, such as the cementoenamel junction (CEJ). The increase in the distance from the CEJ to the base of the periodontal pocket determines disease activity.

72. What is the classic definition of the presence of periodontal disease?
    Attachment loss with the presence of plaque-induced gingival inflammation and radiographic evidence of interproximal bone loss. Generally, there are probing depths ≥ 4 mm.

73. How is the radiographic evidence of bone loss determined?
    In a healthy state, the crestal bone levels are about 2 mm below the CEJ. In periodontitis, crestal bone is below this level with a loss of crestal septal lamina dura (Fig. 6-16).

74. Which radiographs tend to be most accurate in the determination of bone loss?
    Vertical bitewings (Fig. 6-17).

75. What is the most common pattern of bone loss in periodontal disease?
    Horizontal bone loss (Fig. 6-18).

76. What is bone sounding?
    Sounding is used to provide the clinician with additional information regarding the morphology of bony defect. The area in question is anesthetized, and a probe in a sulcus is forced through the epithelium and the connective tissue until it strikes bone. Sounding may facilitate flap design (Figs. 6-19 and 6-20).

77. How is periodontal disease activity described?
    Patterns of periodontal disease activity include random bursts/or and slow continuous processes.

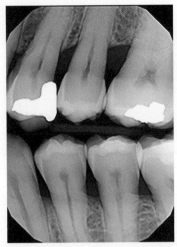

Fig. 6-17. Vertical bitewing captures the crestal bone levels of both maxillary and mandibular teeth.

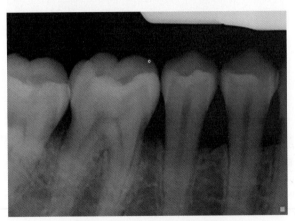

Fig. 6-18. Horizontal bone loss noted on the radiograph.

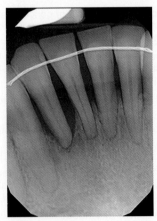

Fig. 6-19. Radiograph showing vertical bone loss of mandibular left lateral incisor.

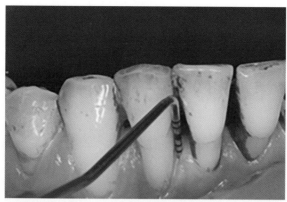

Fig. 6-20. Sounding of the defect following anesthesia provides the clinician additional information regarding the morphology of the bony defect.

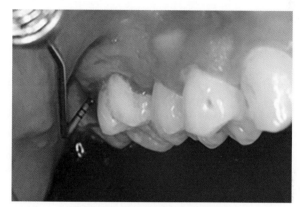

Fig. 6-21. Bleeding on probing around tooth #3.

78. **What is the difference between nonspecific and specific plaque hypothesis?**
The nonspecific hypothesis simply states that it is the quantity and not the quality of the plaque that causes periodontal disease. The specific plaque hypothesis states that specific bacterial pathogens are responsible for periodontal diseases.

79. **What traditional clinical marker (other than an increase in attachment loss) may be significant in determining active periodontal disease?**
Bleeding on probing (BoP), greater the likelihood of breakdown (Fig. 6-21).

80. **What two inflammatory mediators may be indicators of disease activity?**
Interleukin I-beta (IL1-β) and tumor necrosis factor-alpha (TNF-α) may indicate disease activity.

81. **What are the major risk factors for periodontal disease?**
Plaque, smoking, diabetes, and genetics.

82. **What is the effect that open interproximal contact can have on the periodontium?**
Open interproximal can lead to food impaction, caused by plunger cusp activity which can lead to increased alveolar bone loss (Fig. 6-22).

PERIODONTAL DIAGNOSIS

83. **How is a periodontal pocket defined?**
A pathologically deepened sulcus that cannot be accessed by the patient for plaque removal.

84. **What is the difference between suprabony and infrabony pocket?**
   - Infrabony pocket is where the tip of the probe is apical to the crest of the adjacent alveolar bone.
   - Suprabony pocket is where the tip of the probe is at or coronal to the crest of the adjacent alveolar bone.

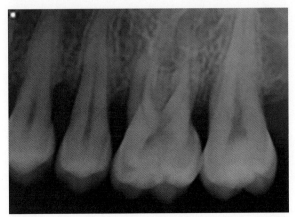

Fig. 6-22. Open contact between the first and second premolars is evident on the radiograph.

85. **What sites are routinely probed during a thorough periodontal examination?**
Six sites are commonly checked: the mesio-, mid-, and distobuccal sites as well as the corresponding lingual/palatal sites. It is recommended to walk the probe continuously (step probing) through the sulcus to get a better feel for the pocket depths as a whole.

86. **What is a pseudopocket?**
It is a pathologically deepened sulcus that is formed by gingival enlargement without attachment loss.

87. **What is clinical attachment loss (CAL)?**
When the most coronal portion of the epithelial attachment is apical to the cementoenamel junction (CEJ).

88. **What is the importance in the progression of periodontal disease relating to attachment loss and periodontal pocketing?**
The periodontal pocket is important because it is a pathologically deepened sulcus that cannot be maintained clean by the patient and can lead to additional attachment loss. Attachment loss signifies the migration of the supracrestal attachment apically.

89. **Which is more important in defining periodontal disease: attachment loss or periodontal pocketing?**
Attachment loss is more important because the depth of the pocket does not necessarily indicate that there is bone loss.

90. **What are the two most significant clinical parameters for the prognosis of a periodontally involved tooth?**
The two most significant clinical parameters are mobility and attachment loss.

91. **What is gingival hypertrophy?**
Gingival hypertrophy indicates that there is an increase in size generally due to edema (Fig. 6-23).

92. **What causes gingival recession?**
The major causes are toothbrush or floss abrasion, periodontal disease, trauma, prominent roots with thin phenotype, and absence of or a minimal zone of attached gingiva (Fig. 6-24).

93. **Which area of the oral cavity has the least amount of attached gingiva?**
The buccal mandibular premolar area commonly has the least amount of attached tissue (Fig. 6-25).

94. **What is a long junctional epithelium?**
After a periodontal pocket has been scaled, root planed, and curetted, a reattachment by epithelial cells to the root surface may occur. This reattachment is called a long junctional epithelium.

95. **What is the term for gingival cells that attach to the root cementum? How do they attach to the root?**
The term is junctional epithelium; the cells attach by a glycocalyx (mucopolysaccharide) secreted by the epithelial cells through hemidesmosomes.

96. **What is a mucogingival defect?**
Mucogingival defects are defined by periodontal pocketing that extends beyond the mucogingival junction with the absence of attached gingiva (Fig. 6-26).

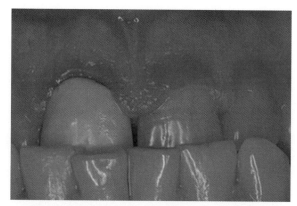

Fig. 6-23. Gingival hypertrophy observed between the central incisors.

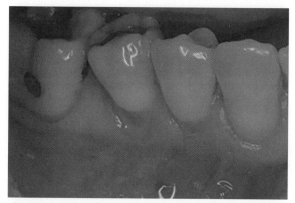

Fig. 6-24. Gingival recessions with cervical abrasions can be observed on the premolars.

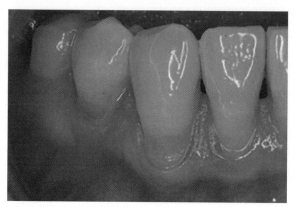

Fig. 6-25. Thin band of attached gingiva around the mandibular first premolar.

97. Is periodontal disease a risk factor for other diseases?
   Epidemiologic evidence indicates that dental plaque-related periodontal diseases negatively affect other chronic systemic diseases as well as other chronic systemic diseases negatively affect the outcome of periodontal diseases (e.g., diabetes, cerebrocardiovascular (CVA) disease, adverse pregnancy outcome).

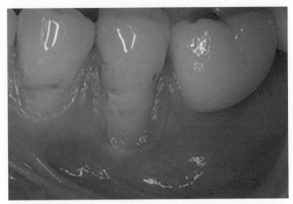

Fig. 6-26. The second premolar has mucogingival defect extending beyond the mucogingival margin with the absence of attached gingiva.

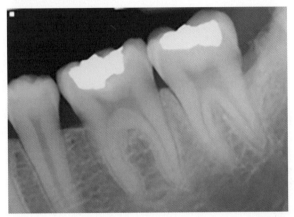

Fig. 6-27. Long tapering roots and long root trunks in multirooted teeth have a more favorable prognosis.

98. **What is the crown-to-root ratio in a healthy dentition?**
As a general rule, the crown-to-root ratio in a healthy dentition is 1:2 (for each tooth). Teeth with unfavorable crown-to-root ratios tend to have a poor prognosis, especially if there is periodontitis and mobility is significant.

99. **What root shapes generally have a favorable prognosis?**
Crown-to-root ratio is very important. Long, tapering roots are usually sturdier than short, conical roots. Long root trunks in multirooted teeth are more favorable than short root trunks (Fig. 6-27).

100. **What is the difference between bony fenestration and bony dehiscence?**
Fenestration refers to a window in the bone, exposing the root. A dehiscence is where denuded areas of teeth extend through the marginal bone. Both are commonly noted in thin periodontium (Figs. 6-28 and 6-29).

101. **What is positive bony architecture?**
Positive bony architecture is when the interproximal marginal bone is coronal to the cervical bone.

102. **What is negative bony architecture?**
Negative bony architecture is when the interproximal marginal bone is apical to the cervical bone (Fig. 6-30).

103. **What is flat bony architecture?**
It is when both the cervical and the interproximal alveolar bone are at the same level.

104. **What is an ideal bony architecture?**
Positive bony architecture is when the interproximal bone level is higher than the cervical bone.

105. **What are the basic classifications of bony defects?**
Bony defects are generally classified according to the number of bony walls that remain. For example, a one-wall defect has only one remaining wall of bone, two-wall defects have two remaining walls, and so on (Fig. 6-31).

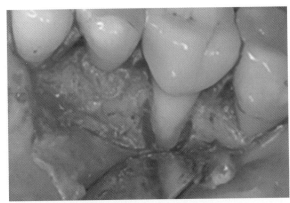

Fig. 6-28. Bone dehiscence noted on the molar.

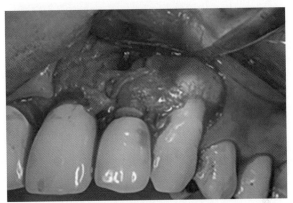

Fig. 6-29. Bone fenestration noted on the lateral incisor.

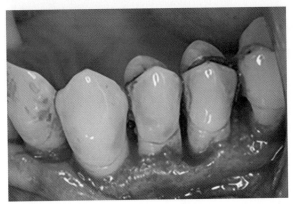

Fig. 6-30. The interproximal marginal bone between the first and second premolars is apical to the cervical bone. This is negative bony architecture.

106. Which bony defect is most likely to repair or fill naturally after treatment?

Narrow three-wall periodontal defects are most likely to repair naturally after therapy because there is less denuded surface of tooth to regenerate.

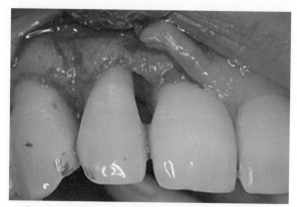

Fig. 6-31. The bony defect on the mesial of tooth #7 is a one-wall defect.

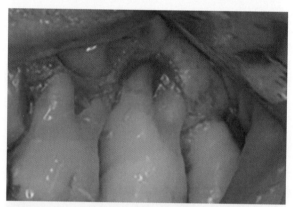

Fig. 6-32. The first molar has a class I buccal furcation involvement while the second molar has a class II buccal furcation involvement.

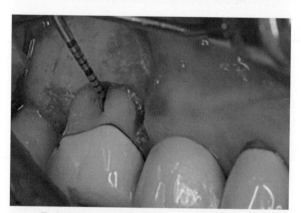

Fig. 6-33. The molar has a buccal class II furcation involvement.

107. **Name different microbiologic methods of assessing bacterial plaque.**
There are numerous ways to assess bacterial plaque. General categories include culturing, microscopic, enzymatic, and genetic methods.

108. **How are furcations classified?**
Furcations are classified according to probing. Class I furcations are incipient furcations; class II, approximately halfway into the furcation; and class III, completely through furcation from the facial to the lingual (Figs. 6-32 and 6-33).

109. **Why do diabetes, Papillon-LeFevre, and Chediak-Higashi disease affect periodontium?**
With all these diseases, the normal cellular immunologic response is impaired. The white cells (PMNs) do not function properly. Therefore, patients are susceptible to periodontal infections.

110. **What is gingival crevicular fluid (GCF)?**
GCF is an ultrafiltrate of serum. Therefore, it contains many of the components of serum, particularly complement and antibody. The flow rates of GCF have been used in attempt to predict disease activity. Furthermore, investigators have been interested in GCF for other markers of periodontal breakdown (e.g., beta-glucuronidase, interleukin, collagenase).

111. **Do links to specific genetic alleles predict risk for periodontitis?**
Yes, variation in the IL-1 beta allele may indicate a risk for periodontitis. This variation has been shown to be especially important in smokers.

112. **Do current smokers have the same levels of periodontitis as nonsmokers?**
Generally, smokers have more attachment loss than nonsmokers.

113. **What is the healing response of current smokers?**
Typically, the response to nonsurgical and surgical therapy is lower in smokers.

114. **What happens to the risk of periodontitis and the healing response if a patient stops smoking?**
When a patient becomes a past smoker, the risk for periodontitis decreases and the healing response improves.

ADJUNCTIVE PERIODONTAL THERAPY

115. **Which antibiotics are used frequently to treat an acute periodontal abscess?**
After the establishment of drainage, penicillin (500 mg every 6 hours for 7 days) provides adequate antibiotic coverage.

116. **What local delivery antibiotics may be advised for the treatment of chronic periodontitis?**
Minocycline or doxycycline.

117. **What is the protocol for systemically treating aggressive periodontitis using antibiotics?**
Localized aggressive periodontitis has a preponderance of *A. actinomycetemcomitans* and is sufficiently treated with the combination of amoxicillin and metronidazole.

118. **In a patient who is allergic to penicillin and erythromycin, what is the next antibiotic to be used for prophylaxis?**
Azithromycin, 500 mg, 1 hour before treatment.

119. **Why are third-generation cephalosporins frequently contraindicated for the treatment of a periodontal abscess?**
Frequently the spectrum of a third-generation cephalosporin becomes so specific that it does not provide adequate antimicrobial coverage. Penicillin should be the first choice; erythromycin or azithromycin may be used in penicillin-allergic patients.

120. **What complication may occur with broad-spectrum antibiotics?**
A major problem is the development of pseudomembranous colitis, which is caused by the overgrowth and toxin production of *Clostridium difficile*.

121. **Why are tetracyclines used in the treatment of periodontal disease?**
Tetracycline is used primarily for antibiotic coverage, but it has advantages over other antibiotics because it concentrates at levels 2 to 4 times higher in the GCF than in the serum, binds to the root surface and can be released over a prolonged time, prevents bacterial reattachment to the root surface, promotes reattachment of fibers to the root surface, and inhibits collagenolytic activity.

122. **What are some of the common guidelines or precautions that should be given to a patient in prescribing tetracyclines?**
Use of any antibiotic involves the potential to upset the natural bacterial flora. Gastrointestinal distress, including nausea, vomiting, and diarrhea, is possible. Women must be advised of the potential of yeast infections. Other side effects include tinnitus, vertigo, and photosensitivity.

123. **Are tetracyclines safe and effective for women who are taking birth control pills?**
In general, a woman who is taking birth control pills should avoid the use of tetracyclines. Clinical studies have shown that tetracyclines may cause abnormal breakthrough bleeding during the menstrual cycle.

124. **What directions should be given to the patient in prescribing oral tetracyclines?**
Tetracyclines should be taken between meals (on an empty stomach) with a tall glass of water. Foods and antacids containing relatively high concentrations of calcium and iron should not be taken with tetracycline. Tetracycline acts as a chelator with these divalent cations, thereby interfering with its own intestinal absorption. Therapeutic dosages, therefore, are not achieved.

125. **What are the major advantages and disadvantages of using local delivery doxycycline or minocycline in the treatment of periodontal disease?**
The spectrum of doxycycline and minocycline may be slightly better than mechanical debridement alone, particularly in covering *P. gingivalis*. Other advantages include less photosensitivity, less chelating, and better patient compliance when compared with systemic antibiotics. Because both antibiotics are fat soluble, the dose is reduced to 50 or 100 mg 2 times/day.

126. **What is the major problem with the use of metronidazole?**
When prescribing metronidazole, you should advise patients that they must refrain from alcohol, or they may become violently ill from the combination (Antabuse effect). Patients should always be advised not to mix any medicine with alcohol.

127. **Why is metronidazole effective in treating a periodontal infection?**
The periodontal pathogens are predominantly anaerobic, and metronidazole is effective in treating anaerobic infections.

128. **What is localized drug delivery?**
Localized drug delivery is being developed to administer drug directly to the site of infection, the periodontal pocket. The advantage of such devices includes the elimination of many of the side effects associated with systemic delivery.

129. **What are the typical indications for locally administered antibiotics?**
This mode of delivery is generally used in periodontal pockets that measure greater than 5 mm that bleed on probing and are resistant to conventional mechanical therapy.

130. **What preparation is required before administering locally delivered antibiotics?**
Teeth should be thoroughly scaled and root planed.

131. **What pathway do nonsteroidal anti-inflammatory drugs (NSAIDs) block?**
NSAIDs block the cyclooxygenase metabolism of arachidonic acids.

132. **Which mouth rinse appears to be most effective in the control of bacterial plaque?**
Chlorhexidine gluconate is the most effective oral rinse for controlling bacterial plaque, particularly because it leaves the greatest residual concentration in the mouth after use.

133. **HIV-positive patients frequently manifest a condition called hairy leukoplakia in their oral cavity. What microbe is commonly associated with hairy leukoplakia? What is the treatment for this condition?**
Candida albicans (yeast) is frequently associated with hairy leukoplakia and should be treated with antifungal medication, including nystatin or fluconazole. Chlorhexidine rinses should be included, because chlorhexidine is also effective against *C. albicans*.

134. **What is the primary symptom of root sensitivity?**
In general, the primary symptom is sensitivity to cold.

135. **What other symptoms are there for dental sensitivity?**
Besides cold, hot, touch (tactile), biting pressure, sweets, and sour foods may cause sensitivity.

136. **What is the cause of root sensitivity?**
Root sensitivity is believed to be caused by the movement of fluid in the dentinal tubules, which stimulates the pain sensation (the hydrodynamic theory).

137. **What factors may contribute significantly to dentinal sensitivity?**
Toothbrush abrasion, periodontal and orthodontic treatment, gingival recession, acidic foods, and bruxism.

138. **How is root sensitivity treated?**
Primary treatment is good plaque control by the patient. In addition, treatment of root sensitivity can involve seal-coating of the root. Substances routinely used are fluoride mouth rinses, fluoride toothpaste, desensitizing toothpaste, and application of composite restoration.

139. **How do root desensitizers work?**
Several methods are used, including protein precipitants (e.g., strontium chloride), dentinal tubule blockers (e.g., fluorides, oxalates), nerve desensitizers (potassium nitrate), and physical agents such as burnishing the root, composites, monomers, and resins.

OCCLUSAL TREATMENT

140. **What is the role of occlusion in periodontal disease?**
Occlusal trauma by itself will not cause attachment loss, however, with preexisting periodontitis, it may exacerbate attachment loss.

141. **What is primary and what is secondary occlusal trauma?**
Primary occlusal trauma refers to excessive force applied to a tooth or teeth with normal supporting structures. Secondary occlusal trauma refers to when normal occlusal forces become excessive due to loss of attachment.

142. **What is fremitus?**
Fremitus is the vibration or movement of a tooth in functional (centric) occlusion. It is premature contact in functional occlusion.

143. **Is trauma from occlusal force reversible?**
Yes, however, if attachment loss occurs as a result of periodontal disease and occlusal trauma, the removal of the force alone will not reverse the attachment loss.

144. **Does traumatic occlusion lead to pockets or recession?**
There is no research to show that occlusal trauma alone leads to pocketing or recession.

145. **When is a nightguard indicated?**
A nightguard is indicated whenever the signs or symptoms of bruxism or parafunctional habits are found. Wear facets on the teeth are usually indicative of bruxism.

146. **What are the clinical signs of bruxism?**
Signs of bruxism may include occlusal/incisal wear facets, temporomandibular joint (TMJ) symptoms, masticatory muscle soreness, tooth mobility, fractured teeth or restorations, and radiographic widened periodontal ligament spaces (on radiographs). These signs may occur in various combinations.

147. **What criteria should be followed in constructing a nightguard for the treatment of bruxism?**
A nightguard should have four characteristics: (1) it should be made of processed acrylic; (2) it should snap gently over the occlusal surfaces of the maxillary teeth; (3) it should occlude evenly with the mandibular teeth in centric occlusion; (4) it should have no interferences in lateral or protrusive excursion; and (5) it should be adjusted so that it is comfortable.

148. **When should the splinting of teeth be considered?**
Splinting of teeth is performed to stabilize mobile teeth, to stabilize teeth that might become more mobile following periodontal therapy, and for patient's comfort. Any fixed splint should allow access for the patient to remove dental plaque from all tooth surfaces.

149. **What types of splints may be fabricated?**
Examples include interproximal application of composite, composite with mesh/wire reinforcement, and splinted fixed prostheses.

150. **What do widened periodontal ligament spaces indicate?**
Widened periodontal ligament spaces may be indicative of occlusal trauma (Fig. 6-34).

151. **Can orthodontic treatment mitigate the forces of occlusion?**
Yes, along with the occlusal adjustment, occlusal guards, and splinting.

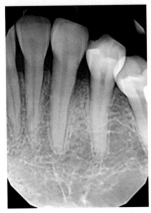

Fig. 6-34. Widened PDL spaces can be observed on the mandibular teeth, particularly around the coronal thirds.

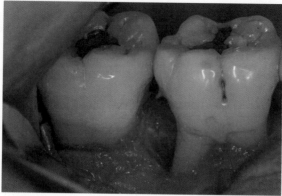

Fig. 6-35. The infrabony defect on the distal of #30 is caused by plaque and occlusal trauma as evident by the wear facets.

152. **What are the etiologic factors causing this defect on #30 distal?**
    - Plaque (primary)
    - Occlusal trauma (adjunctive). Note: wear facets indicating parafunctional habits (Fig. 6-35)

153. **What is the trauma from occlusion?**
    The microscopic changes (hyalinization) in the periodontal ligament as the result of traumatic forces.

INITIAL TREATMENT OF PERIODONTAL DISEASE

154. **What is scaling?**
    Scaling is the removal of hard and soft deposits (plaque, calculus, and stain) from tooth surfaces.

155. **When are scalers used?**
    Scalers are used to remove hard and soft deposits only supragingivally.

156. **What is root planing?**
    Root planing is the smoothing of the subgingival root surfaces with a curette. The objective of root planing is to remove deposits (scaling) as well as exposed cementum, which is rough because it formerly housed Sharpey's fibers of the connective tissue attachment of the gingiva or the periodontal ligament. The purpose is to provide a surface that is commensurate for gingival reattachment.

157. **What is gingival curettage?**
    Curettage is the removal of the epithelium and connective tissue where there is inflammation and a build-up of granulation tissue in the sulcular lining of the periodontal pocket. This procedure is frequently performed along with root planing to promote gingival reattachment. Curettage can reduce the pocket depth and afford a patient improved access to remove subgingival bacterial plaque.

158. **What are the goals of initial periodontal therapy?**
    The objectives of initial therapy are to instruct and motivate and instruct the patient in plaque removal techniques that are evidence-based and effective, to remove hard and soft tissue deposits from tooth/root surfaces, and to achieve pocket reduction with the possibility of reattachment.

159. **What evidence-based plaque removal techniques are best taught to patients?**
    a. Brushing: The stationary bristle tip technique (Bass technique) is a nonabrasive effective technique for displacing bacterial plaque supra- and sub-gingivally.
    b. Flossing: The adapted horizontal vertical flossing technique (AHVFT) used daily has been shown to reduce interproximal bleeding on probing better than when people are uninstructed. This technique is similar to the technique to dry one's back after a bath or a shower.
    c. Interproximal brushes: A number of studies have shown the value of using interproximal brushes.

160. **What is the theory of plaque removal by the patient?**
    Plaque is the product of bacterial metabolism and sticks to any nonshedding surface. It has little mass. The theory of plaque removal is that two objects cannot occupy the same place at the same time and that the object of the greater mass will displace the object of the lesser mass. A toothbrush bristle has greater mass than dental plaque, and thus if the toothbrush bristle is on the tooth, the plaque must be displaced. Dental plaque displaced from a tooth surface will not reattach and will be washed away by the gingival crevice fluid or saliva. Thus, toothbrushes, interproximal brushes, and dental floss have greater mass than bacterial plaque, and they are effective in plaque removal (displacement).

161. When do bacterial populations reach pretreatment levels?

Typically, bacteria repopulate the periodontal pocket as soon as 4 to 6 weeks. Pathogenic bacteria can return to pretreatment levels in approximately 9 to 11 weeks.

162. What is the treatment routinely used for NUG/NUP?

Treatment consists of debridement (scaling and root planing) with an antibiotic. Penicillin VK 500 mg, 4 times/day for 7 days. Pain relievers are prescribed if needed. Rinsing with hydrogen peroxide or chlorhexidine is also recommended. Instructions for oral hygiene should be emphasized; a Stillman's sweep using the sides of the bristles rather than the tips is recommended until the gingiva re-epithelializes.

163. What is nonsurgical therapy for periodontal disease?

Nonsurgical therapy is plaque control technique instruction and scaling and root planing.

164. A patient presents with pain and swelling associated with mandibular anterior teeth. Radiographic evidence of bone loss is seen. What is the ideal initial periodontal treatment for this patient at this visit?

Patient is diagnosed with periodontal abscess, thus mechanical debridement under injectable local anesthesia to establish drainage, and the systemic administration of antibiotic treatment (e.g., Pen VK 500 mg/qid/10 days) are indicated (Figs. 6-36 and 6-37).

SURGICAL TREATMENT OF PERIODONTAL DISEASE

165. What are the advantages of pocket-reducing periodontal surgery over nonsurgical treatment?

The two important reasons for performing periodontal surgery are to provide the clinician with access to thorough scaling and root planing, and other hard tissue therapy and to reduce pockets in order that the patient will have access to perform complete plaque control.

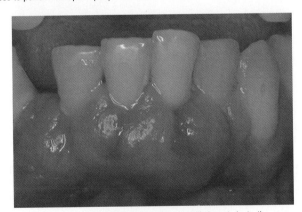

Fig. 6-36. Pain and swelling around the mandibular anterior teeth.

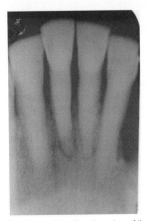

Fig. 6-37. Radiographic evidence of significant bone loss of the mandibular incisors.

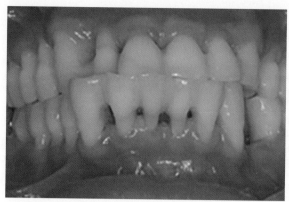

Fig. 6-38. Following periodontal surgery, gingival recession along with exposure of root surfaces led to root hypersensitivity.

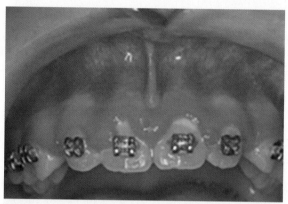

Fig. 6-39. Patient with gingival overgrowth and adequate zone of keratinized gingiva.

166. **What are the major complications that may be associated with periodontal surgery?**
As with any form of surgery, the patient might experience pain, swelling, infection, and bleeding. In addition, gingival recession with root hypersensitivity may occur. A thorough medical history and explanation to the patient of the pros and cons of surgery must be done at the evaluation appointment prior to undertaking any surgical procedure (Fig. 6-38).

167. **When is gingivectomy indicated?**
Gingivectomy is indicated for pocket reduction with normal osseous architecture in the presence of the adequate zone of gingiva (Figs. 6-39 and 6-40).

168. **What drugs may cause gingival hyperplasia?**
Common causative drugs include phenytoin, nifedipine, and cyclosporine A. These medications stimulate proliferation of gingival fibroblasts, causing an overgrowth of the gingiva. Other drugs that may cause gingival hyperplasia include calcium channel blockers (verapamil, felodipine, nisoldipine, diltiazem, amlodipine), antiepileptics (lamotrigine and mephenytoin), the immunosuppressive mycophenolate, the antidepressant sertraline, the antipsychotic pimozide, and interferon alpha 2-b (Figs. 6-41 and 6-42).

169. **In performing gingivectomy, how do you assess the level of initial incision?**
A gingival pocket marker will provide a bleeding point on the facial gingiva at the level of the initial incision.

170. **What instruments are commonly used to perform a gingivectomy?**
Interproximal knives (Orban 1/2) or gingivectomy knives (Kirkland 15/16).

171. **What is a Widman flap?**
A Widman flap is also known as open or flap curettage. Sulcular or submarginal incisions are made initially, and full-thickness flaps are elevated beyond the mucogingival junction for debridement, scaling, and root planing. Flaps are then apically positioned and closed with sutures.

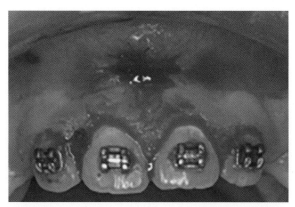

Fig. 6-40. Gingivectomy along with frenectomy was performed with a dental laser.

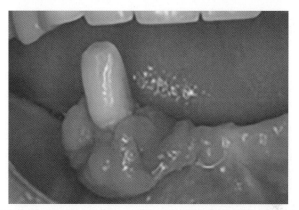

Fig. 6-41. Gingival overgrowth of the mandibular canine. The patient is taking antiepileptics.

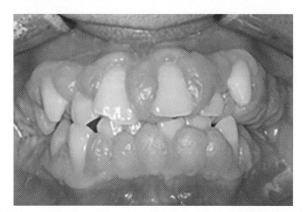

Fig. 6-42. Gingival overgrowth of the maxillary and mandibular incisors. The patient is taking phenytoin for epilepsy.

172. **What is a Modified Widman flap?**

It is similar to the original Widman flap, but the flap is not elevated beyond the mucogingival junction, the non-inflamed gingiva is not removed, and it does not apically displace gingival margin.

173. **What is a full-thickness periodontal flap?**

After the incision is made, a full-thickness flap involves elevation of the entire soft tissue including periosteum exposing the underlying alveolar bone.

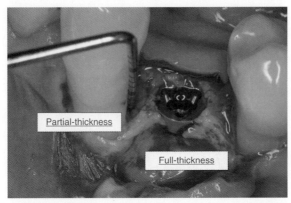

Fig. 6-43. Partial-thickness flap involves sharp dissection, leaving the periosteum attached to the bone.

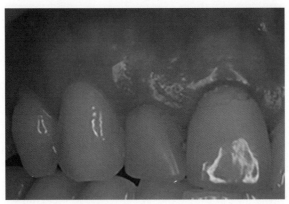

Fig. 6-44. Tooth #7 has a short clinical crown and thus will require a crown lengthening procedure.

174. **What is a partial-thickness periodontal flap?**
Partial-thickness flap involves the splitting (sharp dissection) of the gingival flap, leaving the periosteum adherent to the bone (Fig. 6-43).

175. **Why are inverse bevel incisions frequently used in flap surgery?**
Inverse bevel incisions facilitate degranulation by thinning the flap. Furthermore, the thinning of the flap may promote reattachment of the gingiva to the root by placing connective tissue elements against the root when the flap is closed.

176. **What is an apically positioned flap? When is it most frequently performed?**
After the flap has been elevated and the necessary treatment has been performed, the gingiva is positioned at the crest of bone, which is usually apical to its presurgical position. This procedure is most frequently performed after osseous surgery (e.g., pocket reduction and crown lengthening) and may require vertical releasing incision (Figs. 6-44 and 6-45).

177. **What is osteoplasty?**
Osteoplasty is the reshaping or recontouring of non-supportive bone. An example is the recontouring and eliminating thick bony ledges.

178. **What is ostectomy?**
Ostectomy is the removal of supporting bone. This procedure is usually performed to create positive or flat architecture, which is important for pocket reduction. It is often used to increase the clinical crown length for restorative purposes or for esthetic crown lengthening.

179. **What is odontoplasty? Where is it commonly applied?**
Odontoplasty is the reshaping and smoothing of the root morphology. Teeth with developmental grooves in the roots, such as the premolars and maxillary lateral incisors, may develop localized periodontal defects as bacterial

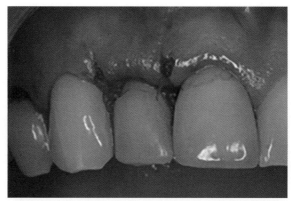

Fig. 6-45. Note the gingival margin of tooth #7 has been displaced and sutured apically to expose more tooth structure.

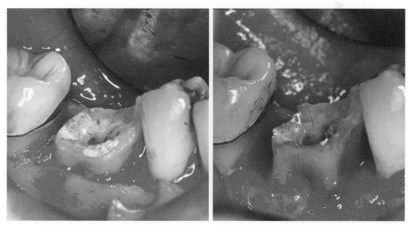

Fig. 6-46. Inadequate tooth structure (>2 mm) coronal to the alveolar crest can be observed on the mandibular first molar (*left*). To maintain a proper supracrestal tissue attachment and adequate tooth structure for proper restoration, a functional crown lengthening procedure was performed. Following the procedure, a 4 to 5 mm tooth structure between the apical extension of the preparation and the alveolar crest can be observed (*right*).

plaque and calculus are found in the defects. Additionally, where there are cementoenamel projections or enamel pearls in furcation areas, odontoplasty is done to remove them.

180. What is the supracrestal tissue attachment?
The supracrestal tissue attachment consists of junctional epithelium and connective tissue attachment. It used to be called the biologic width.

181. When is a functional crown-lengthening procedure indicated?
The procedure is indicated when the clinical crown length is inadequate for the placement of a dental restoration. Generally, there should be 4 to 5 mm between the apical extent of preparation and the crest of bone. This measurement maintains a proper supracrestal attachment width, which is on average 2 mm plus the sulcus depth (Fig. 6-46).

182. A patient presents with grade I furcation involvement on mesial of tooth #14 and no other areas of attachment loss. What is the contributing factor for this?
Violation of supracrestal tissue attachment by plaque retentive overhanging amalgam restoration (Fig. 6-47).

183. A dentist refers you a patient for #19 crown lengthening procedure. What factors need to be considered prior to performing the procedure?
There is a buccal furcation involvement ends at the buccal furcation. Odontoplasty needs to be done to remove the roof of the furcation and the crown needs to be adapted to the new tooth contour with a proper flat emergence profile (Fig. 6-48).

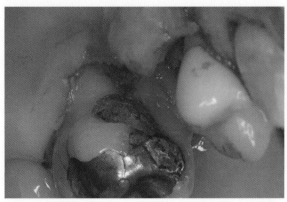

Fig. 6-47. The overhanging amalgam restoration extended to the mesial furcation has violated the supracrestal tissue attachment.

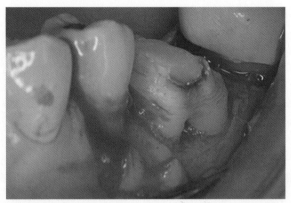

Fig. 6-48. The buccal margin ends almost at the buccal furcation and there is also a buccal furcation involvement.

184. **How are furcation involvements detected clinically?**
Periodontal probe and Nabers periodontal probe are used to detect furcation involvements.

185. **What is a Nabers probe?**
A Nabers probe is a curved probe, which is used to measure the horizontal attachment and bone loss in a furcation.

186. **How are furcations routinely treated?**
The treatment of furcations depends on the extent of bone loss. Therapy ranges from scaling and root planing, curettage, apically positioned flaps with or without osseous recontouring or odontoplasty, or guided tissue regeneration with or without grafting material.

187. **What is the relationship between root trunk lengths and the furcation invasion?**
The longer the root trunk length, the less likelihood of having a furcation invasion (Fig. 6-49).

188. **What is a distal wedge procedure? Where is it commonly found clinically?**
As the name implies, in the distal wedge procedure, a block of soft tissue is removed from the distal aspect of a tooth to reduce the pocket depth. Distal wedge procedures are frequent after the extraction of a third molar (Fig. 6-50).

189. **Why is a palatal flap pocket-reducing procedure done in the maxillary anterior without elevating a labial flap?**
The rationale behind this procedure is to maintain the buccal gingival architecture to minimize recession, which might cause unwanted esthetic changes.

190. **In what location should vertical releasing incision be made?**
It should be made at the line angle to include entire papilla (Fig. 6-51).

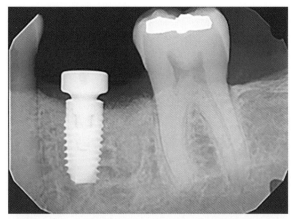

Fig. 6-49. There is a higher chance of furcation involvement in multi-root teeth with short root trunk.

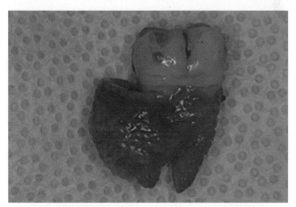

Fig. 6-50. The block of soft tissue resembling a wedge is often removed from the distal of the second molars to reduce pocket depth. The tooth is not extracted. The extracted tooth demonstrated here is only shown for the purpose of demonstrating the soft tissue block.

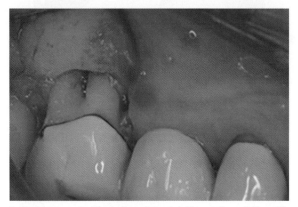

Fig. 6-51. Vertical releasing incisions are made at line angle, as demonstrated here on the mesial-buccal line angle of the first molar.

191. **What is crestal anticipation?**
This term is commonly used to describe the width of submarginal incision technique on palatal tissue in order that flap will be positioned at the crest of the alveolar bone.

192. **When is a root amputation indicated?**
     Stable teeth with a periodontal defect where there is a root proximity problem. The removal of the root will eliminate pocket and allow interradicular space. Additionally, in a stable maxillary molar, in the case of interproximal furcation bone loss, the removal of a root might provide the patient access for plaque removal (Fig. 6-52).

193. **Which teeth are most frequently involved in root amputation procedures?**
     They are generally the maxillary molars (Figs. 6-53 to 6-55).

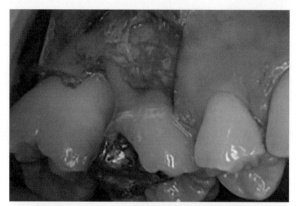

Fig. 6-52. The mesial buccal root of the maxillary molar was amputated, which provided the patient access for plaque removal.

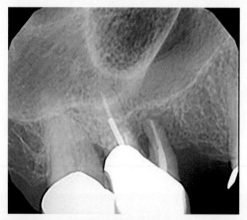

Fig. 6-53. J-shaped radiolucency observed around the mesial buccal root, indicative of a root fracture.

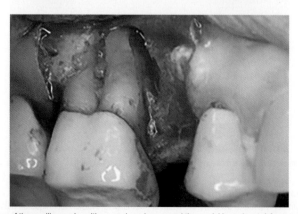

Fig. 6-54. Clinical view of the maxillary molar with severe bone loss around the mesial buccal root. A fracture line can be observed.

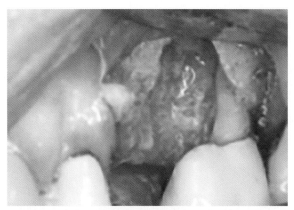

Fig. 6-55. The mesial-buccal root was amputated.

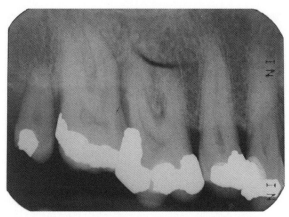

Fig. 6-56. The root proximity between teeth #2 and #3 as well as the overhanging amalgam restoration made it difficult to perform pocket reduction osseous procedure.

194. What is the potential obstacle for performing pocket-reducing osseous surgery for teeth #2-3?
It is root proximity and overhanging amalgam restoration (Fig. 6-56).

195. List common suturing techniques for apically positioned flap.
External vertical mattress suturing technique and simple interrupted technique.

196. A patient presents with a localized osseous defect on mesial of tooth #31. The patient expressed a strong desire to retain the tooth. What is the most ideal surgical periodontal treatment option for this patient?
It is open flap debridement with a possible osseous regeneration procedure (Fig. 6-57).

197. Ideally when and why should a silk suture be removed following periodontal surgery?
It should be removed in 7 to 10 days due to wicking effect of the silk.

198. What surgical periodontal procedure is performed as adjunctive therapy for orthodontic tooth rotation? How successful is it?
Routinely, a fiberotomy is performed to prevent relapse of the tooth rotation. In general, a fiberotomy is insufficient to prevent relapse. The rotated tooth still requires some type of stabilization.

199. What medications may affect salivary flow? How may they affect periodontal health?
Many medicines may influence salivary flow. Prime suspects are tricyclic antidepressants and antihypertensives. Decreased salivary flow diminishes the natural cleansing of the oral cavity, thus increasing the incidence of periodontal disease and caries. Watch for both supra- and subgingival root caries.

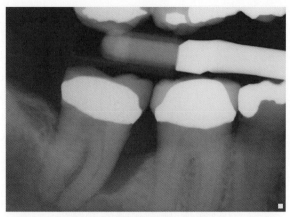

Fig. 6-57. Tooth #31 presented with a deep localized infrabony defect on the mesial.

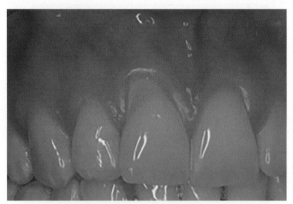

Fig. 6-58. Gingival recession observed on teeth #8 and #9.

MUCOGINGIVAL SURGERY

200. **When should a gingival augmentation be considered as a treatment for a gingival recession?**
Wherever there is an inadequate zone of attached gingiva, there is a progressive recession, and when a patient is concerned about esthetics and root coverage is possible.

201. **What are the most common autogenous soft tissue graft procedures used to treat mucogingival defects?**
The most common grafting procedures are connective tissue and epithelized (free) gingival grafts. Other grafting procedures include the pedicle or lateral sliding flap with or without connective tissue grafting (Figs. 6-58 and 6-59).

202. **How is bleeding controlled after the palate has been used as the donor site for a free gingival graft?**
There are a number of ways to control bleeding at the donor site, including (1) pressure with a moistened gauze, (2) pressure with a tea bag, (3) vasoconstriction (epinephrine in the local anesthetic), (4) suturing (tie off the bleeders), (5) collagen with or without stent, (6) topical thrombin, and (7) chemical/electrical cautery. If bleeding continues, it may be prudent to assess prothrombin time (PT), partial thromboplastin time (PTT), and platelet count.

203. **What is the primary reason for failure of an epithelized gingival graft?**
Inadequate blood supply.

204. **What is the ideal treatment for lack of attached gingiva on tooth #27?**
Epithelized gingival graft (Fig. 6-60).

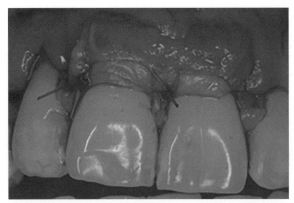

Fig. 6-59. A subepithelial connective tissue grafting procedure was performed to cover the exposed root surfaces.

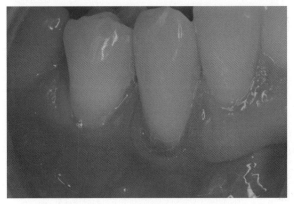

Fig. 6-60. Tooth #27 has a lack of attached gingiva and gingival recession.

205. **What is meant by sloughing of an epithelized gingival graft?**
After an epithelized gingival graft has been placed, the healing involves revascularization of the graft. The superficial layers of the graft are the last to be revascularized; therefore, the layer dies, and the epithelium sloughs.

206. **What type of flap is used at the recipient site of connective tissue or free gingival graft?**
Partial-thickness flaps are used so that the periosteum remains attached to the bone. The reason is that the periosteum is a good blood supply for the graft.

207. **Why does caution need to be taken when placing a free gingival graft in the buccal area of the mandibular premolars?**
Being aware of the location of mental foramen in relation to the apical aspect of the bed preparation in order to avoid injuring the mental nerve.

208. **When does the greatest amount of shrinkage occur with free gingival graft procedure?**
It occurs within the first 6 weeks.

209. **In relationship to gingival recession, when is a frenectomy indicated?**
As the frenum is a mucosal tissue when the attachment of the frenum provides an insufficient zone of attached gingiva, the recession could ensue, and therefore removal of the frenum is indicated (Figs. 6-61 and 6-62).

210. **What procedure may be performed in conjunction with a frenectomy to prevent recurrence?**
An epithelized gingival graft may be performed in conjunction with the frenectomy to prevent the recurrence of fiber attachment to the papilla. Particularly for the maxillary anterior frenum, suturing the labial mucosal tissue and using a periodontal dressing will also prevent a recurrence.

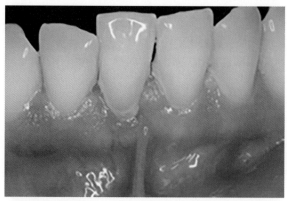

Fig. 6-61. The high frenal attachment on tooth #25 contributed to the recession.

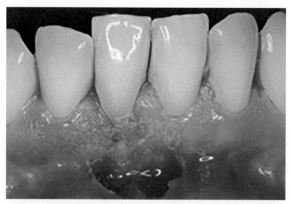

Fig. 6-62. Frenectomy is performed with a dental laser.

211. **What classification systems are used to characterize mucogingival defects?**
Miller's classifications from class I to IV, depend on the width, depth, and location relative to the mucogingival junction.

Cairo's classification: RT 1-3: RT 1 is a facial recession with no interproximal attachment loss; RT 2 is where the facial or lingual recession is greater than the interproximal attachment loss; RT 3 is where the interproximal recession exceeds the facial or lingual attachment loss. There is less likelihood of root coverage with RT 2 than RT 1 and likely no possible root coverage with RT 3.

212. **Which of the Miller's classifications best to root coverage procedure?**
Miller class I and II defects can have excellent results when treated with a connective tissue graft.

213. **Why do certain Miller's classifications have better root coverage predictability?**
The presence of interdental bone provides a better blood supply.

214. **What are the factors that could have contributed to this gingival recession on palatal side of maxillary right posterior teeth?**
Toothbrush abrasion, prominent root, and thin bone (Fig. 6-63).

215. **What is the ideal treatment for facial gingival recession for mandibular right posterior teeth?**
Root coverage procedure using autogenous or allogenic tissue (Fig. 6-64).

216. **What are some of the common reasons for the gingival recession?**
The patient contributed trauma, iatrogenic reasons such as improper (scrubbing) toothbrushing techniques and deep cervical restorative margins, prominent roots, thin phenotype, and orthodontic treatment.

217. **The current evidence suggests that Asian subjects have a thin gingival phenotype compared with white subjects.**
True.

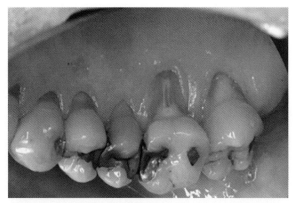

Fig. 6-63. Severe gingival recession on the palatal side of maxillary right posterior teeth.

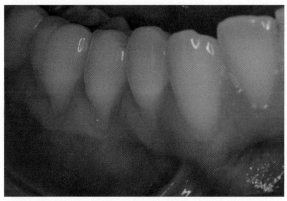

Fig. 6-64. Gingival recessions with a lack of attached gingiva can be observed around the premolars and molars. The condition can be treated with a root coverage procedure with the use of autogenous or allogenic tissue.

218. Which area of the mouth has the greatest gingival thickness?
Maxillary central incisors.

219. Which area has the greatest keratinized tissue gingival width?
Maxillary lateral incisors.

220. Patients with thin tissue and narrow gingival width tend to have more gingival recession.
True.

221. What is the minimal amount of gingiva needed to maintain periodontal health?
Two mm of total gingival width and 1 mm of attached gingiva.

222. What are the clinical indications of gingival augmentation procedures?
Placement of restoration with an intracrevicular margin, impingement of major or minor connectors of removable partial dentures, and overdenture when there is an absence of gingiva associated with retained teeth.

223. What is the optimal graft thickness of an epithelialized gingival graft?
1.5 to 2.0 mm.

REGENERATIVE PROCEDURES

224. What type of bony defect is found on distal of #6?
Infrabony defect (Fig. 6-65).

225. What are the basic types of bone-grafting materials used in the treatment of periodontal defects?
Grafts include autografts (intraoral and extraoral), allografts, alloplasts, and xenografts. The autografts may be harvested from the patient's hip and rib (extraoral) or from a healing extraction socket, the chin, maxillary tuberosity,

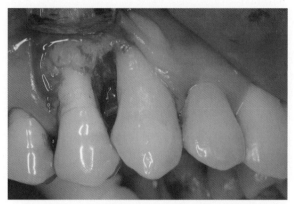

Fig. 6-65. A vertical infrabony defect can be observed on the distal of #6.

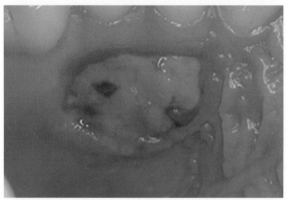

Fig. 6-66. The palatal harvesting site shows areas of bone exposure and necrosis due to secondary wound healing accompanied by pain.

or retromolar areas (intraoral). Allografts consist of freeze-dried bone and freeze-dried decalcified bone from another source (usually cadaver bone). Alloplasts are synthetic materials; the most commonly used are tricalcium phosphate, calcium carbonate, and hydroxyapatite. Xenografts are typically bovine-based and particulate.

226. What is osseous coagulum? Where is it used?
The osseous coagulum is another type of grafting material, normally obtained during osseous surgery. The bone/blood shavings are collected and then packed into the defect in an attempt to promote new bone formation. Because the bone is predominantly cortical, the results are not predictable.

227. What is bone swaging?
Swagging is the bending and breaking of the bony walls into the periodontal defect. It, too, has poor predictability and is not used with great frequency.

228. When should an intraoral autograft from an extraction site be harvested?
As a general guideline, the intraoral autograft should be harvested 6 to 8 weeks after extraction. This gives the extraction site enough time to become organized with osteogenic components.

229. What negative sequelae may occur with autogenous bone grafts when used in periodontal regeneration procedures?
Possible sequelae include ankylosis and root resorption.

230. Why are connective tissue grafts used for soft tissue ridge augmentation?
They are used for esthetic and phonetic reasons to augment an edentulous site that is concave.

231. What sites are commonly used to harvest connective tissue for grafting?
Common sites include the hard palate and maxillary tuberosity.

232. What is a common complication that is seen from the connective tissue graft donor site?
Pain due to secondary wound healing (Fig. 6-66).

233. **What commercially available growth factors may potentially be used to stimulate osseous regeneration?**
Platelet-derived growth factor (PDGF) and bone morphogenetic protein (BMP) have been used in human clinical trials.

234. **What is guided tissue regeneration (GTR)? How is it done? Where is it most successful?**
GTR is a surgical procedure to promote the regeneration of cementum, PDL, and bone around natural teeth. A barrier membrane with and without underlying graft material and/or growth factor is used for this procedure. This procedure is most successful for narrow, three-wall defects.

235. **What is the purpose of a barrier membrane?**
The membrane prevents apical migration of the epithelium and growth of connective tissue into the defect and allows for the proliferation of periodontal ligament along the root surface. It also serves as a space maintainer and stabilizes the graft.

236. **What surgical techniques may be used for hard tissue ridge augmentation?**
Bone graft materials with a barrier membrane are commonly used.

237. **What are the indications for ridge augmentation?**
Basically, it is used whenever more bony mass is indicated. Examples include the future placement of a dental implant and filling a concavity after tooth extraction for esthetic reasons.

238. **When is ridge preservation indicated following tooth extraction?**
When the facial/lingual walls are thin or missing, in the esthetic zone, and when bone remodeling following healing would preclude an adequate volume of bone for the placement of dental implants.

239. **Following the extraction, which bony surface resorbs the most?**
Facial.

240. **What are the Seibert classifications for edentulous ridge defects?**
Class I: Buccolingual loss of ridge contour
Class II: Apicocoronal loss of ridge contour
Class III: A combined loss of both apicocoronal and buccolingual dimensions

241. **What is the Seibert classification for the mandibular anterior edentulous ridge?**
Seibert Class III (Fig. 6-67).

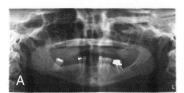

Fig. 6-67. (A) Panoramic view of a Seibert class III ridge defect in the mandibular anterior ridge.

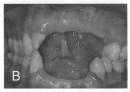

Fig. 6-67. (B) Buccal clinical view of a Seibert class III ridge defect in the mandibular anterior ridge. Note the vertical ridge deficiency.

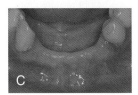

Fig. 6-67. (C) Occlusal clinical view of a Seibert class III ridge defect in the mandibular anterior ridge. Note the horizontal ridge deficiency.

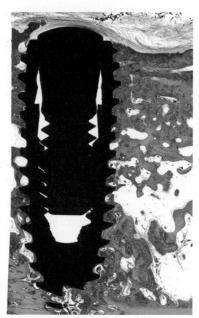

Fig. 6-68. Histological view showing direct bone (pink)-to-implant contact at the light microscopic level.

DENTAL IMPLANTS

242. **Define osseointegration.**
    Osseointegration is defined as direct bone-to-implant contact at the light microscopic level. At the clinical level, bone appears to be fused to the implant (Fig. 6-68).

243. **What is the difference between one-stage and two-stage implant placement?**
    For one-stage implant, a healing abutment is attached at the time of the implant placement. For a two-stage implant, a covers screw is attached to the implant, and soft tissue is placed over the two-stage implant. The second stage is done several months later when the cover screw is exposed surgically, and a healing abutment is then placed.
    A second surgical procedure is required to remove the cover screw and place the healing abutment. This is generally done several months after the implant placement.

244. **Clinically, what determines a successful implant?**
    Clinically a successful implant is one where the peri-implant soft tissue is healthy with no bleeding on probing, and there is a stable bone level surrounding the implant. From a patient's perspective, a successful implant is one that provides comfort, function, and pleasing esthetics.

245. **In which region of the jaws are dental implants the most successful?**
    Dental implants in the anterior mandible have the highest success rate. The highest rate of failure is in the posterior maxilla.

246. **When is a sinus elevation indicated?**
    It is indicated when there is an insufficient volume of bone to place an implant without invading the sinus.

247. **What is the minimum crestal bone height required for osteotome sinus elevation procedure?**
    A minimum of 4 to 5 mm of crestal bone height is necessary to stabilize the implant (Fig. 6-69).

248. **When do you consider doing bone augmentation around a dental implant when it is being placed?**
    Bone augmentation should be considered when implant threads are exposed or the facial or lingual bone is less than 1 mm thick.

249. **What parameter usually indicates a failing implant?**
    It is indicated by radiographic bone loss in combination with soft tissue inflammation (BOP and purulence).

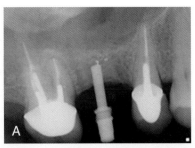

Fig. 6-69. (A) The residual bone height is about 4 to 5 mm. After the first pilot drill, a guide pin is inserted to verify the depth and distance to the sinus floor.

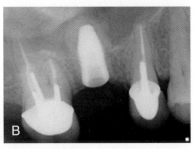

Fig. 6-69. (B) A dental implant was placed following osteotome sinus elevation. Note the dome shape radiopacity around the apex of the implant, which indicated the use of a bone replacement graft.

250. **What parameter indicates a failed implant?**
Mobile implant.

251. **What considerations are important during the surgical placement of implants?**
During the osteotomy, the implant site should be cooled during drilling. In addition, the implant should have primary stability (no movement).

252. **What bacteria are associated with peri-implantitis?**
Many of the same species associated with periimplantitis are also associated with periodontitis, including *A. actinomycetemcomitans, P. gingivalis*, and *P. intermedia*. Other species frequently detected by cultural methods are *Capnocytophaga* species, *C. recta*, and *E. corrodens*.

253. **What can cause a dental implant to fail?**
Dental implant failure can result from occlusal overload, peri-implantitis, or overheating the bone during the osteotomy.

254. **How are implants maintained?**
Implants require maintenance, much like crowns and bridges and natural teeth. The maintenance instruments on the implant or abutment are usually plastic-tipped or titanium so that the surface of the implant and abutment is not scratched. Floss, Superfloss®, braided floss, and appropriately sized interproximal brushes are also handy.

255. **Is keratinized mucosa needed around the implant?**
Yes, studies support the notion that keratinized mucosa will prevent future bone loss around the implant (Fig. 6-70).

256. **What is the most common problem with cemented implant restorations?**
Residual cement.

257. **What is the average amount of vertical ridge augmentation that can be achieved?**
Four to 5 mm.

258. **Which procedure is more predictable? Horizontal ridge augmentation or vertical ridge augmentation?**
Horizontal ridge augmentation.

259. **What is peri-implantitis?**
Characterized by inflammation in the peri-implant mucosa and loss of supporting bone.

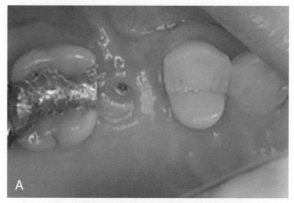

Fig. 6-70. (a) A lack of keratinized mucosa can be observed around the first molar implant.

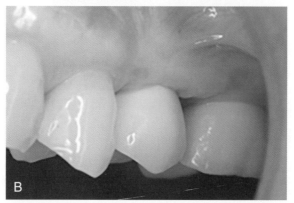

Fig. 6-70. (b) A gingival augmentation procedure has been performed to increase the zone of keratinized mucosa.

260. **What is peri-implant mucositis?**
Characterized by an inflammatory lesion in the soft tissues surrounding an implant in the absence of loss of supporting bone.

261. **Is peri-implantitis reversible?**
No.

262. **Is peri-implant mucositis reversible?**
Yes.

263. **What is the most common dental implant surface?**
Sandblasted, large grit, acid-etched (SLA).

264. **Is it better to have mesial cantilever or distal cantilever?**
Mesial cantilever (Fig. 6-71).

265. **Can dental implants last forever?**
No.

266. **How often do implant patients need to come in for check-up?**
Every 3 to 6 months.

PERIODONTAL MAINTENANCE (PDHT)

267. **What is PDHT?**
PDHT stands for Professional Dental Hygiene Therapy. Often it is called a "cleaning, prophylaxis, or maintenance"; however, it is important to emphasize to the patients that the stain and calculus that clinicians

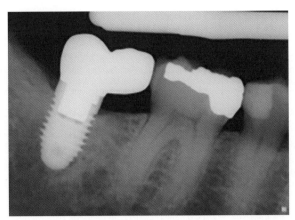

Fig. 6-71. A mesial cantilever was fabricated for the second molar implant crown due to the distal implant placement.

remove are transient, and the value of the visit is the coaching of plaque removal techniques (PRT) that the patients perform daily. It is the patient who prevents caries and periodontal diseases with their PRTs. However, since the patient is unable to see plaque, it is the dental clinician's responsibility to correct the PRTs as needed.

268. **What does the typical periodontal maintenance procedure involve?**
Generally, the appointment involves reviewing medical and dental histories, observing the patient doing their brushing, flossing, and any other plaque removal techniques at the outset of the appointment, evaluation of the periodontal status by comparing probing depths with ones previously done, oral hygiene technique review as and instruction as needed, remove all plaque and stain with air polishing or a rubber cup, scaling, root planing as needed, determining the appropriate interval for the next visit. Radiographs also may be indicated. Many clinicians remove all the stain and plaque prior to calculus removal with air polishing supra-and subgingivally. This allows the clinician to better concentrate on calculus removal and smoothing the root surfaces.

269. **Why is it preferable to review oral hygiene technique prior to doing scaling and root planing during the maintenance visit?**
It is important to reinforce plaque control techniques as plaque removal lasts only a few days, and patients have to maintain themselves following the appointment. Doing the plaque removal techniques at the outset of the appointment underscores its importance, and if the patient has difficulty performing the techniques, it can be reviewed at the end of the appointment.

270. **After periodontal therapy is completed, what should be the recall interval?**
The recall interval should be individualized. Usually, a 3- to 4-month interval is recommended for periodontally compromised patients. A patient with a history of periodontitis, a patient with implants, and a patient with a history of smooth surface caries should never be maintained on an interval longer than 4 months.

271. **How important is periodontal maintenance?**
Regular periodontal maintenance is extremely important to the long-term prognosis of the dentition. If patients fail to adhere to routine maintenance, their periodontal status is likely to deteriorate.

272. **What clinical parameters are generally used to indicate periodontal breakdown?**
Bleeding on probing, increased probing depths, and loss of interproximal density radiographically typically indicate periodontal breakdown.

BIBLIOGRAPHY

Fundamentals of the Periodontium

Kim DM, Bassir SH, Nguyen TT. Effect of gingival phenotype on the maintenance of periodontal health: An American Academy of Periodontology best evidence review. *J Periodontol.* 2020;91:311–338.
Lang NP, Lindhe J. *Clinical Periodontology and Implant Dentistry.* 5th ed. Oxford: Blackwell Munksgaard; 2008.
Newman MG, Takei HH, Klokkevold PR, Carranza FA. *Carranza's Clinical Periodontology.* 10th ed. St. Louis: Saunders Elsevier; 2006.
Rose LF, Mealey BL. *Periodontics: Medicine, Surgery and Implants.* St. Louis: Elsevier Mosby; 2004.

Classification of Periodontal Diseases and Etiologies

Haffajee AD, Socransky SS, Dzink JL, et al. Clinical, microbiological and immunological features of subjects with refractory periodontal diseases. *J Clin Periodontol.* 1988;15:390.
Lang NP, Lindhe J. *Clinical Periodontology and Implant Dentistry.* 5th ed. Oxford: Blackwell Munksgaard; 2008.

Listgarten MA. The role of dental plaque in gingivitis and periodontitis. *J Clin Periodontol.* 1988;15:485–487.

Mandell ID, Gaffar A. Calculus revisited. *J Clin Periodontol.* 1986;13:249–257.

Moore WEC, Moore LH, Ranney RR, et al. The microflora of periodontal sites showing active progression. *J Clin Periodontol.* 1991;18:729–739.

Newman MN, Socransky SS. Predominant microbiota of periodontosis. *J Periodontol Res.* 1977;12:120–128.

Newman MG, Takei HH, Klokkevold PR, Carranza FA. *Carranza's Clinical Periodontology.* 10th ed. St. Louis: Saunders Elsevier; 2006.

Rose LF, Mealey BL. *Periodontics: Medicine, Surgery and Implants.* St. Louis: Elsevier Mosby; 2004.

Sooriyamoorthy M, Gower DB. Hormonal influences on gingival tissue: Relationship to periodontal disease. *J Clin Periodontol.* 1989;16:201–208.

Tanner ACR, Haffer C, Brathall GT, et al. A study of the bacteria associated with advancing periodontitis in man. *J Clin Periodontol.* 1979;6:278.

Zambon JJ, Reynolds HS, Genco RJ. Studies of the subgingival microflora in patients with acquired immunodeficiency syndrome. *J Clin Periodontol.* 1990;61:699–704.

Concepts of Disease Activity

Lang NP, Lindhe J. *Clinical Periodontology and Implant Dentistry.* 5th ed. Oxford: Blackwell Munksgaard; 2008.

Lindhe J, Haffajee AD, Socransky SS. The progression of periodontal disease in the absence of periodontal therapy. *J Clin Periodontol.* 1983;10:433–442.

Newman MG, Takei HH, Klokkevold PR, Carranza FA. *Carranza's Clinical Periodontology.* 10th ed. St. Louis: Saunders Elsevier; 2006.

Rose LF, Mealey BL. *Periodontics: Medicine, Surgery and Implants.* St. Louis: Elsevier Mosby; 2004.

Socransky SS, Haffajee AD, Goodson JM, Lindhe J. New concepts of destructive periodontal disease. *J Clin Periodontol.* 1984;11:21–32.

Periodontal Diagnosis

Cochran DL. Bacteriological monitoring of periodontal disease: cultural, enzymatic, immunological, and nucleic acid studies. *Curr Opin Dent.* 1991;1:37–44.

Goultschin J, Cohen HDS, Donchin M, et al. Association of smoking with periodontal treatment needs. *J Periodontol.* 1990;61:364–367.

Grbic JT, Lamster IB, Celenti RS, Fine JB. Risk indicators for future clinical attachment loss in adult periodontitis: Patient variables. *J Periodontol.* 1991;62:322–329.

Lang NP, Lindhe J. *Clinical Periodontology and Implant Dentistry.* 5th ed. Oxford: Blackwell Munksgaard; 2008.

Newman MG, Takei HH, Klokkevold PR, Carranza FA. *Carranza's Clinical Periodontology.* 10th ed. St. Louis: Saunders Elsevier; 2006.

Rose LF, Mealey BL. *Periodontics: Medicine, Surgery and Implants.* St. Louis: Elsevier Mosby; 2004.

Savitt ED, Keville MW, Peros WJ. DNA probes in the diagnosis of periodontal microorganisms. *Arch Oral Biol.* 1990;35(Suppl):153S–159S.

Schlossman M, Knowler WC, Pettitt DT, Genco RJ. Type 2 diabetes mellitus and periodontal disease. *J Am Dent Assoc.* 1990;121:532–536.

Adjunctive Periodontal Therapy

Bonesville P. Oral pharmacology of chlorhexidine. *J Clin Periodontol.* 1977;4:49–65.

Ciancio SA. Antibiotics in periodontal care. In: Newman MG, Kornman KS, eds. *Antibiotic/Antimicrobial Use in Dental Practice.* Carol Stream, IL: Quintessence; 1990:136–147.

Goodson JM. Drug delivery. In: *Perspectives on Oral Antimicrobial Therapeutics.* Chicago: American Academy of Periodontology; 1987:61–78.

Lang NP, Lindhe J. *Clinical Periodontology and Implant Dentistry.* 5th ed. Oxford: Blackwell Munksgaard; 2008.

Newman MG, Takei HH, Klokkevold PR, Carranza FA. *Carranza's Clinical Periodontology.* 10th ed. St. Louis: Saunders Elsevier; 2006.

Rose LF, Mealey BL. *Periodontics: Medicine, Surgery and Implants.* St. Louis: Elsevier Mosby; 2004.

Southard GL, Boulware RT, Walborn DR, et al. Sanguinarine: a new antiplaque agent. *Compend Cont Educ Dent.* 1984;5(Suppl):72–75.

Williams RC. Non-steroidal anti-inflammatory drugs in periodontal disease. In: Lewis AJ, Furst DE, eds. *Non-steroidal Anti-inflammatory Drugs.* New York: Marcel Dekker; 1987.

Occlusal Treatment

Newman MG, Takei HH, Klokkevold PR, Carranza FA. *Carranza's Clinical Periodontology.* 10th ed. St. Louis: Saunders Elsevier; 2006.

Rose LF, Mealey BL. *Periodontics: Medicine, Surgery and Implants.* St. Louis: Elsevier Mosby; 2004.

Lang NP, Lindhe J. *Clinical Periodontology and Implant Dentistry.* 5th ed. Oxford: Blackwell Munksgaard; 2008.

Initial Treatment of Periodontal Disease

Drisko CL, Killoy WJ. Scaling and root planing: removal of calculus and subgingival organisms. *Curr Opin Dent.* 1991;1:74–80.

Hirshfeld L, Wasserman B. A long term survey of tooth loss in 600 treated periodontal patients. *J Periodontol.* 1978;49:225–237.

Lang NP, Lindhe J. *Clinical Periodontology and Implant Dentistry.* 5th ed. Oxford: Blackwell Munksgaard; 2008.

Pihlstrom B, McHugh RB, Oliphant TH, Ortiz-Campos C. Comparison of surgical and non-surgical treatment of periodontal disease. *J Clin Periodontol.* 1983;10:524–541.

Rose LF, Mealey BL. *Periodontics: Medicine, Surgery and Implants.* St. Louis: Elsevier Mosby; 2004.

Newman MG, Takei HH, Klokkevold PR, Carranza FA. *Carranza's Clinical Periodontology.* 10th ed. St. Louis: Saunders Elsevier; 2006.

Surgical Treatment of Periodontal Disease

Becker BE, Becker W, Caffesse R, et al. Three modalities of periodontal therapy: 5-year final results. *J Dent Res.* 1990;69:219.

Kalkwarf KL. Surgical treatment of periodontal diseases: access flaps, bone resection techniques, root preparation, and flap closure. *Curr Opin Dent.* 1991;1:87–92.

Lang NP, Lindhe J. *Clinical Periodontology and Implant Dentistry.* 5th ed. Oxford: Blackwell Munksgaard; 2008.

Newman MG, Takei HH, Klokkevold PR, Carranza FA. *Carranza's Clinical Periodontology.* 10th ed. St. Louis: Saunders Elsevier; 2006.

Ramfjord SP, Morrison EC, Kerry GJ, et al. Four modalities of periodontal treatment compared over five years. *J Clin Periodontol.* 1987;14:445–452.

Ramfjord SP, Nissle RR, Shick RR, Cooper H. Subgingival curettage versus surgical elimination of periodontal pockets. *J Periodontol.* 1968;39:167–175.

Robertson PB. The residual calculus paradox. *J Periodontol.* 1990;61:65–66.

Rose LF, Mealey BL. *Periodontics: Medicine, Surgery and Implants.* St. Louis: Elsevier Mosby; 2004.

Tarnow DP, Fletcher P. Root resection vs. maintenance of furcated molars. *NY State Dent J 55.* 1989;34(36):39.

Mucogingival Surgery

Allen EP. Use of mucogingival surgery to enhance esthetics. *Dent Clin North Am.* 1988;32:307–330.

Kim DM, Bassir SH, Nguyen TT. Effect of gingival phenotype on the maintenance of periodontal health: An American Academy of Periodontology best evidence review. *J Periodontol.* 2020;91:311–338.

Kim DM, Neiva R. Periodontal soft tissue non-root coverage procedures: a systematic review from the AAP regeneration workshop. *J Periodontol.* 2015;86:S56–S72.

Lang NP, Lindhe J. *Clinical Periodontology and Implant Dentistry.* 5th ed. Oxford: Blackwell Munksgaard; 2008.

Lang NP, Loe H. The relationship between the width of keratinized gingiva and gingival health. *J Periodontol.* 1972;43:623–627.

Miller PD. Regenerative and reconstructive periodontal plastic surgery: Mucogingival surgery. *Dent Clin North Am.* 1988;32:287–306.

Newman MG, Takei HH, Klokkevold PR, Carranza FA. *Carranza's Clinical Periodontology.* 10th ed. St. Louis: Saunders Elsevier; 2006.

Prato GPP, De Sanctis M. Soft tissue plastic surgery. *Curr Opin Dent.* 1991;1:98–103.

Rose LF, Mealey BL. *Periodontics: Medicine, Surgery and Implants.* St. Louis: Elsevier Mosby; 2004.

Gingival augmentation/mucogingival surgery. In: *Proceedings of the World Workshop in Clinical Periodontics.* Chicago: American Academy of Periodontology; 1989. 1989:VII-1–VII-21.

Regenerative Procedures

Becker BE, Becker W. Regenerative procedures: Grafting materials, guided tissue regeneration, and growth factors. *Curr Opin Dent.* 1991;1:93–97.

Branemark PI, Zarb GA, Albrektsson T. Tissue-integrated prostheses. In: *Osseointegration in Clinical Dentistry.* Carol Stream, IL: Quintessence; 1985.

Lang NP, Lindhe J. *Clinical Periodontology and Implant Dentistry.* 5th ed. Oxford: Blackwell Munksgaard; 2008.

Lynch SE, Williams RC, Polson AM, et al. A combination of platelet-derived growth factors enhances periodontal regeneration. *J Clin Periodontol.* 1989;16:545–548.

Magnusson I, Batch C, Collins BR. New attachment formation following controlled tissue regeneration using biodegradable membranes. *J Periodontol.* 1988;59:1–6.

Newman MG, Takei HH, Klokkevold PR, Carranza FA. *Carranza's Clinical Periodontology.* 10th ed. St. Louis: Saunders Elsevier; 2006.

Rose LF, Mealey BL. *Periodontics: Medicine, Surgery and Implants.* St. Louis: Elsevier Mosby; 2004.

Dental Implants

Lang NP, Lindhe J. *Clinical Periodontology and Implant Dentistry.* 5th ed. Oxford: Blackwell Munksgaard; 2008.

Newman MG, Takei HH, Klokkevold PR, Carranza FA. *Carranza's Clinical Periodontology.* 10th ed. St. Louis: Saunders; 2006.

Rose LF, Mealey BL. *Periodontics: Medicine, Surgery and Implants.* St. Louis: Elsevier Mosby; 2004.

Periodontal Maintenance

Lang NP, Lindhe J. *Clinical Periodontology and Implant Dentistry.* 5th ed. Oxford: Blackwell Munksgaard; 2008.

Newman MG, Takei HH, Klokkevold PR, Carranza FA. *Carranza's Clinical Periodontology.* 10th ed. St. Louis: Saunders; 2006.

Rose LF, Mealey BL. *Periodontics: Medicine, Surgery and Implants.* St. Louis: Elsevier Mosby; 2004.

CHAPTER 7

ENDODONTICS

Winna G. Gorham

DIAGNOSIS

1. **What are pulp sensitivity tests and why are they useful in pulpal diagnosis?**
   Cold, heat, and electrical stimulation are used to elicit a response from the pulp tissue to aid in pulpal diagnosis. Cold tests utilize an outward hydrodynamic fluid to stimulate A-delta fibers and Endo-Ice (tetrafluoroethane) and carbon dioxide snow can be used to determine the level of inflammation in the pulp tissue. Heat testing can be done safely and effectively by heating a small piece of gutta-percha with a warming device. Electrical pulp testing causes changes in dentinal fluid, stimulates the A-delta nerve fibers, and tests for pulp vitality. However, it does not test the level of inflammation of the pulp tissue. The information acquired from thermal and electrical testing alone is not enough to make a diagnosis of the true histologic state of the pulp tissue.

2. **What is the importance of percussion sensitivity in endodontic diagnosis?**
   When infection or inflammation extends through the periodontal ligament to the apical tissues, percussion tenderness occurs. While there are conflicting opinions in the literature, research shows that percussion sensitivity may be associated with a diagnosis of symptomatic apical periodontitis. Percussion tests are comparable to mechanical allodynia in that a typically non-noxious stimulus causes pain.

3. **What is the difference between irreversible and reversible pulpitis?**
   Spontaneous pain and lingering cold sensitivity are consistent with irreversible pulpitis. In this diagnosis, the inflamed pulp tissue is incapable of healing and endodontic therapy is indicated. Reversible pulpitis can be characterized by sharp pain to a stimulus such as cold, that is quick and nonlingering. A reversible pulpitis diagnosis indicates that the pulp inflammation will resolve and return to normal. Studies have shown that it is typical to experience postoperative pain after a deep restorative procedure for 1 to 7 days, which may present as transient, nonlingering cold sensitivity.

4. **What are the typical findings associated with a vertical root fracture?**
   Radiographic findings of a vertical root fracture may include a J-shaped or halo radiolucency extending apically from the marginal periodontium and/or a loss of bone mid-root with intact bone coronal and apical to the defect. In addition, cone beam computed tomography (CBCT) imaging may show the absence of buccal plate, or a mid-root radiolucency associated with the location of the inferior border of a post. Finally, a space may be discernable between the buccal or lingual plate and the root surface. Clinical findings may include deep and narrow periodontal pocketing and draining sinus tracts located close to the gingival margin.

5. **Describe the different types of periodontal-endodontic (perio-endo) lesions.**
   True perio-endo lesions occur when an independent periodontal infection extends and joins an independent endodontic lesion. Perio-endo lesions that are primary endodontic infections can present with draining sinus tracts through the periodontium along with deep, narrow probing depths. These can be treated effectively with endodontic therapy. Perio-endo lesions that are primary periodontal lesions occur as result of advance periodontal pathology. They occur if the advancement of periodontal disease exposes lateral/accessory canals to the bacteria of the oral environment. Thus, periodontal disease causes pulp necrosis.

6. **Describe the various radiographic tools that can be useful in endodontic diagnosis.**
   Periapical radiographs examine both the entire tooth and apical tissues and can be used to evaluate for periapical bone loss and periodontal pathology. Bitewing radiographs examine existing restorations, caries, and coronal pulp anatomy. Panoramic radiographs are useful in trauma cases and can rule out alveolar fracture. Cone beam computed tomography (CBCT) can provide a dimensionally accurate evaluation of apical pathology and surrounding structures.

7. **A patient presents with severe pain that began 24 hours ago, followed by rapid swelling in the buccal vestibule of the mandibular posterior right side of his mouth. Tooth #30 was found to have radiographic findings of both a widened apical periodontal ligament (PDL) on both roots and a PFM crown. Cold testing was negative, with significant pain to percussion, palpation, and biting tests. What is your pulpal and periapical diagnosis?**
   Pulp necrosis with acute apical abscess.

8. **What are the indications for cone beam computed tomography (CBCT) in endodontics?**
CBCT provides highly detailed imaging by using a small, focused field. It is invaluable in aiding diagnosis and treatment planning and is beneficial when traditional periapical radiographs cannot be taken. Supported reasons for CBCT imaging include diagnosis, complex anatomy, previous root canal treatment, trauma, resorption, implants, and preoperative planning for endodontic surgery. CBCT has the advantage of providing limited geometric distortion and higher sensitivity useful in determining apical pathology.

9. **What is internal resorption and what are the clinical and radiographic findings?**
Internal resorption can occur following pulpal injury, causing pulpal hemorrhage and inflammation. The exposed dentin tubules from the loss of predentin are thus adjacent to the inflamed tissue. Macrophages then become dentino-clast cells, causing resorption. Internal resorption may present clinically as a coronal pink hue. Radiographic appearance may show an oval uniform lesion within the pulp space. Non-surgical root canal therapy is indicated to halt the resorptive process leading to a high probability for success in the case outcome.

10. **A patient presents with pain in the maxillary left posterior quadrant. She states that "all the teeth hurt," and she cannot pinpoint the source. What could account for this presentation?**
Referred pain. A patient may perceive that pain is coming from a different tooth besides the culprit causing the pain. Pain can also arise from another nondental source due to afferent neurons arising from the trigeminal nerve converging to the same projection neuron. Further, if the inflammatory process has not reached the proprioceptive fibers of the periodontal ligament, pain may not result from percussion or palpation tests.

11. **What are the possible etiological causes of cervical resorption?**
Cervical resorption can mimic class V caries radiographically and can be the result of a developmental or iatrogenic defect in the cementum. This causes the periodontal ligament to come in direct contact with the dentin. Possible etiologies include previous orthodontia or trauma, intracoronal restorations, periodontal therapy, viral causes (feline herpes virus), idiopathic causes, and nonvital bleaching.

12. **A female patient presents to your office with pain to percussion on tooth #30 that was previously treated endodontically 5 years ago. She has been taking ibuprofen, 600 mg every 8 hours for the pain for 2 days. You diagnose tooth #30 with symptomatic apical periodontitis and recommend and complete retreatment endodontic therapy. Twenty-four hours later, the patient contacts your office with severe pain in the mandibular right posterior area of her mouth and localized swelling buccal and apical to tooth #30. What is the cause and what is the treatment?**
This is a flare-up. The Glossary of Endodontic Terms (AAE) defines a flare-up as an acute exacerbation of an asymptomatic pulp/periapical pathosis after the initiation or continuation of root canal treatment. It does not affect the long-term prognosis and can be treated with local anesthesia, incision and drainage, psychological care, and pharmacological treatment with antibiotics and NSAIDs.

13. **A 50-year-old African American female patient presents for consultation of teeth #23, 24, 26. Radiographic examination reveals areas of apical radiolucency on teeth #23 and 24, and an area of mixed radiopacity on tooth #26. Clinical examination reveals that all teeth respond normally to cold and are determined to be vital. What is your likely diagnosis?**
Periapical cemento-osseous dysplasia (PCOD). Differential diagnoses for vital teeth with multiple areas of periapical bone loss should include PCOD, malignancy, neurofibromatosis, and brown tumor. PCOD is a benign condition that often occurs in mandibular incisors and can mimic endodontic pathology in radiographs. It is more common in middle-aged African American women, and often appears radiographically as apical bone loss that is either radiolucent or of mixed radiopacity. Histologically, these lesions contain anastomosing bone trabeculae and cementum-like calcifications in a fibroblast background. There is no treatment indicated other than continued monitoring (Fig. 7-1).

14. **What facial spaces could be involved from a pulpal/periapical infection of a mandibular second molar?**
Extension of any infection is closely tied to the proximity of root apices to cortical bone and muscle attachments. As the apices of mandibular second and third molars are typically below the mylohyoid attachment, infection may spread to the submandibular space. That infection may then spread beyond the pterygomandibular space leading to jugular thrombosis.

15. **What is the lamina dura and how is it used to evaluate for endodontic pathology?**
The lamina dura, also called the alveolar bone proper, is the internal septum that appears as a thin radiopaque border adjacent to the periodontal ligament. Partial or complete loss of lamina dura in one tooth usually indicates localized pathology such as chronic inflammation or infection. This is a result of the byproducts of pulpal disease which cause bone degeneration and the subsequent loss of the radiographic white line surrounding the root structure. Changes to lamina dura that are more generalized can be an identifying factor in nonodontogenic pathology, such as Paget's disease, scleroderma, and leukemia.

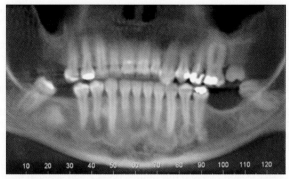

Fig. 7-1. A CBCT scan reveals multiple foci of bone dysplasia in different stages of evolution in the periapical regions of the anterior and posterior teeth. (Delai D, Bernardi A, Felippe GS, da Silveira Teixeira C, Felippe WT, Felippe MCS: Florid cemento-osseous dysplasia: a case of misdiagnosis, J Endod 41(11):1923–1926, 2015.)

16. **Can you diagnose a periapical cyst from a periapical granuloma based on clinical and radiographic evaluation?**
    No. The only way to truly identify these lesions is through histological analysis following a biopsy. An apical cyst has a stratified, squamous epithelial lining and a granuloma which has connective tissue, neutrophils, monocytes, and blood vessels.

17. **A patient presents with severe pain in the entire right maxillary arch that is described as sharp, shooting pain. He tells you that this pain is sometimes brought on by touching his face. What pathology would be suspected after ruling out any endodontic origin for the pain?**
    Trigeminal neuralgia or Tic Douloureux is a neuralgia that affects the fifth cranial nerve, also called the trigeminal nerve. Patients often describe a sharp, shooting, or burning pain which is transient. If no odontogenic pathology can be diagnosed, referral for a neurological consult should be given. If confirmed, treatment is often pharmacologic therapy in the form of anticonvulsant medications such as phenytoin, gabapentin, or carbamazepine.

MICROBIOLOGY/PHARMACOLOGY

18. **What is the significance of bacteria in endodontic disease?**
    Bacteria is key in the development of apical periodontitis. The classic study by Kakehashi demonstrated that bacteria cause apical periodontitis. The study was done by exposing the pulps of germ-free rats and observing no pathological changes. In rats with normal oral flora, pulp exposures lead to pulp necrosis with apical pathology. Bacteria can enter the pulp chamber directly via caries extending into the dentinal tubules or through a fracture. Indirect exposure can also cause pulp necrosis via inflammation reactions and microcracks.

19. **What kind of bacteria are most found in endodontic infections?**
    Most bacteria in endodontic infections are strict anaerobes. Studies have shown that in the initial infection stages, the bacteria are facultative. These are displaced by anaerobic bacteria as infection time increases. Strict anaerobes grow only in the absence of oxygen and lack the enzymes superoxide dismutase and catalase. The bacteria found in periapical lesions have been shown to be polymicrobial and their diversity and abundance vary from individual to individual. The primary isolated BACTERIAL species in root canal infections are *Streptococcus, Enterococcus, Prevotella,* and *Porphyromonas.* In addition, the species *Actinomyces,* as well as fungi, viruses, archaea, and spirochetes have all been isolated in root canal infections.

20. **The role of gram-negative anaerobic bacteria is an established fact in the pathogenesis of endodontic lesions. What role do bacterial endotoxins play?**
    Gram-negative bacteria have lipopolysaccharide (LPS), known as endotoxin, as an integral part of the cell wall. When LPS is released, it causes both the mobilization of an immune response and cytokine production by macrophages in the pulp. Cytokines, such as IL-1beta, IL-8, VEGF, and toll-like receptor-4, have all been shown to have increased expression resulting from endotoxin.

21. ***Enterococcus faecalis* is a facultative anaerobe that has been frequently cultured from previously root-filled teeth with apical periodontitis. It is known for its resistance to intracanal irrigating materials and medications such as calcium hydroxide. What are the virulence factors attributed to *E. faecalis* that allow it to contribute to endodontic failures?**
    1. Survival of glucose starvation
    2. The ability to form biofilms

3. The ability to bind to dentin via the production of serine protease and collagen-binding protein (Ace)
4. Survival in harsh environments

22. Culture studies allow microorganisms to grow in a laboratory with either aerobic or anaerobic environmental conditions. What are the limitations of culture studies that cause bacteria to be unculturable and unidentifiable?
    1. Lack of essential nutrients in artificial mediums
    2. Overfeeding conditions
    3. Toxicity of the culture medium
    4. Substance produced by other bacteria which inhibits the growth of the target organism
    5. Metabolic dependence on other species for growth
    6. Separation of microbiota from culture media prohibiting bacterial communication

23. What are some molecular biological methods that have been employed to investigate the previously uncultivatable microbes?
    1. PCR, or polymerase chain reactions
    2. DNA-DNA hybridization
    3. FISH (fluorescent in situ hybridization), using fluorescently labeled rRNA

24. Why do biofilms form in endodontic infections and what are their unique characteristics?
    Polymicrobial ecosystems are present in endodontic infections and result from the harsh environment in the root canal system. As endodontic infections progress, the root canal system becomes more anaerobic and depleted in nutrition for microbes. These unfavorable conditions encourage the formation of complex organized structures that are more resistant to antimicrobial agents called biofilms. Biofilms are successful in bacterial survival because they are metabolically diverse, capable of genetic exchange, can communicate via signaling molecules, and can increase the concentration gradient of nutrients.

25. What are black-pigmented bacteroides?
    These anaerobic rods are a common isolate in endodontic infections and play a role in the formation of apical abscesses and periodontitis. Black-pigmented bacteria have been associated with both the spread of infection and purulent inflammation in apical periodontitis. These bacteria are classified into two groups: the saccharolytic species *Prevotella* and the asaccharolytic species *Porphyromonas*. *Porphyromonas endodontalis* is implicated in acute periapical inflammation, pain, and exudate.

26. When are antibiotics indicated in endodontic therapy?
    Antibiotics are indicated for rapidly increasing symptoms, systemic involvement, trismus, autoimmune disease, involvement of an anatomic danger zone, lymphadenopathy, a fever more than 100°F, osteomyelitis, and persisting infection.

27. What antibiotic would you choose to prescribe for a patient with a Penicillin allergy?
    The preferred antibiotic for a patient with a penicillin allergy is Azithromycin. Historically, Clindamycin was the preferred medication. This changed due to rising concerns over both antibiotic resistance and the occurrence of *Clostridium difficile* infections. Studies have shown that one single dose of Clindamycin can change the intestinal microbiota causing susceptibility to *C. difficile* and pseudomembranous colitis. This can cause diarrhea, weight loss, and can have up to a 50% mortality rate.

28. What are some contraindications for the use of antibiotics in endodontic therapy?
    1. Irreversible pulpitis
    2. Asymptomatic radiolucency
    3. Pain without signs and symptoms of infection
    4. Drainage through the presence of a sinus tract
    5. Fluctuant swelling

29. What is the antibiotic of choice for dental infections?
    Penicillin is effective against most aerobic and anaerobic bacteria and is therefore the antibiotic of choice for treatment of endodontic/oral infections. Amoxicillin, which has a broader spectrum than penicillin, has been found to be more effective, but may lead to antibiotic resistance. Augmentin (Amoxicillin and Clavulanate) is also more effective than Pen VK and should be employed when there is a persistent infection after the use of a beta-lactam antibiotic. Metronidazole is a bactericidal antibiotic that is effective against anaerobes but not aerobes. Due to the polymicrobial nature of endodontic infections, a combination of Penicillin and Metronidazole can be used if infections do not respond to Penicillin.

30. What cardiac conditions require premedication?
    The following cardiac conditions require premedication:
    1. Prosthetic heart valves
    2. History of infective endocarditis
    3. Unrepaired or incompletely repaired cyanotic heart defect within 6 months of the repair

4. Repaired cyanotic congenital heart defect within 6 months of the repair
5. Repaired cyanotic heart defects with residual defects at the surgical site

31. **Up to 50% of patients will experience postoperative pain within the first 24 hours after endodontic therapy. What pain management protocol would you advise for a patient with no medical contraindications to NSAIDs or acetaminophen?**
NSAIDs are the first-line medication choice for inflammatory postoperative tooth pain. The recommended dose is 400 to 600 mg, every 4 to 6 hours daily with a maximum dose of 3200 mg per day. If a patient is still experiencing pain, a combination of ibuprofen (200-400 mg) and acetaminophen (500-1000 mg) can be utilized. The combination has a greater peak analgesia and more constant analgesia than either medication alone. For severe odontogenic pain or if patients cannot tolerate NSAIDs, an opioid may be prescribed. Percocet (oxycodone 5 mg/acetaminophen 325 mg), Vicodin (hydrocodone 5 mg/acetaminophen 325 mg), acetaminophen with codeine #3 (30 mg codeine/300 mg acetaminophen), and Ultram (Tramadol 50 mg) are typical dental pain medication options.

32. **In patients with cardiovascular risk factors, which antibiotics should you avoid and why?**
Macrolide antibiotics have been shown to be associated with arrhythmia-related effects. Clarithromycin and erythromycin can increase the risk of severe ventricular arrythmias. Azithromycin has been associated with prolonging the QT interval and has been documented to cause an increased risk of cardiac death compared to amoxicillin.

33. **How does local anesthesia work?**
Local anesthesia works by blocking sodium channels in peripheral neurons, thus preventing depolarization of the nerve and propagation of the action potential.

34. **What are some reasons for failure of local anesthetic failures in dentistry?**
Anatomic variations such as cross innervations, accessory innervation, patient anxiety, and unsuccessful administration can lead to anesthetic failure. Pulpal inflammation and infection cause a decrease in tissue pH which favors a shift to a cationic form of the local anesthetic. Permeability through the lipoprotein neural sheath is only possible with the anionic state of the anesthetic, therefore causing anesthesia to be ineffective.

35. **What are some supplemental anesthesia techniques used to attain profound pulpal anesthesia?**
Infiltration following a failed inferior alveolar nerve (IAN) block can provide successful anesthesia. Intraosseous injections can be successful, although caution should be used with a patient with any cardiac history as increased heart rate has been associated with this method. A safe alternative to intraosseous injections is a PDL injection. A PDL injection works by interrupting the pulpal vasculature and is only effective with anesthetics containing epinephrine. Intrapulpal injections may also be employed if no other technique is effective. Any anesthetic may be used as its success is pressure dependent.

36. **Describe the benefits and the dangers in using Septocaine (articaine).**
Septocaine is an amide anesthetic which first became available in the United States after FDA approval in 2000. It contains ester and thiophene rings in place of a traditional benzene ring giving it better tissue penetration (liposolubility). High plasma-protein binding also contributes to its increased effectiveness. It has a 4% concentration and two available formulations with either 1:100,000 or 1:200,000 epinephrine. Though research has been divided, caution should be employed as some studies have shown an increase in the risk of permanent paresthesia when Septocaine is administered as an IAN block.

37. **What are some symptoms of epinephrine toxicity and how can it be avoided?**
Epinephrine is added to local anesthetics to slow diffusion from the site of action. Intravascular injection of epinephrine-containing anesthetics can cause an acute increase in blood pressure or cardiac dysthymias. Toxicity symptoms include tremors, anxiety, headache, perspiration, and palpitations. A cardiac patient can receive a maximum dose of 0.04 mg of epinephrine. Using the minimum effective dose of epinephrine and careful aspiration can reduce the chance of toxicity.

PULP AND PERIAPICAL BIOLOGY

38. **Describe the embryologic origin of dentin and the dental pulp.**
Teeth form by a series of interactions between neural crest-derived mesenchymal and ectodermal cells. The dental pulp arises from the dental papilla which exists within the enamel organ. The enamel organ develops into the inner and outer enamel epithelium, and the cells from the inner epithelium induce the adjacent neuro-mesenchymal cells to form odontoblasts. Odontoblasts form predentin and later, dentin. The mesenchymal cells surrounding the tooth bud condense to form the dental sac which will later become the periodontal ligament and cementum.

39. **What are Tomes processes, and where are they located within the tooth structures?**
The odontoblast cells develop from the mesenchymal cells adjacent to the inner epithelium and form predentin and dentin. As the dentin thickens, the odontoblast regresses toward the dental papilla, leaving its odontoblastic processes, or Tomes processes, embedded in the dentin. There has been much debate as to how much these

processes extend into the dentin. Scanning electron microscope studies have found that these processes extend only into the inner third of the dentin. However, light microscopy and immunofluorescent antibody labeling have found that the odontoblastic processes extend to the dentin-enamel-junction. There is still debate whether these processes extend to the dentin-enamel junction in early development or after development has been completed.

40. **What type of dentin is caused to form by pulpal irritants?**
Tertiary dentin, or reparative dentin, is formed following the death of odontoblasts. Odontoblastic differentiation occurs either by an existing odontoblast or by a newly formed odontoblast around the site of trauma. The dentin formation is irregular and less tubular than primary or secondary dentin and is often formed at sites corresponding to irritation (such as carious exposures). The formation of this type of dentin is rapid but slows over time.

41. **Describe odontoblasts.**
Odontoblasts are cells derived from mesenchyme of the dental papilla. They have the unique quality of forming an unmineralized glycoprotein which mineralizes over time. The cells are highly polarized due to synthesizing and secretion of dentin in the cell body during the odontoblastic process. Odontoblasts appear to be pseudostratified and columnar in the coronal pulp, cuboidal in the radicular pulp, and cuboidal near the apex. Odontoblasts produce dentin which consists of approximately 70% inorganic material, 20% organic material, and 10% water. The dentin is made up of tubules that contain an extracellular fluid and are more dense and larger in size toward the dental pulp.

42. **What is the dental pulp?**
The dental pulp arises from the neuro-mesenchymal dental papilla and contains mostly unmyelinated nerves, fibroblasts, capillaries, undifferentiated mesenchymal cells, immune cells, and extra-cellular matrix (ECM). The peripheral part of the pulp contains a layer of odontoblasts which produce a rigid dentin wall that surrounds the dental pulp. This functions to decrease the reactions to inflammatory and injurious insults. The odontoblast layer connects the pulp to the dentin allowing the dentin-pulp complex. The dental pulp has a highly vascular but isolated circulatory system and is densely innervated by afferent sensory neurons called nociceptors.

43. **Describe the vasculature of the dental pulp.**
The dental pulp has a microcirculatory system which is comprised primarily of arterioles, venules, and lymphatics. Vasculature enters through the apical foramen, eventually forming a dense capillary plexus in the sub-odontoblastic region. Venous and lymphatics exit through the apical foramen. There is evidence that there are blood vessel connections to the pulp via the periodontal ligament. Scanning electron microscope studies have shown three layers to the dense capillary network including a terminal network in the odontoblastic layer, a layer of precapillary and postcapillary cells that run parallel to each other, and a venule network with a lattice appearance. Arterio-venous anastomosis, U-turn loops, and venous-venous anastomosis are all unique features of the dental pulp.

44. **What explains why decreased pulpal blood flow results from stimulation of beta-adrenergic receptors in the dental pulp?**
Blood flow in the dental pulp is regulated by alpha- and beta-adrenergic receptors located on the smooth muscles which coat the walls of the arterioles and venules. Stimulation of a-adrenergic receptors causes vasoconstriction while stimulation of beta receptors causes vasodilation in skeletal muscle. A low compliance system could explain why a beta agonist, which typically causes vasodilation, causes a decreased blood flow in the dental pulp. If the blood flow is initially increased, the venular pressure is high, leading to increased tissue pressure. When the tissue pressure becomes higher than the venule pressure, compression causes ultimate decreased pulpal blood flow.

45. **Explain how the dental pulp becomes necrotic.**
A pulp irritant causes the release of neuropeptides and mediators, leading to vasodilation and vascular leakage. The increase in pulpal pressure and a subsequent decrease in pulp blood flow result in the accumulation of mediators and vessel damage causing pulp inflammation and death.

46. **What theory best explains dentin sensitivity?**
The classic study by Brannstrom demonstrated the hydrodynamic mechanism for dentin sensitivity. This theory describes the process of fluid movement in the dentin tubules, either inward or outward, causing the sensory nerves located in the dental pulp or dentin to be activated. Studies have shown that cold leads to an outward movement of fluid flow caused by contraction of the fluid. Outward movement of fluid causes a higher pain response than inward flow.

47. **What are the classic signs of an aging pulp?**
A decrease in nerve cells and vascularity, decreased odontoblast size and quantity, and a decrease in the size and volume of the pulp tissue are classic signs of an aging pulp. There is also an increase in the quality and quantity of collagen fibers and in the overall cellularity. The apical foramen can also change size and position with age.

48. **What are some of the studied effects of orthodontic movement on the dental pulp?**
Negative changes to the pulp due to orthodontic movement are rarely permanent but can result in an initial pulp hyperemia. There have been documented changes in the pulp tissue including more congested blood cells within

the vessels as well as an increase in inflammatory mediators. Orthodontic movement can cause an increase response to an electric pulp tester that could last for several weeks as well as a decrease in the pulp chamber size.

49. **What is the neurological explanation for sensitivity to heat that causes a constant dull ache?**
The dental pulp is innervated by sensory nerve fibers that are myelinated (a-fibers) and unmyelinated (c-fibers). These sensory fibers arise from the trigeminal nerve ganglion and enter the dental pulp in bundles through the apical foramen. Stimulation of alpha-delta fibers results in the production of fast, sharp pain. C-nociceptive fibers respond to external stimuli that reach the pulp proper, releasing neuropeptides from their peripheral terminals such as CGRP, substance P, neurokinin A, and neuropeptide Y. C-fibers are more resistant to hypoxia and can transmit a dull ache that causes pain after a-delta fibers are inactivated.

50. **What type of cells exist in the dental pulp that indicate the capability of an immune response?**
Histological analysis of the pulp tissue has shown the presence of mast cells, dendritic cells, lymphocytes, leukocytes, and plasma cells.

TREATMENT

51. **What is an electronic apex locator (EAL), and how does it work?**
EALs work based on the principle that there is a consistent resistance measurement between the PDL and the oral mucosa of 6.5 kilo-ohms. As a file nears the periodontal ligament, the resistance drops, and the circuit is complete. The newer EALs are more accurate because they measure impedance which considers both resistance and capacitance.

52. **How can you determine the working length and why is it so important?**
Working length is the distance from the coronal reference point to the point where the canal preparation and obturation should terminate. Canal preparation should terminate at the cemento-dentinal junction (CDJ). Obturation materials and sealers that extend beyond this point can cause inflammation or paresthesia. EALs, like the Root-ZX (Morita), have a high rate of accuracy for determining the working length. Radiographs can also be used, but accuracy may be lower due to the discrepancy between the radiograph and actual lengths. CBCT imaging can be very accurate in gathering this information given there is less chance for geometric distortion.

53. **Can you use the Root-ZX (EAL) for length determination on a patient with a pacemaker?**
It was once thought that EALs were not indicated for patients with cardiac pacemakers or implanted cardiac defibrillators due to the possibility of electrical interference. There are several recent studies that have shown EALs are safe in these situations. Studies have been done both measuring pacemaker function with pace monitoring and measuring cardiac function with electrocardiograms. Both methods have demonstrated that using an EAL will neither inhibit nor interfere with normal pacemaker function. It has been proposed that EALs should be confined to the head and neck region, not cross the chest, and are approximately 10 to 12 inches away from the heart.

54. **Why is rubber dam isolation the standard of care in routine endodontic treatment?**
Rubber dam isolation (RDI) is essential for improving root canal therapy prognosis and patient safety. It provides a sterile, dry environment free of blood and saliva. A rubber dam prevents the patient from swallowing or aspirating caustic chemicals or small files used during endodontic procedures.

55. **Surgical operating microscopes are an important part of the modern endodontic technique. What are the purposes for their use?**
   1. Detection of fractures
   2. Removal of separated instruments and repairing perforations in the case of a complications
   3. Increasing the overall visual field and increasing the ability to locate canals
   4. Removal of obturation materials during nonsurgical retreatment cases
   5. Improving access preparation to allow for conservative removal of mineralized tissue
   6. Use in microsurgery
   7. Documentation purposes in the case of litigation

56. **Minimally invasive access cavity (MIA), or the contracted endodontic access cavity, has been the focus of recent debate. Discuss the minimal access preparation and how it differs from the traditional access preparation.**
Endodontic access should be as small as possible without compromising the biological objectives of root canal therapy. Newly practiced MIA preparations emphasize minimally invasive access to conserve coronal tooth structure. This allows for possible fracture resistance, and may lessen the necessity for a full coverage restoration. Traditional access preparations are larger and allow for straight-line access. These have the advantage of maximal tissue removal and minimal risk of iatrogenic complications such as rotary file separation from cyclic fatigue.

Fracture resistance and proper sterilization in MIA preparations have been debated in the literature. Some studies have found that MIA cavity preparations are inferior in their ability to debride and disinfect the pulp chamber compared to traditional preparations. Ultimately, more research is needed to determine the benefits/risks for each type of access.

57. What guidelines are important in accessing a calcified tooth?
    1. The pulp chamber floor is always darker than the walls
    2. The pulp chamber floor is always in the center of the tooth at the CEJ
    3. The external root surface reflects the internal pulp anatomy
    4. The CEJ is a repeatable landmark for locating the pulp chamber
    5. There is symmetry within the tooth structure
    6. The canals are always located at either the junction, angle, or terminus of the floor-wall junction

58. After determining the working length (WL) and beginning your canal preparation, you pass a patency file through the apex. Why is apical patency important in the cleaning and shaping of the root canal system?
    A patency file is used to pass through the CDJ, or apical constriction, without increasing its width. There are many benefits for maintaining patency during the cleaning and shaping of the root canal system. Having patent canals will decrease the chance of losing working length, transportations, ledges, or other accidents. Achieving patency improves the tactile sensation for the clinician during apical shaping and allows for easier irrigation in the apical third. Finally, maintaining patency allows the anatomy of the apical constriction to remain intact. Caution should be exercised as studies have shown the risk of apical extrusion of bacteria-laden debris and postoperative pain when using patency files. Some research has shown that apical perforation, or translocation, could occur if the patency file is wider than that of the apical constriction.

59. What is internal bleaching and what are the associated treatment risks?
    Internal bleaching, or walking bleach, is a method of internally whitening the coronal tooth structure. A mixture of Superoxyl (30% hydrogen peroxide) and sodium perborate is placed in the access cavity with a 2 mm temporary seal to prevent leakage into the oral cavity. Typically, the bleaching agents are left in place for 4 to 7 days. There is a risk of invasive cervical root resorption (ICRR) in internal bleaching that can range from 6% to 8%, or up to 25%. The use of heat activation and a history of trauma are predisposing risk factors for the occurrence of ICRR. The presumed mechanism involves the exposure of open dentinal tubules and cementum defects to the irritating chemicals used in bleaching. This leads to inflammation of the cementum and periodontal ligament which can cause root resorption. As ICRR can be detrimental to the prognosis of the tooth, it is important to protect the open dentinal tubules at the CEJ with a base material that is 2 mm in thickness. This base can be made of a glass ionomer cement.

60. What is the smear layer, and should it be removed?
    The smear layer is dentinal debris created from canal preparation which can block access to the dentinal tubules, preventing the antibacterial effects of irrigation materials. Given the smear layer harbors bacteria and causes microleakage after obturation, it should be removed. Removal of the smear layer with the chelating agent ethylenediaminetetraacetic acid, or EDTA 17% in combination with 5.25% sodium hypochlorite has been shown to facilitate the disinfection of the root canal system. Other materials that can remove the smear layer are citric acid, SmearClear, and Biopure MTAD. Biopure MTAD contains doxycycline, an antibiotic that has a high binding affinity for dentin allowing possible increased antimicrobial activity. Leaving the smear layer intact has been debated in the literature. One in vivo study demonstrated that bacteria in the root canal system could be higher without the smear layer, postulating that this blockage prevents bacteria from invading and infecting the dentinal tubules.

61. What is the standard irrigation material widely accepted in endodontics, and why is it so effective?
    Sodium hypochlorite, or NaOCl, at a 5.25% preparation is the most widely accepted and used irrigant. Sodium hypochlorite dissolves necrotic tissue and eliminates a broad range of bacteria including those typically found in biofilms. Sodium hypochlorite can eliminate bacteria at a small distance into the dentinal tubules but cannot remove the smear layer. In addition, it can achieve tissue toxicity at certain concentrations.

62. What is an alternative irrigation material to sodium hypochlorite?
    Chlorhexidine gluconate (CHX) is a good alternative to sodium hypochlorite. It is not irritating to the periapical tissues and is antimicrobial against gram-positive and gram-negative microorganisms. CHX is also effective against fungus and E. faecalis and can work for several days following treatment if left in contact with root dentin. However, it is usually not preferred over sodium hypochlorite primarily because it does not dissolve necrotic or vital tissue. CHX should be avoided in combination with sodium hypochlorite as it will produce a brown precipitate called para-chloroaniline (PCA). PCA has been shown to be carcinogenic and can cause cyanosis due to methemoglobin formation. CHX can also be used as an intracanal medicament between visits. An in vivo study examining the periapical immune response with CHX as an intracanal medicament revealed that it reduces the proinflammatory and immunoregulatory cytokines after treatment.

63. What are the ideal qualities for a root canal irrigant?
    1. Dissolves necrotic tissue
    2. Antimicrobial against broad-spectrum bacteria, such as facultative and anaerobic microorganisms
    3. Low potential for cytotoxicity or allergic reaction
    4. Inactivates endotoxin
    5. Prevents the development of a smear layer, or can remove it once it is formed

64. The root canal system is complex, with isthmuses, accessory canals, and lateral canals. What are some irrigation techniques that can increase the level of disinfection when there are anatomical difficulties?
    Agitation of the irrigation material shows an increase in effectiveness in terms of the disinfecting abilities of the irrigant. Newer irrigation techniques have been marketed and used in endodontics to eliminate microorganisms from parts of the root canal system that are difficult to address with mechanical instrumentation. The Endovac is an apical negative pressure irrigation system that can result in less bacteria 1 mm from the working length, as well as decrease the smear layer left following treatment. Passive ultrasonic irrigation improves the cleanliness of both the isthmuses and the main canal. However, caution must be taken to avoid perforation, transportation, and abnormally shaping the canals. The Endoactivator, a sonically driven activator of irrigation materials, and is comparable to the Endovac regarding removal of the smear layer.

65. Is prognosis affected by the obturation technique during root canal therapy?
    Lateral condensation uses cold gutta-percha laterally compacted with spreaders allowing for the addition of accessory cones. Vertical obturation condenses warmed gutta-percha to potentially fill more lateral and accessory canals. It is technique sensitive because an apical stop is essential in the prevention of an overfill. There have been no differences in overall outcomes in terms of bacterial leakage between lateral condensation and vertical condensation. Contrastingly, carrier-based systems, which were thought to be easier to use than other approaches, have been shown to have increased bacterial leakage compared to lateral and vertical condensation.

66. Describe the chemical and physical characteristics of gutta-percha (GP).
    GP is the most widely used obturation material and succeeds in fulfilling many of the obturation material ideals. It possesses low cytotoxicity, especially when not extruded into the apical tissues. It is derived from the sap of a tropical tree found in Southeast Asia and is a trans-isomer of polyisoprene, closely related to natural rubber. GP cones are composed of approximately 20% GP, 50% zinc oxide, 11% barium sulfate, and 3% waxes and resins. They have two phases consisting of the alpha crystalline phase, which is brittle at room temperature and less viscous, and beta crystalline phase, which is stable and flexible at room temperature and more viscous. GP cones are available primarily in the beta crystalline phase as they can be melted into a thermoplastic alphaphase.

67. What are some of the requirements for an ideal obturation material?
    An obturation material should be easily introduced to the canal, radiopaque, and nontoxic to the periapical tissues. It should be easy to sterilize and be removable from the canal. It should seal the canal both laterally and apically, not shrink, and not be affected by moisture. Finally, it should be bacteriostatic.

68. What are the predisposing factors that increase the likelihood of a flare-up?
    A large retrospective study found that several factors influence the probability of a flare-up.
    1. Patients between 40 and 59 are most likely to have a flare-up
    2. Females are more likely than males to experience a flare-up
    3. Systemic conditions or a medical history that includes allergies
    4. Mandibular teeth are more likely to flare up than maxillary teeth
    5. Psychological factors such as anxiety about postoperative pain
    6. Retreatment endodontic therapy
    7. Presence of a periapical radiolucency
    8. Over instrumentation or overfilling of a canal

69. Describe cracked tooth syndrome, or cracked tooth, and the recommended treatment plan.
    A patient with cracked tooth syndrome may present with pain to bite and to bite release along with acute temperature sensitivity. Incomplete tooth fractures can be defined as a fracture plane of unknown depth and direction that passes through tooth structure and may communicate with the pulp or periodontal ligament. Cold tests, bite tests with the tooth sleuth, transillumination, methylene blue dye, and use of a surgical operating microscope are tools that can be utilized to diagnose fractures. Guidelines for treatment depend on the previously determined pulpal diagnosis. If a tooth is diagnosed with irreversible pulpitis or pulp necrosis, non-surgical endodontic therapy would be recommended. In the case of reversible pulpitis, restoring the tooth with a temporary crown can be considered. If the pain does not resolve, endodontic treatment would be recommended. There is a low percentage chance that a cracked tooth with reversible pulpitis will eventually require endodontic therapy if it is restored with a full coverage restoration (Fig 7-2).

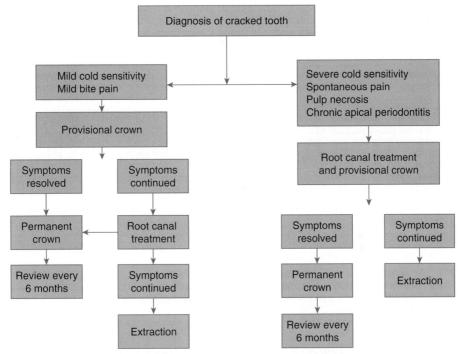

Fig. 7-2. Flow chart for determination of treatment plan for cracked/fractured teeth. (Kim SY, Kim SH, Cho SB, Lee GO, Yang SE: Different treatment protocols for different pulpal and periapical diagnoses of 72 cracked teeth, J Endod 39(4):449–452, 2013.)

70. **What is the guideline and appropriate treatment for a 9-year-old patient with a complicated, bleeding crown fracture of tooth #8?**

A complicated crown fracture involves injury to the enamel and dentin, resulting in a pulp exposure. Given the patient is 9 years old, it is likely that the root of tooth #8 has not completely formed. For treatment of mechanical or traumatic pulp exposures for unformed roots, either a pulp cap or pulpotomy is recommended. In the case of bleeding at the site of exposure, a Cvek, or partial pulpotomy is advised. A portion of the coronal pulp tissue is removed and mineral trioxide aggregate (MTA) or calcium hydroxide is used to cover the tissue. Cvek pulpotomies have a high success rate (96%) and preserve the remaining coronal and radicular pulp tissue, allowing the roots to form naturally. Monitoring at 6 to 8 weeks and 1 year is indicated.

71. **What is MTA and what are its defining characteristics?**

MTA is a material used in surgical root end filling, perforation repair, regeneration, and vital pulp therapy. It is comprised of tricalcium aluminate, tricalcium oxide, and bismuth oxide. It has the unique ability to set in the presence of water and is antimicrobial as it provides an alkaline environment. It has been shown to provide a good apical seal and stimulates the formation of a dentinal bridge by ultimately providing the growth of cementum adjacent to it. Newer materials have been developed to improve some of the negative qualities of MTA, including a long setting time, and difficult manipulation based on its sand-like consistency.

72. **What is apexification and when is it indicated?**

Apexification is the process of performing endodontic therapy to address a necrotic pulp while also creating an apical barrier for obturation. It is performed when the pulpal diagnosis of an immature tooth is necrotic or has irreversible pulpitis. There are two methods of apexification: calcium hydroxide and MTA apexification. In calcium hydroxide apexification, calcium hydroxide is placed in the canal allowing antimicrobial action and an apical calcific bridge to form over a long period of time. It is suggested that calcium hydroxide is changed every 3 months until bridge formation is complete. Patient compliance may be difficult to achieve given several office visits are necessary for up to 2 years. The alternative, MTA apexification, allows for a one- or two-visit approach. MTA can set in the presence of moisture and creates an artificial apical barrier to obturate against. While outcomes have been shown to be equal between the two methods in terms of resulting inflammation and amount of calcified tissue, there is a higher chance of root fracture with calcium hydroxide apexification.

73. **Is there a difference in outcome in one-visit vs. two-visit endodontic therapy?**
While some studies have found an increase in disinfection with multiple visits using calcium hydroxide as an intracanal medicament, no difference in postoperative pain or overall prognosis has been established in the research between the one and two-visit treatment plans.

74. **What is the rationale for the use of calcium hydroxide as an intracanal medicament?**
Calcium hydroxide is alkaline and has a high pH, making it antimicrobial. It dissolves necrotic tissue, allowing for an increase in the solubilizing action of sodium hypochlorite. It also neutralizes the biological activity of LPS. Some studies have proposed that the disinfection of apical isthmuses and portions of the root canal system that may not be able to be cleaned and shaped mechanically benefit from a multiple-visit approach with calcium hydroxide.

75. **What are the objectives of a temporary restoration?**
A temporary restoration should seal the tooth from bacteria and saliva and provide protection until the permanent restoration is placed. It should be easily placed and removed and be esthetically perfunctory. Cavit, which provides better sealing ability than intermediate restorative material, is widely used as a temporary restoration in endodontics. It is a premixed material made of zinc oxide, calcium sulfate, glycol, polyvinyl acetate, polyvinyl chloride, and triethanolamine. 3 mm of Cavit should be placed to ensure a good seal and to avoid fracture.

76. **When a post is indicated, how much gutta-percha (GP) should remain after creating the post space?**
There should be at least 5 to 7 mm of gutta-percha in the canal to prevent apical leakage. Removing too much GP can result in a poor apical seal. In addition, an excessively long post space may remove too much dentin and result in a future root fracture.

77. **Does preparation of the post space immediately after obturation improve the apical?**
Some studies have found a decrease in apical seal if post spaces were delayed and others found no difference. Ultimately, if the apical seal is intact, it makes sense to create the post space at the time of obturation.

78. **What are the pros and cons of post placement?**
Posts are placed for the purpose of retaining a core, providing support for full coverage restorations. Post placement has been shown to decrease the overall prognosis for endodontically treated teeth and studies have demonstrated that endodontically treated teeth with posts are not more resistant to fracture.

79. **What is ankylosis or replacement resorption?**
In cases of significant trauma where there is damage to more than 20% of the root surface, the injured surface becomes devoid of cementum. Without this protection, cells in the area move in to populate the surface. Precursor cells to bone formation connect with the denuded root surface allowing for bone to contact the root. The progressive replacement of root with bone is called replacement resorption, or ankylosis. The pathognomonic clinical finding of ankylosis is a metallic tone on percussion.

80. **What is an intrusive subluxation injury and what are the findings and treatment recommendations?**
Displacement of a tooth inward and into the alveolar bone can be defined as intrusive subluxation. The tooth may appear partially or fully infra-occluded and will be immobile and locked into this position. While the tooth may be painful to percuss, cold tests will likely be negative. Generally, if the patient is an adult with a fully formed root, and if the intrusion is 3mm or less, one can allow the tooth to re-erupt for 2 to 3 weeks. If re-eruption does not occur, then orthodontic or surgical intervention will be needed to reposition the tooth before ankylosis occurs.

81. **Why is sealer necessary in obturation with gutta-percha?**
Limitations of gutta-percha cause voids to occur which can be filled with the proper sealer. Sealers both hold the obturation material together using cohesive strength and bond well with the dentin using adhesive strength. Studies have shown that gutta-percha by itself does not bind to dentin. Without a sealer a hermetic seal, necessary for long-term success, would not be achieved.

82. **What are some important qualities a good sealer must have?**
    1. Tacky when mixed
    2. Provides an adequate seal
    3. Radiopaque
    4. Easily mixable
    5. Does not shrink
    6. Does not stain the tooth
    7. Does not encourage the growth of bacteria
    8. Biocompatible
    9. Insoluble in tissue fluids
    10. Slow setting time
    11. Not carcinogenic

83. **What is the course of treatment for a fully formed, avulsed tooth with more than 60 minutes of extraoral dry time, and what are the concerns regarding the prognosis?**
There is a high probability of both pulpal necrosis and ankylosis with a dry time of more than 60 minutes. The goal upon reimplantation is to encourage alveolar bone growth which will surround the root structure of the tooth. The tooth should be cleaned and debrided then treated with a 2% fluoride solution for 20 minutes. The socket should be irrigated with saline and the alveolar bone should be inspected for fractures. The tooth is then reimplanted, and any lacerations are sutured. A periapical radiograph should be taken to confirm the proper placement of the tooth before a flexible splint is placed for 1 to 2 weeks. As necrosis of the pulp is inevitable, endodontic therapy is recommended. This can be done either prior to reimplantation or within 7 to 10 days of reimplantation. Some studies have shown that performing pulp extirpation at the time of implantation will increase periapical inflammation, negatively impacting the periodontal ligament. This suggests performing endodontic therapy after 7 to 10 days prior to splint removal. Ankylosis is also inevitable, and one should consider decoronation in the case of infraocclusion in children under 15 years old. Decoronation involves removal of the coronal tooth structure while leaving the root in the socket. This will help to maintain the alveolar bone in a buccal to lingual direction and allow for future vertical bone growth, improving the future success of an implant.

84. **How long does it take for the periodontal fibers to heal following reimplantation of permanent mature tooth?**
Approximately 1 to 2 weeks. A flexible splint is used for 1 to 2 weeks to allow for healing and should be flexible to decrease the chance of ankylosis occurrence.

85. **What are some benefits of a zinc oxide-eugenol sealer?**
Zinc oxide-eugenol (ZOE) sealers are commonly used sealers in endodontics. The powder component, zinc oxide, has antimicrobial properties which provide cytoplasmic protection to the tissue cells. Eugenol is the liquid component and is derived from clove oil. It can be anti-inflammatory at low doses and has an analgesic effect by blocking the sodium channels. Eugenol is cytotoxic to tissue at high doses.

86. **Resin-based sealers were developed as an alternative to ZOE sealers and calcium hydroxide-containing sealers. What are some of its characteristics?**
Epoxy resin sealers, such as AH Plus, Epiphany, and Diaket, have good handling, good flow, seal to dentin walls, and can have high biocompatibility. Newly developed resin sealers also have lower working times and increased radiopacity. It is important to note that AH26, an epoxy resin sealer that preceded the development of AH Plus, gives off formaldehyde as it sets. It is very toxic during the preparation process. Newer versions of this sealer allow for polymerization without formaldehyde formation.

87. **What is the ideal storage option for an avulsion of a tooth for the time between the trauma and reimplantation?**
Attachment damage is inevitable in the case of an avulsed tooth. To prevent additional damage to the periodontal ligament cells and physiologic metabolism, dry time should be limited. Hank's Balanced Salt Solution (HBSS) found in the "Save-A-Tooth," preserving system is the ideal storage material. It has ideal pH and osmolality and can keep the PDL cells viable prior to implantation. It is often stored in schools and at the site of sporting events. If HBSS is not available, a good alternative is milk which allows for 3 hours of cell vitality. Milk has a pH comparable to vital cells and is usually free of bacteria. If necessary, the tooth can be stored in the mouth using saliva as the storage medium given the pH is close to that of vital cells.

88. **What is regenerative endodontics?**
Regeneration procedures can be used to treat a necrotic tooth with an immature root to allow development of the apical hard tissues. Regeneration has been described as tissue engineering as it uses the blood clot beneath an MTA plug to serve as a scaffold for dental pulp stem cells and growth factors. The requirements for regeneration cases include a tooth with a necrotic pulp, no requirement for a post/core or final crown, a compliant patient and parent, and no known allergies to medicines used during the procedure. The goal of regeneration procedures is both the elimination of apical pathosis and increases in both root length and width.

89. **How can you tell the difference between internal inflammatory root resorption (IRR), external inflammatory root resorption (ERR), and replacement resorption (ankylosis) radiographically?**
IRR appears radiographically as an oval or round shape within the canal and is continuous with the root canal space. IRR is treatable if it has not perforated the root structure with root canal therapy. ERR presents radiographically with a moth-eaten appearance, and the canal is often visible through the defect. It may be treated in the early stages with root canal therapy, or with newly developed protocols using bioceramic sealers and putty materials (Figs. 7-3 and 7-4).

90. **What is BRONJ (bisphosphonate-related osteonecrosis of the jaw) and how does it affect dental treatment planning in endodontics?**
BRONJ is defined as exposed bone in the maxillofacial region for more than 8 weeks in someone who has not undergone radiation therapy and who is currently or has been treated with bisphosphonates. It is important to take into consideration both the amount of time a patient has been receiving these

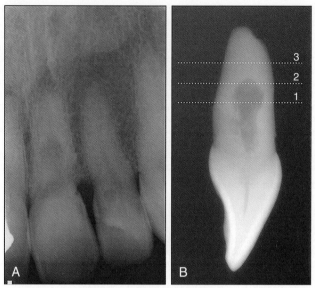

Fig. 7-3. Internal root resorption. (Patel S, Ricucci D, Durak C, Tay F: Internal root resorption: a review, J Endod 36(7):1107–1121, 2010.)

medications and the route of administration. IV Bisphosphonates have an increased chance of causing BRONJ compared to oral preparations. To decrease the risk, oral surgery, including extractions, should be avoided if patients are receiving IV bisphosphonates. Performing endodontic therapy on nonrestorable teeth that may have otherwise been recommended for extraction may be a safer treatment option for these patients.

91. What is the likelihood of two canals in the mesial buccal root of a first molar?
    Newer studies that utilize CBCT imaging have found that they exist up to 92% of the time.

92. Describe the current protocol for regeneration procedures.
    The first appointment should include standard local anesthetic, isolation, and access, with gentle debridement of the pulp tissue. A nontoxic but antibacterial irrigation system of diluted 1.5% to 3% sodium hypochlorite followed by an EDTA, or saline rinse is used to disinfect the canal. An intracanal medicament is placed for 2 to 4 weeks. Earlier methods employed a triple antibiotic paste between visits to disinfect the root canal system; however, newly accepted protocols utilize calcium hydroxide as it is less damaging to apical stem cells. At the second appointment, an endodontic file is used to over instrument into the apical tissues to induce bleeding. This causes an influx of blood and apical papilla stem cells into the canal. MTA is placed over the blood clot at the level of the CEJ, and a 3 to 4 mm layer of glass ionomer is used to close. Follow-up appointments to monitor healing should occur at 6, 12, and 24 months.

93. Describe K-files and Hedstroms?
    K-files are stainless steel, ground-twisted files machined on a lathe. They are either a triangular, square, or rhombus in shape and are machine twisted to create the sharp cutting edges called the rake angle. K-files are the strongest files and cut the least aggressively. They can be used in a watch-winding motion or a rasping motion. Hedstroms are also made of stainless steel but differ from K-files as they visually appear to resemble a screw. They have high cutting efficiency based on the high rake angle. Hedstroms can be used only in a retracting motion as they are impossible to withdraw from the canal once locked into the dentin.

94. Discuss nickel-titanium instruments and their properties, function, and application in cleaning and shaping the root canal system.
    Nickel-titanium (Ni-Ti) alloy has clinical applications in endodontics as it has a low elastic modulus and a wide elastic working range which allows for improved negotiation of curved canals. The Ni-Ti alloy used in endodontic files is conditioned to have superplastic behavior and shape memory. It consists of 55% weight nickel and 45% weighted titanium. Ni-Ti exists in three phases: the austenite phase exists at high temperatures and low stresses, the martensite phase exists at lower temperatures and higher stresses, and the R phase exists during transformation from the austenite to the martensite phase. Ni-Ti in the martensite phase is more stable and fracture resistant, and newer "M-wire" rotary files have been developed to exist in the martensite phase at room

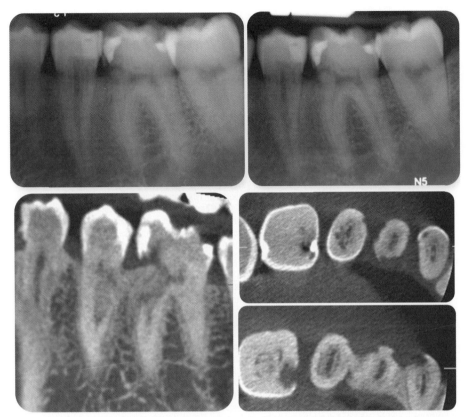

Fig. 7-4. External root resorption, top row: PA radiographs showing mesial external resorption #19, and distal external resorption #20. Botton row: CBCT images showing extent of resorptive defects. (Patel K, Mannocci F, Patel S: The assessment and management of external cervical resorption with periapical radiographs and cone-beam computed tomography: a clinical study, J Endod 42(10):1435–1440, 2016.)

temperature. The risk of instrument separation occurs during transformation from one crystalline phase to the other due to a change in rotational speed and resistance while instrumenting curved canals.

95. **How does filing differ from a reaming action and watch-winding motion?**
A filing action works by removing dentin as the file is withdrawn from the canal. The file is placed inside the canal and pressed laterally while withdrawing it to scrape the canal wall. No rotational motion is applied to the file. Reaming involves placing the file in the canal and rotating it clockwise before it is withdrawn. A watch-winding action can be used to negotiate canals and work files into place. This involves placing the file in the canal and reciprocating it back and forth with light pressure in a clockwise-counterclockwise direction.

96. **Why is it so important to tell your patient that a permanent restoration is needed following endodontic therapy?**
Permanent restorations are necessary to prevent bacterial leakage into the root canal system from the oral cavity. Studies have shown that a permanent restoration which properly seals the tooth is just as important as a high-quality endodontic procedure. Without a permanent restoration, bacterial leakage can occur in addition to coronal tooth structure loss, caries, or fracture. As endodontically treated teeth have been shown to be more stiff than untreated teeth, full coverage restorations should be considered to reduce the likelihood of fracture in molars and premolars. The overall prognosis for an endodontically treated tooth is decreased without the proper follow-up restorative care.

97. **What are some properties and advantages of the newly marketed bioceramic cements?**
New bioceramic sealers improve the dilemma of toxicity to the apical tissues in the instance of extrusion. They have the desired effect of modulating the apical tissues by diffusion of molecules following endodontic treatment. They were designed to increase the process of osteogenesis in the apical area to enhance remineralization.

Studies show that bioceramic sealers have increased biocompatibility and increased ability for differentiation of osteoblast precursor cells, leading to increased mineralization of bone in the apical area.

98. **What are the factors that affect the overall prognosis of a perforation complication?**
Perforations are holes in the root structure created by either iatrogenic events or by biological processes such as caries or resorption. Unrepaired perforations may result in downgrowth of the epithelial attachment, leading to periodontal bone loss. Several factors influence the prognosis for a repaired perforation. Perforations in the furcation, or in the cervical area of the root, have a worse prognosis due to the potential for the periodontium to become compromised. The size of the perforation is significant as the larger the perforation, the poorer the prognosis will be. It is important to choose MTA, or a similar Bioceramic material, as they are less inflammatory and seal better than other materials. MTA further allows for the formation of cementum and ultimately, normal bone. Immediate perforation repair with MTA allows for a favorable long-term prognosis.

99. **What is the overall prognosis for separated file in a tooth that was previously disinfected properly?**
The prognosis may not be affected at all. Studies have shown that there is no change to the overall prognosis if the canal was previously disinfected prior to the separation. When an instrument breaks, removal may be attempted with ultrasonics or a cannula system such as the Endo-Extractor. If the file cannot be removed without traumatizing the surrounding structures, it is best to attempt to bypass it or just to leave it in its place and obturate around it as best as possible. The patient should be monitored for any developing apical pathology. An apicoectomy or extraction may be advised in the future if pathology persists or develops.

100. **What are the treatment recommendations for endodontic therapy during pregnancy?**
Failure to properly manage endodontic infections in a pregnant patient could place the fetus at significant risk. Treatment considerations include the use of anesthetics, analgesics, and antibiotics. It is widely accepted that lidocaine, a category B medication, is safe for pregnant patients. While the use of epinephrine should be limited to avoid decreased uterine blood flow, it is considered safe in small quantities. Bupivacaine, articaine, and mepivacaine are all category C medications and are considered less safe than lidocaine. While Citanest, or prilocaine, is a category B medication, it may cause methemoglobinemia, a potentially hypoxic event. It should be noted that if the maximum recommended dose is not exceeded, there is a low risk of methemoglobinemia. Benzocaine, typically found in most topical anesthetic preparations, is a category C medication and may cause methemoglobinemia. Topical lidocaine can be substituted for benzocaine for pregnant patients to reduce this risk. In the case of significant infection where an antibiotic is necessary, penicillin is the drug of choice during pregnancy. According to the FDA, there have been no adverse outcomes using a medication in the penicillin family during pregnancy. Acetaminophen is an analgesic medication and considered safe during pregnancy. NSAIDs are contraindicated in pregnancy as they pose a risk of birth defects and increased risk of miscarriage in the third trimester. When possible, dental treatment should be performed in the second trimester and radiographs should be limited.

101. **What are the causes of failure resulting in file separation when using rotary nickel-titanium files?**
Fatigue failure can result from overuse with prolonged rotation in a curved canal. Torsional failure can result from forcing and rotating the instrument into a narrow space. Corrosive failure is a combination of fatigue and torsional failure.

102. **Discuss the crown-down, or step-down method.**
The crown-down method involves cleaning the coronal two-thirds of the root structure before apical instrumentation. This method allows for the apical foramen to be reached more easily when determining the working length. Also, there may be less separation of rotary files as the step-down method avoids overloading these instruments with frictional wall contact. This technique also provides straight-line access to the canals and can minimize the extrusion of infected debris beyond the apex. Gates Glidden burs and orifice opening file, such as the SX in the Protaper system, can be used in initial coronal to preflare the canal.

103. **In the case of a traumatic root fracture in the mid-root area where the coronal segment has been displaced, what is the course of action?**
Reposition the segment as soon as possible and confirm its proper placement radiographically. Splinting is indicated for 4 weeks or up to 4 months if the fracture is in the cervical area. Follow-up should be done at 4 to 6 weeks to remove the splint and re-evaluate clinically and radiographically, then again at 6 to 8 weeks. Finally, 6-month and 1-year follow-ups are indicated to assess the healing. If at any point during follow-up the pulp is determined to be necrotic, endodontic therapy is recommended.

104. **What are some potential causes of endodontic failure?**
Persisting or new bacteria in the root canal system following endodontic therapy can cause failure. Failure to properly debride microbes, such as E. faecalis and fusobacterium and biofilms, cause persistent endodontic infections. Studies have shown that biofilms, which have the increased capacity to survive endodontic disinfection, exist in many infected root canal systems and are highly associated with the presence of abscesses,

granulomas, and cysts. Bacterial leakage during or following treatment, such as failure to use a rubber dam, or not placing a sufficient permanent restoration could lead to failure. Bacterial leakage from the saliva has been found to cause contamination of the root canal system in as little as 3 days. Other possible causes of endodontic failure include complications such as separated files, perforations, obturation material that extends beyond the apex, and failure to locate and treat all canals.

105. How is gutta-percha removed during retreatment endodontic procedures?
Following access, the coronal gutta-percha can be removed with Gates Glidden burs or a heated plugger. Solvents, such as chloroform, can be placed in the canal space to soften the obturation material aiding in its removal. Chloroform solvent should be used with care or avoided as it is carcinogenic. Hedstroms, files, and rotary systems can be used to pull gutta-percha toward the canal orifice. It is important to avoid ledging and apical perforation during retreatment cases.

106. What is dens invaginatus, and how should these cases be treated?
Dens invaginatus (DI), or dens in dente, is a dental anomaly that is caused by invagination of the enamel into the dental papilla during osteogenesis. It appears radiographically as a tooth within a tooth and most commonly occurs in maxillary lateral incisors. DI can be categorized as type I, II, or III and varies by the degree to which it penetrates the affected tooth and root structure. Depending on the stage of root development, endodontic therapy, pulpotomy, apexification, or regeneration is indicated when either irreversible pulpitis or pulp necrosis is diagnosed. DI that is found in a healthy tooth should be treated with a sealant or a small restoration. CBCT imaging can be useful in correct diagnosis and treatment plan decisions.

SURGERY

107. What are some indications for an apical surgery?
1. Failure of nonsurgical retreatment endodontic therapy
2. Failure of nonsurgical endodontic treatment where retreatment would not be possible, or improve the outcome
3. When a biopsy is necessary

108. Epinephrine is the most effective and widely used medicine for vasoconstriction in dentistry. Explain why and how it can be utilized in apical surgical techniques.
Epinephrine works on the alpha-adrenergic receptors which predominate in the oral mucosa. Stimulation of the alpha receptors results in the contraction of smooth muscle cells in the microvasculature which then reduces the blood flow. Anesthetics with a higher concentration of epinephrine, such as lidocaine, with 1:50,000 instead of 1:100,000 can reduce blood flow resulting in increased visibility, postoperative hemostasis, and shorter working time. Hemostatic cotton pellets that contain 0.55 mg racemic epinephrine can be used locally to reduce bleeding without any adverse changes to cardiac status.

109. What flap design would be best utilized in the apicoectomy of an anterior maxillary incisor with a porcelain crown?
A full mucoperiosteal flap should be avoided in this case. It is intrasulcular and involves the reflection of the marginal and interdental gingival tissues causing a higher chance of postoperative recession affecting the esthetics. The alternative and better option is a submarginal incision, or Oschenbein-Luebke technique, which preserves the marginal and interdental papilla. The practitioner must be cautious to make sure the flap is made and repositioned over solid bone, thus requiring the need for careful periodontal evaluation. Increased bleeding, flap shrinkage, and possible scar formation are potential postoperative issues.

110. What is the proper size for the osteotomy, or surgical window?
The osteotomy should be as conservative as possible to improve outcomes. However, it is important that the window is large enough to allow for proper visualization and access for the retro-preparation and retro-sealing portions of the surgery.

111. What are some advantages of endodontic microsurgery vs. traditional surgical procedures that were used previously?
Surgical microscopes and illumination have allowed for a smaller osteotomy. Microsurgical instruments have been developed to better fit the decreased size bone window while maintaining ideal comfort and handling. Ultrasonic use in microsurgery has allowed for properly cleaned isthmuses and retro-preparations that are in line with the canal. Finally, the use of MTA as a root end material has contributed to the improved success rates of apical surgery.

112. Why is MTA an ideal root-end material?
MTA has many advantages over the previously used root-filling materials, such as amalgam and S-EBA. MTA is biocompatible, radiopaque, and hydrophilic, which is important as it must provide an excellent apical seal in the presence of blood. It forms hard tissues with the formation of new cementum, and it provides better surgical

outcomes compared to other root-filling materials. Newer bioceramic materials are being used in apical surgery that offer easier handling but similar biocompatibility properties of traditional MTA.

113. **What is the purpose of a scalloped horizontal incision in a mucogingival flap?**
A scalloped horizontal incision provides a guide for repositioning the flap during suturing. The scalloping should replicate the shape of the corresponding gingival margin.

114. **What is the purpose of root resection, and what are the guidelines?**
Root resection is done to remove the maximum number of accessory and lateral canals in the apical root structure without compromising crown-root ratio. 3 mm of root resection has been found to reduce these anatomic entities often leading to failure. The resection should be done perpendicular to the angle of the root with no bevel angle. Older methods suggested that beveled root resections would improve visibility and provide ease in the placement of the retro filling material. Presently, guidelines depict a zero-degree bevel to avoid periodontal-endodontic communications, to limit the amount of buccal plate removal which impacts healing, and to expose fewer dentinal tubules, thus improving leakage and contamination.

115. **How is methylene blue dye used in apical surgery?**
Methylene blue dye is a biocompatible dye that can stain vital tissue, allowing for clear visualization of the periodontal ligament following resection of the apical root structure. Methylene blue dye can also be used to better visualize fractures or to identify isthmuses in resection and retro-preparation.

116. **What is the purpose of the apicoectomy procedure?**
An apicoectomy is a surgical procedure performed to address endodontic failure, where retreatment endodontic therapy either cannot be performed or will not allow for resolution of the infection. Poor obturation, remnants of necrotic tissue in the accessory canals of the apical delta, and tissue that has been left in the canal during nonsurgical treatment are potential causes of endodontic failure and subsequent infection. This procedure also addresses the apical lesion and calls for curettage and biopsy of the tissue. Resecting and resealing the apical portion of the canal ensures protection from future bacterial leakage and the recurrence of the apical lesion. MTA and bioceramic materials are used in root end fillings to allow cementum reformation, a reestablished PDL, and apical bone repair.

117. **What are the advantages of piezo ultrasonics in apical surgery?**
The goal of retro-preparation is to clean and shape the apical portion of the canal so that a retro-filling material can be placed, providing an apical seal. Piezo Ultrasonic tips are an improvement to traditional burs in high-speed handpieces as they allow for better access to the surgical site and better removal of tissue and debris. Ultrasonics create conservative preparations that are in line with the canal anatomy and extend to the proper depth and they can better prepare the isthmus if one is present.

118. **What are the three principles of microsurgery?**
The three principles of endodontic microsurgery are magnification, illumination, and instruments. Surgical operating microscopes with bright focused light allow for smaller osteotomies, resulting in less removal of healthy buccal bone. Less removal of the buccal cortical plate results in faster and less painful healing. New surgical instruments reduced in size have been developed to fit in a smaller osteotomy. Mirrors, pluggers, curettes, and ultrasonic tips have been fabricated so that the handles are the traditional size, but the working ends can function easily in the 4- to 5-mm osteotomy site.

119. **What is the importance of cleaning the apical isthmus?**
Isthmuses are defined as connections between two canals that usually contain tissue. They are part of the root canal anatomy which must be disinfected and sealed and are often difficult to clean in traditional nonsurgical root canal procedures. The incidence of isthmuses is highest in the mesial root of mandibular first molars and the mesial buccal root of maxillary first molars. With the use of ultrasonics in microsurgery, one can prepare the isthmus to connect the two canals and remove tissue that may otherwise cause a potential failure.

120. **What is the ideal suture material available for apical surgery?**
A monofilament synthetic suture is the optimal choice for apical surgery. They have no wicking effect and have the flexibility of silk but cause less inflammation and plaque buildup. Chromic gut or resorbable sutures can be used if the patient cannot return for suture removal. However, they are less ideal as they can cause inflammation to the tissues until they are resorbed completely or removed. Nonresorbable suture removal is recommended between 48 and 96 hours post-op.

121. **When performing an apicoectomy on the mesial buccal root of a first molar, the sinus floor is perforated. How do you manage this complication?**
Perforation of the Schneiderian membrane which covers the sinus floor can be perforated during apical surgery due to anatomic proximity or extent of the periapical pathology. It is important to keep the sinus free of materials during treatment. Postoperatively, the patient is advised not to blow or force air through their nose. A decongestant such as Sudafed is recommended for 1 week. Traditionally, a prophylactic antibiotic such as Augmentin is prescribed for 1 week following the complication, but some newer studies disagree with this practice.

122. **Guided tissue regeneration (GTR) techniques have been studied to improve outcomes in the cases of lesions that evade both the buccal and palatal bone and large periapical defects. Describe GTR and how it works.**

GTR is a form of tissue engineering that has been theorized to improve healing outcomes in apical endodontic infections. The placement of a membrane in periodontal surgery functions to prevent the downgrowth of epithelial cells on the denuded root surface. It allows and guides PDL progenitor stem cells to form PDL and cementoblasts on the root surface. It has not been shown in periapical surgery to be beneficial to place a membrane for the loss of only one bony wall. However, it may be advantageous to use a resorbable membrane in the case of a through-and-through defect. While it is still unclear if the long-term prognosis will improve in the case of GTR for periapical lesions, endodontic-periodontal lesions with apicomarginal defects that communicate with the alveolar crest may benefit the most from membrane placement. The use of bone grafts may serve as a scaffold in periapical healing, but they have not been shown to induce the regeneration of apical tissues on their own.

123. **What mistake is most often made when performing apical surgery on the mesial buccal root of maxillary first molars?**

It is critical to look for and treat the second mesial buccal canal, if present. The canal lies lingual to the mesial buccal canal and proper resection that extends to cover the entire root surface is necessary. Methylene blue dye can be used to identify the PDL and ensure the entire root end has been removed, revealing the possibly untreated mesial lingual canal.

124. **What type of scalpel is best used for intraoral incision and drainage of an endodontic abscess?**

A no. 11 or 12 blade is preferred to a no. 5 blade.

BIBLIOGRAPHY

American Association of Endodontics. *Glossary of Endodontic Terms*. 7th ed. Chicago; 2003.

American Association of Endodontics. *The Recommended Guidelines of the American Association of Endodontists for The Treatment of Traumatic Dental Injuries*. 2016;21. https://www.aae.org/specialty/clinical-resources/treatment-planning/traumatic-dental-injuries/.

American Association of Endodontists: *Clinical Considerations for a Regenerative Procedure*. Revised 5/18/21. https://www.aae.org/specialty/wp-content/uploads/sites/2/2021/08/ClinicalConsiderationsApprovedByREC062921.pdf.

American Association of Endodontists: *AAE and AAOMR Joint Position Statement Use of Cone Beam Computed Tomographic in Endodontics*. 2015/2016 Update. https://www.asds.ca/uploads/source/resources/conebeamstatement.pdf.

American Association of Endodontists. *AAE Position Statement. Scope of Endodontics: Regenerative Endodontics*. 2013. Revised by Regenerative Endodontics Committee. https://www.aae.org/specialty/wp-content/uploads/sites/2/2017/06/scopeofendo_regendo.pdf.

American Association of Endodontists. *Endodontics Colleagues of Excellence: Use and Abuse of Antibiotics*; 2012. https://www.aae.org/specialty/wp-content/uploads/sites/2/2017/06/ecfewinter12final.pdf.

American Association of Endodontists. *Endodontics Colleagues of Excellence: AAE Guideline on Antibiotic Prophylaxis for Patients at Risk for Systemic Disease*. 2017. https://www.aae.org/specialty/wp-content/uploads/sites/2/2017/06/aae_antibiotic-prophylaxis.pdf.

American Association of Endodontists: *Glossary Contemporary Terminology for Endodontics*, 10th ed. Revised 3/2020. https://www.aae.org/specialty/clinical-resources/glossary-endodontic-terms.

American Association of Endodontists. *Use of Microscopes and Other Magnification Devices*. 2012. https://www.aae.org/specialty/wp-content/uploads/sites/2/2017/06/microscopesstatement.pdf.

American Association of Oral and Maxillofacial Surgeons. *Position Paper on Bisphosphonate-Related Osteonecrosis of the Jaw*. Update 2009. https://www.aae.org/specialty/wp-content/uploads/sites/2/2017/07/bonj_aaoms_statement.pdf.

American Dental Association-Appointed Members of the Expert W. Voting Panels Contributing to the Development of American Academy of Orthopedic Surgeons Appropriate Use Criteria: American Dental Association guidance for utilizing appropriate use criteria in the management of the care of patients with orthopedic implants undergoing dental procedures. *J Am Dent Assoc*. 2017;148:57–59.

Andersson L, Andreasen JO, Day P, et al. Guidelines for the management of traumatic dental injuries: 2. Avulsion of permanent teeth. *Pediatr Dent*. 2018;40(6):424–431.

Andreasen JO, Borum MK, Jacobsen HL, Andreasen FM. Replantation of 400 avulsed permanent incisors. 1. Diagnosis of healing complications. *Dent Traumatol*. 1995;11(2):51–58.

Appelbe OK, Sedgley CM. Effects of prolonged exposure to alkaline pH on Enterococcus faecalis survival and specific gene transcripts. *Oral Microbiol Immunol*. 2007;22(3):169–174.

Ather A, Zhong S, Rosenbaum AJ, Quinonez RB, Khan AA. Pharmacotherapy during pregnancy: an endodontic perspective. *J Endod*. 2020;46(9):1185–1194.

Attin T, Paque F, Ajam F, Lennon AM. Review of the current status of tooth whitening with the walking bleach technique. *Int Endod J*. 2003;36(5):313–329.

Barkhordar RA, Stark MM. Sealing ability of intermediate restorations and cavity design used in endodontics. *Oral Surg Oral Med Oral Pathol*. 1990;69(1):99–101.

Basrani BR, Manek S, Sodhi RN, Fillery E, Manzur A. Interaction between sodium hypochlorite and chlorhexidine gluconate. *J Endod*. 2007;33(8):966–969.

Baumgardner KR, Taylor J, Walton R. Canal adaptation and coronal leakage: lateral condensation compared to Thermafil. *J Am Dent Assoc*. 1995;126(3):351–356.

Baumgartner JC, Ibay AC. The chemical reactions of irrigants used for root canal debridement. *J Endod*. 1987;13(2):47–51.

Baumgartner JC, Xia T. Antibiotic susceptibility of bacteria associated with endodontic abscesses. *J Endod*. 2003;29(1):44–47.

Baumgartner JC, Watkins BJ, Bae KS, Xia T. Association of black-pigmented bacteria with endodontic infections. *J Endod*. 1999;25(6):413–415.

Bender IB. Pulpal pain diagnosis-a review. *J Endod*. 2000;26:175–179.

Bergenholtz G, Lindhe J. Effect of soluble plaque factors on inflammatory reactions in the dental pulp. *Scand J Dent Res.* 1975;83:153.

Blair HA. Evaluation of sealing properties of endodontic filling materials and techniques. A preliminary study. *J Ky Dent Assoc.* 1972;24(3):36–38.

Blicher B, Pryles R, Lin J. *Endodontics Review, A Study Guide.* Hanover Park: Quintessence Publishing Co, Inc; 2016.

Blicher B. *American Association of Endodontists. Differentiating Resorption.* 2021. https://www.aae.org/specialty/communique/differentiating-resorption/.

Blomlöf L, Lindskog S, Andersson L, Hedström KG, Hammarström L. Storage of experimentally avulsed teeth in milk prior to replantation. *J Dent Res.* 1983;62(8):912–916.

Botero TM, Mantellini MG, Song W, Hanks CT, Nör JE. Effect of lipopolysaccharides on vascular endothelial growth factor expression in mouse pulp cells and macrophages. *Eur J Oral Sci.* 2003;111(3):228–234.

Botero TM, Shelburne CE, Holland GR, Hanks CT, Nör JE. TLR4 mediates LPS-induced VEGF expression in odontoblasts. *J Endod.* 2006;32(10):951–955.

Bourgeois RS, Lemon RR. Dowel space preparation and apical leakage. *J Endod.* 1981;7(2):66–69.

Bramante CM, Berbert AA. A critical evaluation of some methods of determining tooth length. *Oral Surg Oral Med Oral Pathol.* 1974;37(3):463–473.

Brannstrom M, Astrom A. The hydrodynamics of the dentine: its possible relationship to dentinal pain. *Int Dent J.* 1972;22:219–227.

Brannstrom M. Sensitivity of dentin. *Oral Surg.* 1966;21:517.

Brännström M, Garberoglio R. The dentinal tubules and the odontoblast processes a scanning electron microscopic study. *Acta Odontol Scand.* 1972;30(3):291–311.

Brothman P. A comparative study of the vertical and lateral condensation of gutta-percha. *J Endod.* 1981;7:27.

Buchanan LS. Management of the curved root canal: Predictably treating the most common endodontic complexity. *J Calif Dent Assoc.* 1989;17:40–45.

Buckley JA, Ciancio SG, McMullen JA. Efficacy of epinephrine concentration in local anesthesia during periodontal surgery. *J Periodontol.* 1984;55(11):653–657.

Buffie CG, Jarchum I, Equinda M, et al. Profound alterations of intestinal microbiota following a single dose of clindamycin results in sustained susceptibility to *Clostridium difficile*-induced colitis. *Infect Immun.* 2012;80(1):62–73.

Byers MR, Sugaya A. Odontoblast processes in dentin revealed by fluorescent Di-I. *J Histochem Cytochem.* 1995;43(2):159–168.

Caldwell DE, Atuku E, Wilkie DC, et al. Germ theory vs. community theory in understanding and controlling the proliferation of biofilms. *Adv Dent Res.* 1997;11(1):4–13.

Caliskan MK, Turken M. Prognosis of permanent teeth with internal resorption: a clinical review. *Endod Dent Traumatol.* 1997;13:75–81.

Cambruzzi JV, Marshall FJ, Pappin JB. Methylene blue dye: an aid to endodontic surgery. *J Endod.* 1985;11(7):311–314.

Cave SG, Freer TJ, Podlich HM. Pulp-test responses in orthodontic patients. *Aust Orthod J.* 2002;18(1):27–34.

Chang J, Zhang C, Tani-Ishii N, Shi S, Wang CY. NF-κB activation in human dental pulp stem cells by TNF and LPS. *J Dent Res.* 2005;84(11):994–998.

Chhabra RS, Huff JE, Haseman JK, Elwell MR, Peters AC. Carcinogenicity of p-chloroaniline in rats and mice. *Food Chem Toxicol.* 1991;29(2):119–124.

Chugal NM, Clive JM, Spångberg LS. Endodontic treatment outcome: effect of the permanent restoration. *Oral Surg Oral Med Oral Pathol Oral Radiol Endod.* 2007;104(4):576–582.

Cohen B. *Pathways of the Pulp.* 8th ed. St. Louis, Missouri: Mosby; 2002.

Crump MC, Natkin E. Relationship of broken root canal instruments to endodontic case prognosis: a clinical investigation. *J Am Dent Assoc.* 1970;80(6):1341–1347.

Cvek M. A clinical report on partial pulpotomy and capping with calcium hydroxide in permanent incisors with complicated crown fracture. *J Endod.* 1978;4(8):232–237.

Delai D, Bernardi A, Felippe GS, da Silveira Teixeira C, Felippe WT, Felippe MCS. Florid cemento-osseous dysplasia: a case of misdiagnosis. *J Endod.* 2015;41(11):1923–1926.

Deveaux E, Hildelbert P, Neut C, Romond CB. Bacterial microleakage of Cavit, IRM, TERM, and Fermit: a 21-day in vitro study. *J Endod.* 1999;25(10):653–659.

Diogenes A, Ruparel NB, Shiloah Y, Hargreaves KM. Regenerative endodontics: a way forward. *J Am Dent Assoc.* 2016;147(5):372–380.

DiRenzo A, Gresla T, Johnson BR, Rogers M, Tucker D, BeGole EA. Postoperative pain after 1-and 2-visit root canal therapy. *Oral Surg Oral Med Oral Pathol Oral Radiol Endod.* 2002;93(5):605–610.

Doyle SL, Hodges JS, Pesun IJ, Baisden MK, Bowles WR. Factors affecting outcomes for single-tooth implants and endodontic restorations. *J Endod.* 2007;33(4):399–402.

Drake DR, Wiemann AH, Rivera EM, Walton RE. Bacterial retention in canal walls in vitro: effect of smear layer. *J Endod.* 1994;20(2):78–82.

Dutner J, Mines P, Anderson A. Irrigation trends among American Association of Endodontists members: a web-based survey. *J Endod.* 2012;38(1):37–40.

Ellis SGS. Incomplete tooth fracture–proposal for a new definition. *Br Dent J.* 2001;190(8):424–428.

Emilson CG. Susceptibility of various microorganisms to chlorhexidine. *Eur J Oral Sci.* 1977;85(4):255–265.

Evans M, Davies JK, Sundqvist G, Figdor M. Mechanisms involved in the resistance of *Enterococcus faecalis* to calcium hydroxide. *Int Endod J.* 2002;35(3):221–228.

Fayad MI, Ashkenaz PJ, Johnson BR. Different representations of vertical root fractures detected by cone-beam volumetric tomography: a case series report. *J Endod.* 2012;38(10):1435–1442.

Ford TRP, Torabinejad M, McKendry DJ, Hong CU, Kariyawasam SP. Use of mineral trioxide aggregate for repair of furcal perforations. *Oral Surg Oral Med Oral Pathol Oral Radiol Endod.* 1995;79(6):563–567.

Fors UG, Berg JO, Sandberg H. Microbiological investigation of saliva leakage between the rubber dam and tooth during endodontic treatment. *J Endod.* 1986;12(9):396–399.

Frank AL. Therapy for the divergent pulpless tooth by continued apical formation. *J Am Dent Assoc.* 1966;72(1):87–93.

Friedman S. Prognosis of initial endodontic therapy. *Endod Dent Topics.* 2002;2:59–98.

Friedman CE, Sandrik JL, Heuer MA, Rapp GW. Composition and physical properties of gutta-percha endodontic filling materials. *J Endod.* 1977;3(8):304–308.

Fuss Z, Trowbridge H, Bender IB, Rickoff B, Sorin S. Assessment of the reliability of electrical and thermal pulp testing agents. *J Endod.* 1986;12(7):301–305.

Garberoglio R, Brännström M. Scanning electron microscopic investigation of human dentinal tubules. *Arch Oral Biol.* 1976;21(6):355–362.

Garofalo RR, Ede EN, Dorn SO, Kuttler S. Effect of electronic apex locators on cardiac pacemaker function. *J Endod.* 2002;28(12):831–833.

Gartner LP, Seibel W, Hiatt JL, Provenza DV. A fine-structural analysis of mouse molar odontoblast maturation. *Cells Tissues Organs.* 1979;103(1):16–33.

Giacomino CM, Wealleans JA, Kuhn N, Diogenes A. Comparative biocompatibility and osteogenic potential of two bioceramic sealers. *J Endod.* 2019;45(1):51–56.

Giard JC, Hartke A, Flahaut S, Boutibonnes P, Auffray Y. Glucose starvation response in *Enterococcus faecalis* JH2-2: survival and protein analysis. *Res Microbiol.* 1997;148(1):7–35.

Gilheany PA, Figdor D, Tyas MJ. Apical dentin permeability and microleakage associated with root end resection and retrograde filling. *J Endod.* 1994;20(1):22–26.

Goerig AC, Michelich RJ, Schultz HH. Instrumentation of root canals in molar using the step-down technique. *J Endod.* 1982;8(12):550–554.

Gonzalez Sanchez JA, Duran-Sindreu F, Albuquerque Matos M. Apical transportation created using three different patency instruments. *Int Endod J.* 2010;43(7):560–564.

González-Martín M, Torres-Lagares D, Gutiérrez-Pérez JL, Segura-Egea JJ. Inferior alveolar nerve paresthesia after overfilling of endodontic sealer into the mandibular canal. *J Endod.* 2010;36(8):1419–1421.

Goodman A, Schilder H, Aldrich W. The thermomechanical properties of gutta-percha: II. The history and molecular chemistry of gutta-percha. *Oral Surg Oral Med Oral Pathol.* 1974;37(6):954–961.

Grossman LI. *Root Canal Therapy.* Philadelphia: Lea and Febiger; 2008:p189.

Grossman LI. Physical properties of root canal cements. *J Endod.* 1976;2(6):166–175.

Gunraj MN. Dental root resorption. *Oral Surg Oral Med Oral Pathol Oral Radiol Endod.* 1999;88(6):647–653.

Gutarts R, Nusstein J, Reader A, Beck M. In vivo debridement efficacy of ultrasonic irrigation following hand-rotary instrumentation in human mandibular molars. *J Endod.* 2005;31(3):166–170.

Gutmann JL, Harrison JW. Posterior endodontic surgery: anatomical considerations and clinical techniques. *Int Endod J.* 1985;18(1):8–34.

Haapasalo M, Ranta HE, Ranta K, Shah HR. Black-pigmented *Bacteroides* spp. in human apical periodontitis. *Infect Immun.* 1986;53(1):149–153.

Haas DA, Lennon DA. A 21 year retrospective study of reports of paresthesia following local anesthetic administration. *J Can Dent Assoc.* 1995;61(4):319–320.

Hancock III HH, Sigurdsson A, Trope M, Moiseiwitsch JB. Bacteria isolated after unsuccessful endodontic treatment in a North American population. *Oral Surg Oral Med Oral Pathol Oral Radiol Endod.* 2001;91(5):579–586.

Hargreaves KM, Cohen S. *Pathways of the Pulp.* 10th ed. St. Louis: Elsevier; 2011.

Hargreaves KM, Keiser K. Development of new pain management strategies. *J Dent Educ.* 2002;66:113–121.

Hargreaves KM, Keiser K. Local anesthetic failure in endodontics: mechanisms and management. *Endod Dent Top.* 2002;1(1):26–39.

Hargreaves KM. *American Associates of Endodontics. Colleagues of Excellence. A 3-D approach to treating acute pain. Winter 2015 Endodontics.* Colleagues for Excellence Newsletter; 2015.

Harnden DG. Tests for carcinogenicity and mitogenicity 1. *Int Endod J.* 1981;14(1):35–61.

Harrington GW, Natkin E. External resorption associated with bleaching of pulpless teeth. *J Endod.* 1979;5:344–348.

Heithersay GS, Dahlstrom SW, Marin PD. Incidence of invasive cervical resorption in bleached root filled teeth. *Aust Dent J.* 1994;39:82.

Heithersay GD. Clinical, radiographic, and histopathologic features of cervical root resorption. *Quint Int.* 1999;30(1):27–37.

Hennessey TD. Some antibacterial properties of chlorhexidine. *J Periodontol Res.* 1973;8:61–67.

Hepworth MJ, Friedman S. Treatment outcome of surgical and non-surgical management of endodontic failures. *J Can Dent Assoc.* 1997;63(5):364–371.

Hiebert BM, Abramovitch K, Rice D, Torabinejad M. Prevalence of second mesiobuccal canals in maxillary first molars detected using cone-beam computed tomography, direct occlusal access, and coronal plane grinding. *J Endod.* 2017;43(10):1711–1715.

Himel VT, Brady Jr J, Weir Jr J. Evaluation of repair of mechanical perforations of the pulp chamber floor using biodegradable tricalcium phosphate or calcium hydroxide. *J Endod.* 1985;11(4):161–165.

Hosoya S, Matsushima K. Stimulation of interleukin-1β production of human dental pulp cells by *Porphyromonas endodontalis* lipopolysaccharide. *J Endod.* 1997;23(1):39–42.

Hsu YY, Kim S. The resected root surface. The issue of canal isthmuses. *Dent Clin North Am.* 1997;41(3):529–540.

Huang GTJ, Liu J, Zhu X, et al. Pulp/dentin regeneration: It should be complicated. *J Endod.* 2020;46(9):S128–S134.

Hubble TS, Hatton JF, Nallapareddy SR, Murray BE, Gillespie MJ. Influence of *Enterococcus faecalis* proteases and the collagen–binding protein, Ace, on adhesion to dentin. *Oral Microbiol Immunol.* 2003;18(2):121–126.

Iqbal M, Kim S, Yoon F. An investigation into differential diagnosis of pulp and periapical pain: A PennEndo Database Study. *J Endod.* 2007;33(5):548–551.

Iqbal MK, Kratchman SI, Guess GM, Karabucak B, Kim S. Microscopic periradicular surgery: perioperative predictors for postoperative clinical outcomes and quality of life assessment. *J Endod.* 2007;33(3):239–244.

Jacobovitz M, De Lima RKP. Treatment of inflammatory internal root resorption with mineral trioxide aggregate: a case report. *Int Endod J.* 2008;41(10):905–912.

Jansson L, Ehnevid H. The influence of endodontic infection on periodontal status in mandibular molars. *J Periodontol.* 1998;69:1392.

Jansson L, Ehnevid J, Lindskog SF, Blomlof L. The influence of endodontic infection on progression of marginal bone loss in periodontitis. *J Clin Periodontol.* 1995;22:729.

Jew RC, Weine FS, Keene Jr JJ, Smulson MH. A histologic evaluation of periodontal tissues adjacent to root perforations filled with Cavit. *Oral Surg Oral Med Oral Pathol.* 1982;54(1):124–135.

Jiang LM, Lak B, Eijsvogels LM, Wesselink P, van der Sluis LW. Comparison of the cleaning efficacy of different final irrigation techniques. *J Endod.* 2012;38(6):838–841.

Johnson MD. *American Association of Endodontists. Endodontics Colleagues of Excellence: Fall 2019 ENDODONTICS: Colleagues for Excellence newsletter. Endodontics and Antibiotics update.* 2019.

Johnson BR, Remeikis NA. Effective shelf-life of prepared sodium hypochlorite solution. *J Endod.* 1993;19(1):40–43.

Johnson EM, Flannagan SE, Sedgley CM. Coaggregation interactions between oral and endodontic *Enterococcus faecalis* and bacterial species isolated from persistent apical periodontitis. *J Endod.* 2006;32(10):946–950.

Kaffe I, Tamse A, Schwartz Y, Buchner A, Littner MM. Changes in the lamina dura as a manifestation of systemic diseases: report of a case and review of the literature. *J Endod.* 1982;8(10):467–470.

Kakehashi S, Stanley HR, Fitzgerald RJ. The effects of surgical exposures of dental pulps in germ-free and conventional laboratory rats. *Oral Surg Oral Med Oral Pathol.* 1965;20(3). 340–334.

Kamberi B, Bajrami D, Stavileci M, Omeragiq S, Dragidella F, Koçani F. The antibacterial efficacy of biopure MTAD in root canal contaminated with *Enterococcus faecalis. Int Sch Res Not.* 2012:1–5.

Kanaa M, Whitworth J, Meechan JG. A prospective randomized trial of different supplementary local anesthetic techniques after failure of inferior alveolar nerve block in patients with irreversible pulpitis in mandibular teeth. *J Endod.* 2012;38(4):421–425.

Kapetanaki I, Dimopoulos F, Gogos C. Traditional and minimally invasive access cavities in endodontics: a literature review. *Restor Dent Endod.* 2021;46(3):e46.

Keenan JV, Farman AG, Fedorowicz Z, Newton JT. A Cochrane systematic review finds no evidence to support the use of antibiotics for pain relief in irreversible pulpitis. *J Endod.* 2006;32(2):87–92.

Kim S, Pecora G, Rubenstein R. *Color Atlas of Microsurgery in Endodontics.* Philadelphia: W.B. Saunders Company; 2001.

Kim S. Neurovascular interactions in the dental pulp in health and inflammation. *J Endod.* 1990;16(2):48–53.

Kim S. Principles of endodontic microsurgery. *Dent Clin North Am.* 1997;41(3):481–497.

Kim S, Kratchman S. Modern endodontic surgery concepts and practice: a review. *J Endod.* 2006;32(7):601–623.

Kim S, Liu M, Simchon S, Dörscher-Kim JE. Effects of selected inflammatory mediators on blood flow and vascular permeability in the dental pulp. *Proc Finn Dent Soc [Suomen Hammaslaakariseuran toimituksia].* 1992;88:387–392.

Kim SY, Kim SH, Cho SB, Lee GO, Yang SE. Different treatment protocols for different pulpal and periapical diagnoses of 72 cracked teeth. *J Endod.* 2013;39(4):449–452.

Kishi Y, Shimozato N, Takahashi K. Vascular architecture of cat pulp using corrosive resin cast under scanning electron microscope. *J Endod.* 1989;15(10):478–483.

Kowalski WJ, Kasper EL, Hatton JF, Murray BE, Nallapareddy SR, Gillespie MJ. *Enterococcus faecalis* adhesin, Ace, mediates attachment to particulate dentin. *J Endod.* 2006;32(7):634–637.

Kramer IR. The vascular architecture of the human dental pulp. *Arch Oral Biol.* 1960;2(3):177–189.

Krasner P, Rankow HJ. Anatomy of the pulp-chamber floor. *J Endod.* 2004;30(1):5–16.

Krasner P, Rankow HJ. New philosophy for the treatment of avulsed teeth. *Oral Surg Oral Med Oral Pathol Oral Radiol Endod.* 1995;79(5):616–623.

Kvist T, Rydin E, Reit C. The relative frequency of periapical lesions in teeth with root canal-retained posts. *J Endod.* 1989;15(12):578–580.

Lanza R, Langer R, Vacanti JP, Atala A, eds. *Principles of Tissue Engineering.* 5th ed. London, UK: Academic Press; 2020.

Laplace JM, Thuault M, Hartke A, Boutibonnes P, Auffray Y. Sodium hypochlorite stress in *Enterococcus faecalis*: influence of antecedent growth conditions and induced proteins. *Curr Microbiol.* 1997;34(5):284–289.

Law A, Lilly J. Trigeminal neuralgia mimicking odontogenic pain: a report of two cases. *Oral Surg Oral Med Oral Pathol Oral Radiol Endod.* 1995;80(1):96–100.

Lazzaretti DN, Bortoluzzi GS, Fernandes LFT, Rodriguez R, Grehs RA, Hartmann MSM. Histologic evaluation of human pulp tissue after orthodontic intrusion. *J Endod.* 2014;40(10):1537–1540.

Lee KW, Williams MC, Camps JJ, Pashley DH. Adhesion of endodontic sealers to dentin and gutta-percha. *J Endod.* 2002;28(10):684–688.

Leonardo MR, da Silva LAB, Tanomaru Filho M, da Silva RS. Release of formaldehyde by 4 endodontic sealers. *Oral Surg Oral Med Oral Pathol Oral Radiol Endod.* 1999;88(2):221–225.

Lilly GE. Reaction of oral tissues to suture materials. *Oral Surg Oral Med Oral Pathol.* 1968;26(1):128–133.

Lin CP, Chou HG, Kuo JC, Lan WH. The quality of ultrasonic root-end preparation: a quantitative study. *J Endod.* 1998;24(10):666–670.

Lin JC, Lu JX, Zeng Q, Zhao W, Li WQ, Ling JQ. Comparison of mineral trioxide aggregate and calcium hydroxide for apexification of immature permanent teeth: a systematic review and meta-analysis. *J Formos Med Assoc.* 2016;115(7):523–530.

Lin L, Chen MYH, Ricucci D, Rosenberg PA. Guided tissue regeneration in periapical surgery. *J Endod.* 2010;36(4):618–625.

Lin PY, Huang SH, Chang HJ, Chi LY. The effect of rubber dam usage on the survival rate of teeth receiving initial root canal treatment: a nationwide population-based study. *J Endod.* 2014;40(11):1733–1737.

Linsuwanont P, Wimonsutthikul K, Pothimoke U, Santiwong B. Treatment outcomes of mineral trioxide aggregate pulpotomy in vital permanent teeth with carious pulp exposure: the retrospective study. *J Endod.* 2017;43(2):225–230.

Loftag-Hansen S, Huumonen S, Grohndahl K, Grondahl HG. Limited cone-beam CT and intra-oral radiography for the diagnosis of periapical pathology. *Oral Surg Oral Med Oral Pathol Oral Radiol Endod.* 2007;103:114–119.

Luebke RG, Ingle JI. Geometric nomenclature for mucoperiosteal flaps. *Periodontics.* 1964;2:301–303.

Malamed SF. *Handbook of Local Anesthesia.* 6th ed. St. Louis: Mosby; 2012.

Malhotra N, Kundabala M, Acharaya SA. A review of root fractures: diagnosis, treatment and prognosis. *Dent Update.* 2011;38(9):615–628.

Mancini M, Cerroni L, Iorio L, Armellin E, Conte G, Cianconi L. Smear layer removal and canal cleanliness using different irrigation systems (EndoActivator, EndoVac, and passive ultrasonic irrigation): field emission scanning electron microscopic evaluation in an in vitro study. *J Endod.* 2013;39(11):1456–1460.

Marion D, Jean A, Hamel H, Kerebel LM, Kerebel B. Scanning electron microscopic study of odontoblasts and circumpulpal dentin in a human tooth. *Oral Surg Oral Med Oral Pathol.* 1991;72(4):473–478.

Markowitz K, Moynihan M, Liu M, Kim S. Biologic properties of eugenol and zinc oxide-eugenol: a clinically oriented review. *Oral Surg Oral Med Oral Pathol.* 1992;73(6):729–737.

Marshall F.J., Pappin J.B. *A crown-down pressureless preparation root canal enlargement technique, [technique manual].* Portland, Oregon; 1980.

Martin E, Nimmo A, Lee A, Jennings E. Articaine in dentistry: an overview of the evidence and meta-analysis of the latest randomised controlled trials on articaine safety and efficacy compared to lidocaine for routine dental treatment. *Br Dent J Open.* 2021;7:27.

Mattison GD, Delivanis PD, Thacker Jr RW, Hassell KJ. Effect of post preparation on the apical seal. *J Prosthet Dent.* 1984;51(6):785–789.

Mehlhaff DS, Harshall JG, Baumgartner JC. Comparison of ultrasonic and high-speed-bur root-end preparations using bilaterally matched teeth. *J Endod.* 1997;23(7):448–452.

Mente J, Leo M, Panagidis D, Saure D, Pfefferle T. Treatment outcome of mineral trioxide aggregate: repair of root perforations—long-term results. *J Endod.* 2014;40(6):790–796.

Meschi N, Patel B, Ruparel NB. Material pulp cells and tissue interactions. *J Endod.* 2020;46(9):S150–S160.

Möller ÅJ, Fabricius L, Dahlen G, Öhman AE, Heyden GUY. Influence on periapical tissues of indigenous oral bacteria and necrotic pulp tissue in monkeys. *Eur J Oral Sci.* 1981;89(6):475–484.

Mona M, Abbasi Z, Kobeissy F, Chahbandar A, Pileggi RA. A bioinformatics systems biology analysis of the current oral proteomic bio-markers and implications for diagnosis and treatment of external root resorption. *Int J Mol Sci.* 2021;22(6):3181.

Montagner F, Jacinto RC, Signoretti FG, Sanches PF, Gomes BP. Clustering behavior in microbial communities from acute endodontic infections. *J Endod.* 2012;38(2):158–162.

Moore PA, Dunsky JL. Bupivacaine anesthesia—a clinical trial for endodontic therapy. *Oral Surg Oral Med Oral Pathol.* 1983;55(2):176–179.

Murray PE, Garcia-Godoy F, Hargreaves KM. Regenerative endodontics: a review of current status and a call for action. *J Endod.* 2007;33(4):377–390.

Nagle D, Reader A, Beck M, Weaver J. Effect of systemic penicillin on pain in untreated irreversible pulpitis. *Oral Surg Oral Med Oral Pathol Oral Radiol Endod.* 2000;90(5):636–640.

Nair PNR, Pajarola G, Schroeder HE. Types and incidence of human periapical lesions obtained with extracted teeth. *Oral Surg Oral Med Oral Pathol Oral Radiol Endod.* 1996;8:93.

Nair M, Rahul J, Devadathan A, Mathew J. Incidence of endodontic flare-ups and its related factors: a retrospective study. *J Int Soc Prev Communit Dent.* 2017;7(4):175.

Naoum HJ, Chandler NP. Temporization for endodontics. *Int Endod J.* 2002;35(12):964–978.

Närhi M, Jyväsjärvi E, Virtanen A, Huopaniemi T, Ngassapa D, Hirvonen T. Role of intradental A- and C-type nerve fibres in dental pain mechanisms. *Proc Finn Dent Soc.* 1992;88(Suppl 1):507–516.

Neville BW, Damm DD, Allen CM, Bouquot JE. *Oral and Maxillofacial Pathology.* 2nd ed. Philadelphia: Saunders; 2002.

Nguyen TN. Obturation of the root canal system. *Pathways Pulp.* 1994;6:219–271.

Nielsen BA, Baumgartner JC. Comparison of the EndoVac system to needle irrigation of root canals. *J Endod.* 2007;33(5):611–615.

Nixon CE, Saviano JA, King GJ, Keeling SD. Histomorphometric study of dental pulp during orthodontic tooth movement. *J Endod.* 1993;19(1):13–16.

Nyman S. Bone regeneration using the principle of guided tissue regeneration. *J Clin Periodontol.* 1991;18(6):494–498.

Oguntebi BR, DeSchepper EJ, Taylor TS, White CL, Pink FE. Postoperative pain incidence related to the type of emergency treatment of symptomatic pulpitis. *Oral Surg Oral Med Oral Pathol.* 1992;73(4):479–483.

Owatz B, Khan A, Schindler W, Schwartz S, Keiser K, Hargreaves K. The incidence of mechanical allodynia in patients with irreversible pulpitis. *J Endod.* 2007;33(5):552–556.

Pak JG, White SN. Pain prevalence and severity before, during, and after root canal treatment: a systematic review. *J Endod.* 2011;37(4):429–438.

Paredes-Vieyra J, Enriquez FJJ. Success rate of single-versus two-visit root canal treatment of teeth with apical periodontitis: a randomized controlled trial. *J Endod.* 2012;38(9):1164–1169.

Parirokh M, Torabinejad M. Mineral trioxide aggregate: a comprehensive literature review—part I: chemical, physical, and antibacterial properties. *J Endod.* 2010;36(1):16–27.

Park CK, Li HY, Yeon KY, et al. Eugenol inhibits sodium currents in dental afferent neurons. *J Dent Res.* 2006;85(10):900–904.

Patel S, Dawood A, Mannocci F, Wilson R, Pitt Ford T. Detection of periapical bone defects in human jaw using cone beam computed tomography and intraoral radiography. *Int Endod J.* 2009;42(6):507–515.

Patel S, Durack C, Abella F, Shemesh H, Roig M, Lemberg K. Cone beam computed tomography in endodontics—a review. *Int Endod J.* 2015;48:3–15.

Patel S, Rhodes J. A practical guide to endodontic access cavity preparation in molar teeth. *Br Dent J.* 2007;203:133–140.

Patel K, Mannocci F, Patel S. The assessment and management of external cervical resorption with periapical radiographs and cone-beam computed tomography: a clinical study. *J Endod.* 2016;42(10):1435–1440.

Patel S, Ricucci D, Durak C, Tay F. Internal root resorption: a review. *J Endod.* 2010;36(7):1107–1121.

Patel S, Saberi N, Pimental T, Teng PH. Present status and future directions: root resorption. *Int Endod J.* 2022;55(Suppl 4):892–921.

Peciuliene V, Balciuniene I, Eriksen HM, Haapasalo M. Isolation of *Enterococcus faecalis* in previously root-filled canals in a Lithuanian population. *J Endod.* 2000;26(10):593–595.

Pécora JD, Capelli A, Guerisoli DMZ, Spanó JCED, Estrela C. Influence of cervical preflaring on apical file size determination. *Int Endod J.* 2005;38(7):430–435.

Persaud M. *Before We Are Born. Essentials of Embryology and Birth Defects.* Philadelphia: Saunders; 2003.

Polson AM, Garrett S, Stoller NH, et al. Guided tissue regeneration in human furcation defects after using a biodegradable barrier: a multi-center feasibility study. *J Periodontol.* 1995;66(5):377–385.

Portell FR, Bernier WE, Lorton L, Peters DD. The effect of immediate versus delayed dowel space preparation on the integrity of the apical seal. *J Endod.* 1982;8(4):154–160.

Prada I, Micó-Muñoz P, Giner-Lluesma T, Micó-Martínez P, Collado-Castellano N, Manzano-Saiz A. Influence of microbiology on endodontic failure. Literature review. *Medicina oral, patologia oral y cirugia bucal.* 2019;24(3):e364.

Pulyodan MK, Mohan SP, Valsan D, Divakar N, Moyin S, Thayyil S. Regenerative endodontics: a paradigm shift in clinical endodontics. *J Pharm Bioall Sci.* 2020;12(Suppl 1):S20.

Rafter M. Apexification: a review. *Dent Traumatol.* 2005;21(1):1–8.

Rahn R, Zegelman M, Brief I, Kreuzer J, Frenkel G. Susceptibility of frequency adapted cardiac pacemakers to dental treatment. *Deutsche Zahnärztliche Zeitschrift.* 1989;44(4):244–247.

Ray HA, Trope M. Periapical status of endodontically treated teeth in relation to the technical quality of the root filling and the coronal restoration. *Int Endod J.* 1995;28(1):12–18.

Ray WA, Murray KT, Hall K, Arbogast PG, Stein CM. Azithromycin and the risk of cardiovascular death. *N Engl J Med.* 2012;366(20):1881–1890.

Rickoff B, Trowbridge H, Baker J, Fuss Z, Bender IB. Effects of thermal vitality tests on human dental pulp. *J Endod.* 1988;14(10):482–485.

Ricucci D, Siqueira Jr JF. Biofilms and apical periodontitis: study of prevalence and association with clinical and histopathologic findings. *J Endod.* 2010;36(8):1277–1288.

Ricucci D, Siqueira Jr JF, Loghin S, Berman LH. The cracked tooth: histopathologic and histobacteriologic aspects. *J Endod.* 2015;41(3):343–352.

Roahen JO, Marshall FJ. The effects of periodontal ligament injection on pulpal and periodontal tissues. *J Endod.* 1990;16(1):28–33.

Roland DD, Andelin WE, Browning DF, Hsu GH, Torabinejad M. The effect of preflaring on the rates of separation for 0.04 taper nickel titanium rotary instruments. *J Endod.* 2002;28(7):543–545.

Rotstein I, Lehr T, Gedalia I. Effect of bleaching agents on inorganic components of human dentin and cementum. *J Endod.* 1992;18:290.

Rotstein I, Torek Y, Misgav R. Effect of cementum defects on radicular penetration of H_2O_2 during intracoronal bleaching. *J Endod.* 1991;17:230.

Rotstein I, Friedman S, Mor C, Katznelson J, Sommer M, Bab I. Histological characterization of bleaching-induced external root resorption in dogs. *J Endod.* 1991;17(9):436–441.

Rotstein I, Torek Y, Misgav R. Effect of cementum defects on radicular penetration of 30% H_2O_2 during intracoronal bleaching. *J Endod.* 1991;17(5):230–233.

Rotstein I, Zalkind M, Mor C, Tarabeah A, Friedman S. In vitro efficacy of sodium perborate preparations used for intracoronal bleaching of discolored non–vital teeth. *Dent Traumatol.* 1991;7(4):177–180.

Ruddle CJ. Nonsurgical retreatment. *J Endod.* 2004;30(12):827–845.

Russell AD, Day MJ. Antibacterial activity of chlorhexidine. *J Hosp Infect.* 1993;25(4):229–238.

Saber SM, Hayaty DM, Nawar NN, Kim HC. The effect of access cavity designs and sizes of root canal preparations on the biomechanical behavior of an endodontically treated mandibular first molar: a finite element analysis. *J Endod.* 2020;46(11):1675–1681.

Safavi KE, Nichols FC. Alteration of biological properties of bacterial lipopolysaccharide by calcium hydroxide treatment. *J Endod.* 1994;20(3):127–129.

Santosh SS, Ballal S, Natanasabapathy V. Influence of minimally invasive access cavity designs on the fracture resistance of endodontically treated mandibular molars subjected to thermocycling and dynamic loading. *J Endod.* 2021;47(9):1496–1500.

Sathorn C, Parashos P, Messer H. The prevalence of postoperative pain and flare–up in single–and multiple–visit endodontic treatment: a systematic review. *Int Endod J.* 2008;41(2):91–99.

Schein B, Schilder H. Endotoxin content in endodontically involved teeth. *J Endod.* 1975;1(1):19–21.

Schilder H. Filling root canals in three dimensions. *Dent Clin North Am.* 1967;11(3):723–744.

Seltzer S, Bender IB, Ziontz M. The dynamics of pulp inflammation: correlations between diagnostic data and actual histologic findings in the pulp. *Oral Surg Oral Med Oral Pathol.* 1963;16:969–971.

Seltzer S, Bender IB, Nazimov H. Differential diagnosis of pulp conditions. *Oral Surg Oral Med Oral Pathol Oral Radiol Endod.* 1965;19:383–391.

Seltzer S, Naidorf IJ. Flare ups in endodontics. I. Etiological factors. *J Endod.* 2004;30(7):476–481.

Seltzer S. Long-term radiographic and histological observations of endodontically treated teeth. *J Endod.* 1999;25(12):818–822.

Sessle BJ, Hu JW, Amano N, Zhong G. Convergence of cutaneous, tooth pulp, visceral, neck and muscle afferents onto nociceptive and non-nociceptive neurones in trigeminal subnucleus caudalis (medullary dorsal horn) and its implications for referred pain. *Pain.* 1986;27(2):219–235.

Seto BG, Nicholls JI, Harrington GW. Torsional properties of twisted and machined endodontic files. *J Endod.* 1990;16(8):355–360.

Shabahang S, Torabinejad M, Boyne PP, Abedi H, McMillan PA. A comparative study of root-end induction using osteogenic protein-1, calcium hydroxide, and mineral trioxide aggregate in dogs. *J Endod.* 1999;25(1):1–5.

Sigurdsson A. Decoronation as an approach to treat ankylosis in growing children. *Pediatr Dent.* 2009;31(2):123–128.

Simard-Savoie S. New method for comparing the activity of local anesthetics used in dentistry. *J Dent Res.* 1975;54(5):978–981.

Simon JH, Glick DH, Frank AL. The relationship of endodontic-periodontic lesions. *J Clin Periodontol.* 1972;43:202.

Simon JHS. Incidence of periapical cysts in relation to the root canal. *J Endod.* 1980;6:845.

Siqueira Jr JF. Microbial causes of endodontic flare–ups. *Int Endod J.* 2003;36(7):453–463.

Siqueira Jr JF. Reaction of periradicular tissues to root canal treatment: benefits and drawbacks. *Endodont Topics.* 2005;10(1):123–147.

Siqueira Jr JF, Rôças IN. Exploiting molecular methods to explore endodontic infections: part 1—current molecular technologies for microbiological diagnosis. *J Endod.* 2005;31(6):411–423.

Siqueira Jr JF, Rôças IN, Hernández SR, et al. Dens invaginatus: clinical implications and antimicrobial endodontic treatment considerations. *J Endod.* 2021;48(2):161–170.

Sirén EK, Haapasalo MP, Waltimo TM, Ørstavik D. In vitro antibacterial effect of calcium hydroxide combined with chlorhexidine or iodine potassium iodide on *Enterococcus faecalis. Eur J Oral Sci.* 2004;112(4):326–331.

Sjogren U, Hagglund B, Sudqvist G, Wing K. Factors affecting the long-term results of endodontic treatment. *J Endod.* 1990;16:498.

Sjögren ULF, Hägglund B, Sundqvist G, Wing K. Factors affecting the long-term results of endodontic treatment. *J Endod.* 1990;16(10):498–504.

Sjögren U, Figdor D, Spångberg L, Sundqvist G. The antimicrobial effect of calcium hydroxide as a short–term intracanal dressing. *Int Endod J.* 1991;24(3):119–125.

Skinner RL, Himel VT. The sealing ability of injection-molded thermoplasticized gutta-percha with and without the use of sealers. *J Endod.* 1987;13(7):315–317.

Sollecito TP, Abt E, Lockhart PB, et al. The use of prophylactic antibiotics prior to dental procedures in patients with prosthetic joints: evidence-based clinical practice guideline for dental practitioners—a report of the American Dental Association Council on Scientific Affairs. *J Am Dent Assoc.* 2015;146. 11-6.e8.

Sorensen JA, Martinoff JT. Intracoronal reinforcement and coronal coverage: a study of endodontically treated teeth. *J Prosthet Dent.* 1984;51(6):780–784.

Spångberg LS, Barbosa SV, Lavigne GD. AH26 releases formaldehyde. *J Endod.* 1993;19(12):596–598.

Stein TJ, Corcoran JF. Anatomy of the root apex and its histologic changes with age. *Oral Surg Oral Med Oral Pathol.* 1990;69(2):238–242.

Steiner DR, West JD. A method to determine the location and shape of an intracoronal bleach barrier. *J Endod.* 1994;20(6):304–306.

Sunada I. New method for measuring the length of the root canal. *J Dent Res.* 1962;41(2):375–387.

Sunde PT, Olsen I, Debelian GJ, Tronstad L. Microbiota of periapical lesions refractory to endodontic therapy. *J Endod.* 2002;28(4):304–310.

Sundqvist G. Ecology of the root canal flora. *J Endod.* 1992;18(9):427–430.

Sundqvist G. *Bacteriological studies of necrotic dental pulps (Doctoral dissertation, Umeå University)*; 1976.

Sundqvist G, Figdor D, Persson S, Sjögren U. Microbiologic analysis of teeth with failed endodontic treatment and the outcome of conservative re-treatment. *Oral Surg Oral Med Oral Pathol Oral Radiol Endod.* 1998;85(1):86–93.

Sundqvist G, Johansson E, Sjögren U. Prevalence of black-pigmented bacteroides species in root canal infections. *J Endod.* 1989;15(1):13–19.

Suter B. A new method for retrieving silver points and separated instruments from root canals. *J Endod.* 1998;24(6):446–448.

Svensäter G, Bergenholtz G. Biofilms in endodontic infections. *Endodont Topics.* 2004;9(1):27–36.

Tabassum S, Khan FR. Failure of endodontic treatment: The usual suspects. *Eur J Dent.* 2016;10(01):144–147.

Takahashi K, Kishi Y, Kim SA. A scanning electron microscope study of the blood vessels of dog pulp using corrosion resin casts. *J Endod.* 1982;8(3):131–135.

Taschieri S, Corbella S, Tsesis I, Bortolin M, Del Fabbro M. Effect of guided tissue regeneration on the outcome of surgical endodontic treatment of through-and-through lesions: a retrospective study at 4-year follow-up. *Oral Maxillofac Surg.* 2011;15(3):153–159.

Tavares WLF, de Brito LCN, Henriques LCF, et al. The impact of chlorhexidine-based endodontic treatment on periapical cytokine expression in teeth. *J Endod.* 2013;39(7):889–892.

Tidmarsh BG, Arrowsmith MG. Dentinal tubules at the root ends of apicected teeth: a scanning electron microscopic study. *Int Endod J.* 1989;22(4):184–189.

Torabinejad M, Walton RE. *Endodontics Principles and Practice.* 4th ed. St. Louis: Saunders Elsevier; 2009.

Torabinejad M, Ford TRP, McKendry DJ, Abedi HR, Miller DA, Kariyawasam SP. Histologic assessment of mineral trioxide aggregate as a root-end filling in monkeys. *J Endod.* 1997;23(4):225–228.

Torabinejad M, Higa RK, McKendry DJ, Ford TRP. Dye leakage of four root end filling materials: effects of blood contamination. *J Endod.* 1994;20(4):159–163.

Torabinejad M, Hong CU, Ford TP, Kettering JD. Cytotoxicity of four root end filling materials. *J Endod.* 1995;21(10):489–492.

Torabinejad M, Hong CU, McDonald F, Ford TP. Physical and chemical properties of a new root-end filling material. *J Endod.* 1995;21(7):349–353.

Tronstad L. Root resorption—etiology, terminology and clinical manifestations. *Dent Traumatol.* 1988;4:241–252.

Trope M. Flare–up rate of single–visit endodontics. *Int Endod J.* 1991;24(1):24–27.

Trope M. Root resorption due to dental trauma. *Endodont Topics.* 2002;1(1):79–100.

Trope M, Maltz DO, Tronstad L. Resistance to fracture of restored endodontically treated teeth. *Dent Traumatol.* 1985;1(3):108–111.

Trowbridge HO, Franks M, Korostoff E, Emling R. Sensory response to thermal stimulation in human teeth. *J Endod.* 1980;6:405–412.

Trowbridge H, Edwall L, Panopoulos P. Effect of zinc oxide-eugenol and calcium hydroxide on intradental nerve activity. *J Endod.* 1982;8(9):403–406.

Tsesis I, Rosen E, Tamse A, Taschieri S, Kfir A. Diagnosis of vertical root fractures in endodontically treated teeth based on clinical and radiographic indices: a systematic review. *J Endod.* 2010;36(9):1455–1458.

Tsesis I, Amdor B, Tamse A, Kfir A. The effect of maintaining apical patency on canal transportation. *Int Endod J.* 2008;41(5):431–435.

Tsesis I, Rosen E, Tamse A, Taschieri S, Del Fabbro M. Effect of guided tissue regeneration on the outcome of surgical endodontic treatment: a systematic review and meta-analysis. *J Endod.* 2011;37(8):1039–1045.

Türp JC, Gobetti JP. The cracked tooth syndrome: an elusive diagnosis. *J Am Dent Assoc.* 1996;127(10):1502–1507.

Udoye CI, Jafarzadeh H, Abbott PV. Transport media for avulsed teeth: a review. *Aust Endod J.* 2012;38(3):129–136.

Velvart P, Peters CI. Soft tissue management in endodontic surgery. *J Endod.* 2005;31(1):4–16.

Venkatesh S, Ajmera S, Ganeshkar SV. Volumetric pulp changes after orthodontic treatment determined by cone-beam computed tomography. *J Endod.* 2014;40(11):1758–1763.

Vertucci FJ. Root canal anatomy of the human permanent teeth. *Oral Surg Oral Med Oral Pathol.* 1984;58(5):589–599.

Vickers FJ, Baumgartner JC, Marshall G. Hemostatic efficacy and cardiovascular effects of agents used during endodontic surgery. *J Endod.* 2002;28(4):322–323.

Von Arx T, Schawalder P, Ackermann M, Bosshardt D. Human and feline invasive cervical resorptions: the missing link? Presentation of four cases. *J Endod.* 2009;35(6):904–913.

von Arx T, Salvi GE. Incision techniques and flap designs for apical surgery in the anterior maxilla. *Eur J Esthet Dent.* 2008;3(2):110–126.

Von Arx T, Walker III WA. Microsurgical instruments for root–end cavity preparation following apicoectomy: a literature review. *Dent Traumatol (Review article).* 2000;16(2):47–62.

von Arx T, Fodich I, Bornstein MM, Jensen SS. Perforation of the sinus membrane during sinus floor elevation: a retrospective study of frequency and possible risk factors. *Int J Oral Maxillofac Implants.* 2014;29(3):718–726.

Sunitha VR, Emmadi P, Namasivayam A, Thyegarajan R, Rajaraman V. The periodontal—endodontic continuum: a review. *J Conserv Dent.* 2008;11(2):54–62.

Wade W. Unculturable bacteria—the uncharacterized organisms that cause oral infections. *J R Soc Med.* 2002;95(2):81–83.

Walton R. Interappointment flare-ups: incidence, related factors, prevention, and management. *Endodontic Topics.* 2002;3(1):67–76.

Warfvinge J, Bergenholtz G. Healing capacity of human and monkey dental pulps following experimentally–induced pulpitis. *Dent Traumatol.* 1986;2(6):256–262.

Webber RT, Carlos E, Brady JM, Segall RO. Sealing quality of a temporary filling material. *Oral Surg Oral Med Oral Pathol.* 1978;46(1):123–130.

Weller RN, Niemczyk SP, Kim S. Incidence and position of the canal isthmus. Part 1. Mesiobuccal root of the maxillary first molar. *J Endod.* 1995;21(7):380–383.

Wesiman MI. The use of a calibrated percussion instrument in pulpal and periapical diagnosis. *Oral Surg Oral Med Oral Pathol Oral Radiol Endod.* 1984;57(3):320–322.

Whitcomb M, Drum M, Reader A, Nusstein J, Beck M. A prospective, randomized, double-blind study of the anesthetic efficacy of sodium bicarbonate buffered 2% lidocaine with 1:100,000 epinephrine in inferior alveolar nerve blocks. *Anesth Prog.* 2010;57(2):59–66.

White JH, Cooley RL. A quantitative evaluation of thermal pulp testing. *J Endod.* 1977;3:453–457.

Wilson BL, Broberg C, Baumgartner JC, Harris C, Kron J. Safety of electronic apex locators and pulp testers in patients with implanted cardiac pacemakers or cardioverter/defibrillators. *J Endod.* 2006;32(9):847–852.

Wood M, Reader A, Nusstein J, Beck M, Padgett D, Weaver J. Comparison of intraosseous and infiltration injections for venous lidocaine blood concentrations and heart rate changes after injection of 2% lidocaine with 1:100,000 epinephrine. *J Endod.* 2005;31(6):435–438.

Wuchenich G, Meadows D, Torabinejad M. A comparison between two root end preparation techniques in human cadavers. *J Endod.* 1994;20(6):279–282.

Xia J, Wang W, Li Z, Lin B, Zhang Q, Jiang Q, Yang X. Impacts of contracted endodontic cavities compared to traditional endodontic cavities in premolars. *BMC Oral Health.* 2020;20(1):1–8.

Yingling NM, Byrne BE, Hartwell GR. Antibiotic use by members of the American Association of Endodontists in the year 2000: report of a national survey. *J Endod.* 2002;28(5):396–404.

Younis O, Hembree Jr JH. Leakage of different root canal sealants. *Oral Surg Oral Med Oral Pathol.* 1976;41(6):777–784.

Zehnder M. Root canal irrigants. *J Endod.* 2006;32(5):389–398.

CHAPTER 8

RESTORATIVE DENTISTRY

Pamela J. Linder, Jennifer A. Magee

CARIOLOGY

1. **What is the definition of dental caries?**
   Over the decades, a number of definitions for dental caries have evolved, depending on the perspective of the author. A few are presented here.
   1. Dental caries is an infectious, communicable disease, resulting in destruction of tooth structure by acid-forming bacteria found in dental plaque, an intraoral biofilm, in the presence of sugar.
   2. Dental caries is an infectious, communicable, transmissible disease caused by bacterial invasion resulting in the breakdown of the tooth structure.
   3. Dental caries is a microbial disease of the calcified tissues of the teeth, characterized by demineralization of the inorganic portion and destruction of the organic substance of the tooth. The former constitutes the acidogenic theory and the latter the proteolytic theory.

2. **List five key facts about dental caries.**
   1. Dental caries, otherwise known as tooth decay, is one of the most prevalent chronic diseases of people worldwide; individuals are susceptible to this disease throughout their lifetime.
   2. Dental caries forms through a complex interaction over time between acid-producing bacteria and fermentable carbohydrates and many host factors related to teeth and saliva.
   3. The disease develops in the crowns and roots of teeth; it can arise in early childhood as an aggressive tooth decay that affects the primary teeth of infants and toddlers.
   4. Risk for caries includes physical, biologic, environmental, behavioral, and lifestyle-related factors (e.g., high numbers of cariogenic bacteria, inadequate salivary flow, insufficient fluoride exposure, poor oral hygiene, inappropriate methods of feeding infants, malnutrition).
   5. The approach to primary prevention should be based on common risk factors. Secondary prevention and treatment should focus on management of the caries process over time for individual patients, with a minimally invasive, tissue-preserving approach.

3. **According to the CDC (Centers for Disease Control and Prevention), what is one of the most common chronic diseases among children, specifically those aged 5 to 11 years?**
   Dental caries is now considered an epidemic in the United States. Approximately one-fifth of all children in the 5 to 11 age range have at least one untreated area of active caries. Furthermore, for youths aged 6 to 19, dental disease remains one of the most chronic diagnoses.

4. **What are some prevalence statistics related to dental caries from the CDC?**
   - 20% of children age 5 to 11 years have untreated decay.
   - Children and adolescents from low-income households are twice as likely to have decay than those from higher-income families.
   - Nearly half (45.8%) of youth aged 2 to 19 years old have experienced caries (both treated and untreated) in either dentition group (primary and/or permanent).
   - Total caries, defined as treated and/or untreated lesions, are highest among Hispanic youth. Lesions left untreated are most prevalent in non-Hispanic black youth (Fig. 8-1).

5. **What is the dental plaque biofilm?**
   A biofilm is any group of microorganisms in which cells stick to each other on a surface. These adherent cells are frequently embedded within a self-produced matrix. Dental plaque is structurally and functionally an organized biofilm. The community of microorganisms remains stable over time, with pathogenic organisms present in low numbers. In dental caries, there is a shift toward community dominance by acidogenic and acid-tolerating species. Evidence shows that conditions that foster a low pH select for the cariogenic species *Streptococcus mutans* and lactobacilli. The result is a higher acid level in the biofilm of acid production and demineralization of tooth structure.

6. **Describe the bacterial elements of the biofilm community that contribute to dental caries.**
   S. mutans and *Lactobacillus* are the dominant species.
   - Aciduric—survive in an acid environment

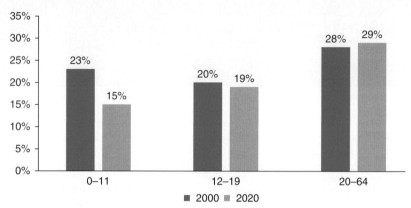

Fig. 8-1. Untreated dental caries prevalence by age—a 20-year comparison. (Data adapted from U.S. Department of Health and Human Services: Oral Health in America: Advances and Challenges Executive Summary, Rockville, December 2021, National Institutes of Health, National Institute of Dental and Craniofacial Research.)

- Acidogenic—produce higher amounts of acid from sugars
- Produce extracellular polysaccharides to thicken plaque and aid in adherence within the biofilm
- Use high levels of adenosine triphosphate (ATP) to maintain an intracellular neutral pH and pump out acids

7. What is generally accepted as a standard of dental care for preventing dental disease and managing a patient's risk?
   According to the American Dental Society and American Academy of Pediatric Dentistry, an individual caries risk assessment analysis should be part of a complete dental examination. Disease indicators and risk factors will determine the probability that a specific patient will become susceptible to dental caries, and early intervention therapies may be implemented.

8. What does the acronym CAMBRA stand for, and what is its value in caries prevention?
   CAMBRA stands for *ca*ries *m*anagement *b*y *r*isk *a*ssessment. Using a written form or oral interview, specific elements that could lead to a bacterial imbalance of dental pathogens can be assessed. Dental treatments and restoration recommendations are formulated from this data.

9. List the elements of CAMBRA.
   - Current decay levels (number of decayed teeth)
   - Current bacterial challenge (measured by testing levels)
   - Decay history (e.g., decay-missing-filled [DMF] index, missing filled teeth)
   - Dietary habits (food types, degree of snacking)
   - Current medications
   - Saliva status (e.g., amount, buffering capacity)
   - Medical conditions
   - Oral appliances present (e.g., braces)
   - Oral hygiene habits

10. What is the cariogram?
    Developed in Sweden, the cariogram is a simple software program that generates a pie graph representation of the elements of a risk assessment survey (Fig. 8-2).

11. How are dental caries classified?
    1. Anatomic site, G.V. Black Classification
    2. Pit and fissure: class I
    3. Smooth surface: interproximal: class II posterior, class III anterior
    4. Involvement of the incisal edge: class IV
    5. Cervical and root surface: class V
    6. Rate of progression—incipient (early enamel surface or white spot lesion)
    7. Acute or rampant (rapid progression and widespread)
    8. Chronic or arrested (demineralization has ceased)
    9. Recurrent (new decay at sites of previous lesions or restorations)
    10. Hard tissue involved—enamel, dentin, cementum
    11. Cause—radiation caries, early childhood caries (ECC), baby bottle caries, xerostomia/reduced salivary flow
    The GV Black classification system is illustrated in Fig. 8-3.

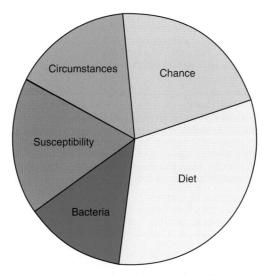

High-risk patient with 25% "chance" of avoiding caries

Fig. 8-2. Example of a cariogram. (Adapted from Bratthall D, Hänsel Petersson G, Stjernswärd JR: Cariogram—Evaluation of the Caries Risk Assessment, Malmö Sweden, 2004, Malmö University.)

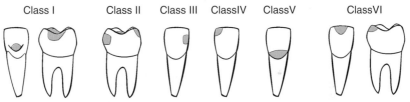

Fig. 8-3. Black classification. Various tooth defects are categorized into six classes based on the specific location of the lesions. (From Shen J: Advanced Ceramics for Dentistry. Waltham, MA, 2014, Butterworth-Heinemann.)

12. Outline the caries susceptibility of teeth in the dental arches.
    Maxillary > mandibular arch
    Tooth type: first molars (upper and lower) > second molars (upper and lower) > second bicuspids (upper) > first bicuspids (upper) and second bicuspids (lower) > central and lateral incisors (upper) > canine (upper) and first bicuspids (lower) > lower anteriors
    Tooth surface: occlusal >> mesial > distal > buccal > lingual

13. List the key risk factors associated with dental caries.
    • Susceptible tooth surface that can maintain plaque and bacteria
    • Presence of acidogenic bacteria
    • Steady supply of dietary fermentable carbohydrates
    • Inadequate salivary flow or buffering capacity
    • Low exposure to topical or dietary fluoride
    • Social determinants of health

14. What organisms are responsible for caries formation?
    S. mutans and lactobacilli are the most cariogenic, with contributions from *Streptococcus sanguis* and *Streptococcus salivarius*. These organisms metabolize sucrose to form acidic byproducts destructive to enamel surfaces. Root surface caries are initiated by *Actinomyces viscus* on accumulated plaque deposits.

15. What are the properties of cariogenic bacteria?
    Specifically unique are their ability to survive at low pH and metabolize simple sugars to form acid byproducts. During the process, extracellular polysaccharides are produced, which aid in adhesion within the plaque biofilms.

16. What is the role of saliva in caries susceptibility?
    • Adequate flow reduces plaque accumulation on tooth surfaces and rate of clearance of carbohydrates.

- Diffusion of the salivary components calcium, phosphate, hydroxyl, and fluoride ions into plaque can reduce the solubility of enamel and promote remineralization of early carious lesions.
- The bicarbonate-buffering ability of saliva can reduce or limit the fall in pH when bacteria metabolize sugars.
- Salivary proteins form the protective acquired pellicle, which retards the flow of ions out of enamel.
- The salivary components of secretory immunoglobulin A (IgA), lysosomes, lactoperoxidase, and lactoferrin have antibacterial activity.

17. **Describe the role of fluoride in preventing dental caries.**
    - The anticaries effects of fluoride are primarily topical for children and adults.
    - Fluoride inhibits demineralization at enamel crystal surfaces inside teeth.
    - Fluoride enhances the remineralization of the enamel crystal surface after demineralization and increases acid resistance.
    - The systemic benefits of fluoride in caries prevention are minimal.
    - Fluoride is an essential adjunct preventative measure in populations with low salivary flow due to disease state (i.e., Sjögren) or sequelae secondary to medical therapies/treatments (i.e., oncologic radiation therapy)

18. **What is the effect of fluoride on bacteria?**
    Fluoride can enter the bacterial cell only as hydrogen fluoride (HF), where it can dissociate and inhibit bacterial enzymes (enolases). As acid production proceeds, some H^+ and F^- ions form HF, which can enter the bacterial cell. At neutral pH, within the bacterial cell, it dissociates, and the fluoride ion is free to act on bacterial enzymes as an inhibitor (Fig. 8-4).

19. **How does fluoride aide in remineralization of tooth structure?**
    Fluoride present in saliva or plaque fluid will become incorporated into a new crystal surface during remineralization. It competitively displaces OH^- ions and then acts topically, from the surface inward, exerting its effects against acid dissolution of the crystal surface. Present in plaque fluid, it will travel into the subsurface enamel with the acids, adsorb to the crystal, and protect it from dissolution. In summary, fluoride present in solution from topical sources enhances remineralization by speeding up the growth of a new surface on the partially demineralized subsurface crystals of the carious lesion. The new crystal surface is fluorapatite-like, with much lower solubility than the original carbonated apatite tooth mineral (Fig. 8-5).

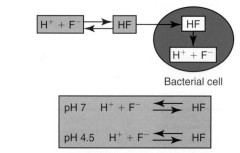

Bacterial cell

Fig. 8-4. Fluoride's effect on bacteria.

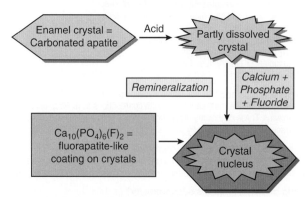

Fig. 8-5. Demineralization and remineralization processes. (Adapted from Featherstone JDB: Prevention and reversal of dental caries: Role of low level fluoride, Community Dent Oral Epidemiol 27:31–40, 1999.)

20. Express the caries risk factors in a functional relationship.

Functional Relation In Dental Caries

$$C_A \quad f \; [(\text{Bacteria}) \; (\text{CHO})] \quad \left[\dfrac{1}{(S)(F)} \right]$$

C_A = Caries activity

Bacteria = *S. mutans/Lactobacillus* activity

CHO = Fermentable carbohydrate substrate

F = Fluoride availability

S = Saliva (flow/buffering capacity/components)

Dental caries occurs when the process of demineralization is faster than the process of remineralization and there is a net loss of tooth mineral into the environment. If the acid production is reduced by removing plaque accumulation or reducing dietary sugar substrates, tooth mineral dissociation will cease (decrease in caries activity [C_A]). The presence of topical fluoride increases enamel resistance to dissolution (forming fluorapatite) and enhances remineralization. It also inhibits bacterial metabolism. Thus, increases in fluoride relate inversely to C_A. Finally, a high salivary buffering capacity decreases caries activity, whereas low flow rates tend to increase C_A.

21. What are the three main tooth mineral complexes and their relative solubilities?

The enamel and dentin of a tooth are composed of tiny crystals embedded in a protein/lipid matrix. The mineral formed during tooth germination is a highly substituted carbonated apatite. It is related to hydroxyapatite but is more acid soluble, as well as calcium-deficient (replaced by sodium, magnesium, and zinc) and contains 3% to 6% carbonate replacing phosphate ions in the crystal lattice. During demineralization, carbonate is preferentially lost, and during remineralization, it is excluded and replaced by OH^- or F^- ions, thereby decreasing the acid solubility. This is the maturation cycle. Mature enamel is mostly hydroxy or fluorapatite.

Tooth Mineral

Carbonated apatite (most soluble)

$$Ca_{10-x}(Na)_x(PO_4)_{6-y}(CO_3)_z\,(OH)_{2-u}(F)_u$$

Hydroxy apatite (less soluble)

$$Ca_{10}(PO_4)_{10}(OH)_2$$

Fluorapatite (least soluble)

$$Ca_{10}(PO_4)10(F)_2$$

22. What is a Stephan plot?

The classic experimental measurement of pH changes on tooth enamel surfaces during exposure to fermentable carbohydrates in the presence of acidogenic bacteria (in plaque) over time is called a Stephan plot. It demonstrates the acid production of bacteria (pH decrease) with a glucose swallow, and the gradual rise caused by salivary buffering. At position #3, after left side brushing, the unbrushed side pH drops, whereas the left brushed side #4 remains above the critical pH (Fig. 8-6).

23. What is the critical pH for enamel dissociation?

The critical pH for enamel (hydroxyapatite) is 5.3 to 5.5; for fluorapatite, it is 4.5. Carbonated beverages (e.g., sodas or sparkling waters) have a pH of about 3.5.

24. What are the pH values of some common beverages?

Knowing that the critical pH of enamel demineralization is 5.5, carbonated beverages can be very destructive (Fig. 8-7). The titratable acidity (TA) is the equivalent to titrate to neutral pH. Energy drinks and sports drinks showed the greatest degree of enamel surface dissolution. Possible explanations for the higher degree of enamel dissolution by sports and energy drinks is the addition of high concentrations of refined carbohydrates (e.g., sucrose, glucose) by the manufacturer, which promotes greater degrees of acid production and, in turn, higher

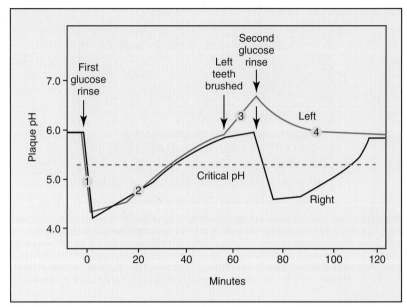

Fig. 8-6. Stephan plot.

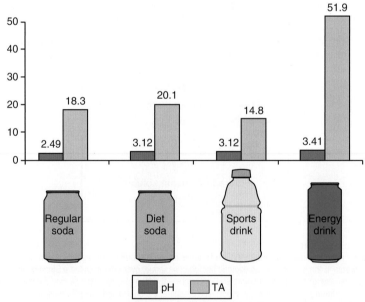

Fig. 8-7. Comparison of pH and TA in common beverages.

buffering capacities. In addition, beverages containing citric acids have the ability to irreversibly chelate (bind) calcium at higher pH values, with the net effect of an accelerated loss of calcium from tooth structure; this maintains the pH of the beverage below the threshold level (pH = 5.5) for enamel erosion to occur (Fig. 8-8).

25. **What is the term for the earliest observable enamel caries lesion?**
The term *white spot lesion* is applied to the earliest visually observable or macroscopic lesion in enamel. It represents dissolution of the surface structure, with increased porosity, and takes on a dull appearance when air-dried because of the differences in light scattering (refractive index) from the surrounding enamel. These lesions may maintain their surface integrity, become stained and arrested, or progress to frank cavitation lesions.

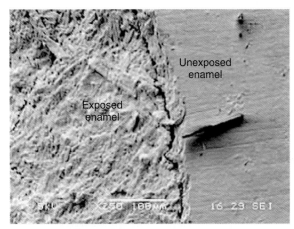

Fig. 8-8. Scanning electron microscope image of enamel before and after exposure to cola.

26. **What are the differences in the mechanisms of enamel and dentinal caries?**
Enamel caries is primarily an acidogenic or physiochemical progression of tooth mineral dissolution, whereas dentinal caries involves acid decalcification followed by proteolytic or enzymatic degeneration of the organic matrix.

27. **What is the current thinking about treating early enamel caries or the incipient lesion?**
Most early enamel lesions are capable of remineralization, or arresting, if the risk factors are reduced and there is adequate fluoride content in the microenvironment. Risk factor assessment (including diet, bacterial, and salivary analysis), followed by fluoride supplements from topical sources, is thus the first line of therapy.

28. **What are the histologic zones of enamel caries?**
Four zones of alternating levels of demineralization illustrate the dynamic nature of caries. The surface zone blocks passage of calcium ions into the body of the lesion. It is well mineralized by replacement ions from plaque and saliva. The body of the lesion is poorly mineralized. The dark zone has some remineralization, whereas the translucent zone has high demineralization (Fig. 8-9).

29. **What are the histologic zones of cavitated dentinal caries?**
There are two distinct layers.
   1. Outer layer—dentin heavily infected with bacteria; organic matrix and mineral are lost and cannot be repaired; liquefaction foci and clefts form.
   2. Inner layer—dentin affected by plaque acids and demineralized; few bacteria, damage reversible.
   A barrier layer of sclerotic (translucent), well-mineralized dentin may be formed by odontoblast deposits into intratubular spaces. Finally, a layer of secondary reactionary-reparative dentin forms at the dentin-pulp junction. These preceding two layers are dependent on a vital pulp's reaction to noxious stimuli (Fig. 8-10).

30. **Describe the progression of caries in dentin.**
Because dentin is a vital tissue, it shows reactivity with bacterial invasion. Caries generally spreads laterally along the dentoenamel junction (DEJ), involving dentinal tubules. At the **infected layer** of dentin, bacteria enter the dentinal tubules and decalcify the matrix by acid and proteolytic dissociation (microscopic liquefaction foci and clefts are present). The inner **affected layer** is demineralized but contains few bacteria. The damage here is reversible if the bacterial metabolism is halted by excavation of the infected layer. Under the affected layer is the **sclerotic** or microscopic **translucent layer,** followed by a layer of **reparative or reactionary dentin** produced by odontoblasts at the dentopulpal boundary.

31. **Identify the labeled structures in this cavitated carious lesion shown in** *Fig. 8-11.*
Carious dentin fills most of the slide, on the right. At the far left is the **pulp**; the faint blue dots are lymphocytes (chronic inflammation). To its right is a band of **reparative dentin** that protected the pulp from infection for a time. Next, progressing right, is a thin band of **sclerotic dentin**, followed by a layer of **affected dentin**, and at the far right is **infected dentin**.

32. **Identify structures shown in** *Fig. 8-12.*
Note that zones of destruction coalesce to form clefts and liquefaction foci. These are filled with necrotic debris. These advancing bacteria seem to have acidogenic and proteolytic properties, resulting in the enzymatic destruction of the organic dentin matrix. Horizontal clefting is typical of dentinal caries. The process of beading, coalescence, and clefting typifies progression of dental caries.

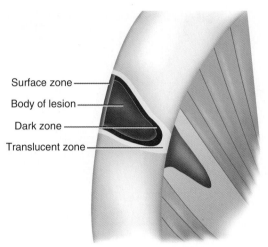

Fig. 8-9. Microscopic zones of enamel caries. (From Sapp JP, Eversole, LR, Wysocki GP: Contemporary Oral and Maxillofacial Pathology, ed 2, St. Louis, 2004, Mosby.)

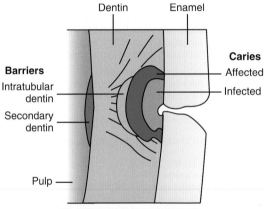

Fig. 8-10. Sclerotic and reparative dentin.

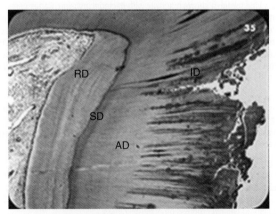

Fig. 8-11. Cavitated carious lesion. *AD,* Affected dentin; *ID,* infected dentin; *P,* pulp; *RD,* reparative dentin; *SD,* sclerotic dentin.

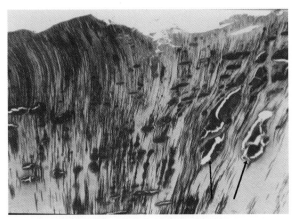

Fig. 8-12. Arrows indicate liquefaction foci filled with necrotic debris.

33. Describe the elements shown in *Fig. 8-13*.

Fig. 8-13A—small, smooth-surfaced enamel caries in water with polarized light; lesion is cone-shaped; body appears dark beneath intact surface layer.

Fig. 8-13B—same section in quinolin (same refractive index as enamel) with polarized light.

1. Translucent zone visible as porous, less mineralized leading zone in enamel
2. Dark zone thought to be area of redeposition of mineral
3. Body is demineralized, with striae of Retzius evident
4. Surface zone (SZ) intact because of constant demineralization (destruction) and remineralization (repair) if fluoride present

34. Clinically, how are the different types of carious dentin treated?

All infected dentin must be removed for successful tooth viability. Because affected dentin has undergone only early demineralization, removal may not be necessary. Topical bonded dentin sealants containing fluoride affect a barrier under restorations.

35. Explain the differences between smooth and pit and fissure caries.

Because **smooth surface caries** (interproximal or cervical) have a wide enamel surface pattern that converges with the anatomic form of the enamel rods toward the DEJ, fewer dentinal tubule are affected, enamel undermining is generally less, and the rate of progression is slow. These lesions have a high success of remineralization with adequate fluoride exposure and reduction in risk factors.

Pit and fissure caries are narrow at the enamel surface and spread widely as the caries progresses to the DEJ, involving many dentin tubules and creating extensive undermining. The progression is often more rapid than that of smooth surface caries. Because of the anatomic sheltering of bacterial plaque, remineralization is not easy, and fissurotomy followed by sealants is necessary for early lesions.

36. Develop a decision tree for the management of pit and fissure tooth surfaces.

See Fig. 8-14 for an example of a decision tree for the management of pit and fissure tooth surfaces.

37. How may caries be diagnosed?

Caries may be detected by a combination of techniques. The most commonly accepted criteria for identifying infected tooth structure are the following: (1) discolored, softened tooth structure; (2) frank cavitation; and (3) areas of radiolucency on radiographs. Direct visual inspection of pits and fissures, root surfaces, and interfaces of restorations and tooth with a sharp explorer and air-drying with the use of magnification are the first steps of the examination. This procedure is supplemented by evaluating properly angulated bitewing and periapical radiographs. Finally, the use of transillumination from a visible light curing wand can reveal shadowing and discoloration on occlusal and interproximal tooth surfaces.

38. What are the objectives of operative treatments in carious teeth?

1. To remove bacterially infected enamel and dentin
2. To protect the dental pulp
3. To preserve healthy tooth structure, occlusion, and restore missing structure
4. To remove the sources of cariogenic bacteria by facilitating plaque control
5. To provide minimal fluoride concentrations in the microenvironment

39. List logical steps to stabilize dentition with active and multiple caries.

1. Carry out a thorough medical and dental history and examination to assess caries risk factors.
2. Initiate appropriate preventive measures.

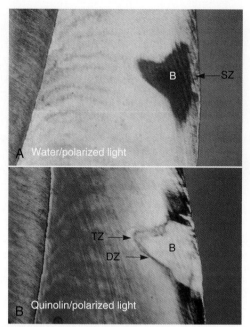

Fig. 8-13. Small, smooth-surface enamel caries. (**A**) In water (polarized light). (**B**) In quinolin (polarized light). *B,* Body; *DZ,* dark zone; *SZ,* surface zone; *TZ,* translucent zone.

3. Plan extraction of nonsalvageable teeth.*

4. Evaluation of caries in vital teeth and protection with pulp-capping agents such as $Ca(OH)_2$ sealed with bonded and flowable resins or resin-reinforced glass ionomers. Use glass ionomer build-up materials for the temporary filling.

5. In frank pulpal exposures, removal of the pulpal tissues is advisable to prevent potential pain, followed by temporization with a suitable glass ionomer material and endodontic treatment.

6. In very deep carious lesions, whether symptomatic or not, if pulpal exposure is to be expected, it is probably best to go directly to endodontic treatment rather than try an intermediate step of excavation and temporary stabilization. However, there is a place for consideration of stabilizing materials such as silver diamine fluoride in populations who may not be able to tolerate a definitive restoration (medically complex, geriatric, or patients with intellectual and/or development disability) or for space maintenance prior to imminent exfoliation (pediatric population).

7. Finalize a treatment plan with permanent restorations for the existing teeth and make suitable provisions for replacement of missing teeth.

40. **What are caries detector solutions? How are they used?**
Caries detector solutions are usually a colored dye (red, green, blue) in a propylene glycol base; they help distinguish between infected and affected dentin. The dye bonds to the denatured collagen in the infected dentin that is part of the decay process. The affected dentin, which may be slightly softer than sound dentin, is not infused with bacteria and is not stained, but still may show a dye-stained haze (pink haze with red dye). This dentin should not be removed. The caries detector solution is applied for 10 seconds and then rinsed off. Any deeply stained tooth structure is then removed. The materials also help identify cracks in tooth structure.

   NOTE: Some products may decrease the bond strength to dentin and careful consideration of their use is necessary when high bonding requirements are needed.

41. **Are cavity disinfectants useful?**
Some current restorative approaches reflect the goal of cleaning a preparation before bonding or placing a restoration with the addition of a bactericidal agent to reduce sensitivity and bacterial growth under a restoration. It is thought that bacteria reaching the pulp may contribute to sensitivity. Current products contain benzalkonium chloride and EDTA or 2% chlorhexidine gluconate.

42. **What supplemental sources of topical fluoride may be used for caries prevention?**
   • Public water supplies: 1 ppm sodium fluoride (NaF)

---

* **NOTE:** This step may be resequenced in the apprehensive patient until full trust and compliance are achieved because extractions may be too traumatic as an initial treatment phase.

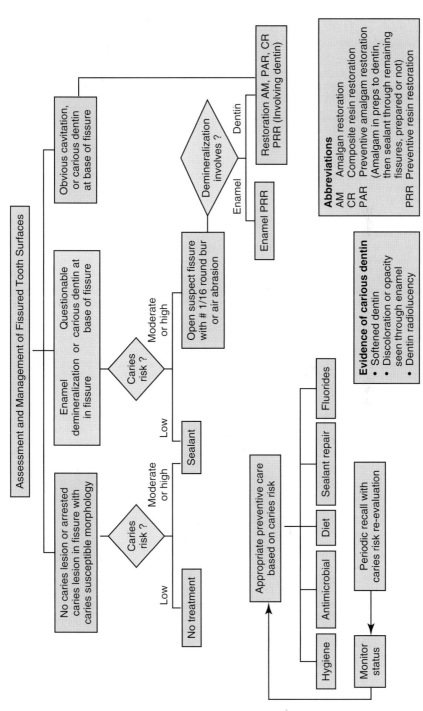

Fig. 8-14. Example of a decision tree. (Adapted from Summitt JB: Conservative cavity preparations, Dent Clin North Am 46:171–184, 2002.)

- Toothpaste: OTC (over-the-counter) regular brands contain 0.10% to 0.15% NaF
- Prescription: 1.1% NaF
- Mouth rinses: 0.2% to 0.5% NaF
- Brush-on gels, fluoride trays: 1.1% NaF, neutral pH

43. **What is a contraindication to the use of acidulated or stannous fluoride preparations?**

$$0.4\% \text{ stannous fluoride (pH, 3.0)} = 0.2\% \text{ sodium fluoride (pH, 7.0)}$$

Acidulated fluoride (APF) solutions and topical 0.4% stannous gels remove the glaze from porcelain, glass ionomer, and composite restorations. It is best to use neutral pH supplements if these restorations are present. Always check the product specifications.

44. **Describe a medical model of caries treatment.**
The medical model attempts to shift the caries balance toward no caries by using medical and behavioral components. The key elements are:
1. Control bacteria.
   a. Surgical antimicrobial treatment: fill or temporize cavitated lesions.
   b. Chemotherapeutic antimicrobial treatment: use chlorhexidine, cetylpyridinium, fluoride varnish, xylitol chewing gum.
2. Reduce risk level of at-risk patients.
   a. Diet
   b. Oral hygiene
   c. Sealants
3. Reverse active sites (remineralization) with fluoride supplements via gels, rinses, or toothpastes.
4. Carry out long-term follow-up and maintenance (Fig. 8-15).

45. **Describe light-based methods of diagnosing dental caries.**
1. **Fiberoptic transillumination (FOTI)** uses light transmission through the tooth to measure surface scattering on the outside of the lesion. Digitized fiberoptic transillumination (DIFOTI) is a light-based tool that captures images of transilluminated visible light on a digital CCD camera and sends them to a computer, where analyses of the decreased densities due to demineralization are shown as images.
2. **Optical coherence tomography (OCT)** can create cross-sectional images of biologic tissues using nonionizing imaging techniques. When a carious tooth is illuminated with infrared light, OCT provides two- or three-dimensional (3D) images and a quantitative image of the subsurface lesion to the depth of the enamel.
3. **Quantitative light-induced fluorescence (QFL)** measures the scattering of light produced by the degree of enamel demineralization.

46. **What about caries vaccines?**
Studies have focused on anticaries vaccines for *S. mutans*. These vaccines have antibodies against bacteria surface receptors Ag I and II, preventing microorganism adhesion to tooth structure. Newer investigations have targeted intranasally administered anticaries DNA vaccines to produce mucosal and systemic responses and protection against caries. However, there is still not an approved modality of caries prevention through commercially available vaccination.

47. **What are some indications for fluoride gel applications using a custom tray?**
Patients who exhibit high caries incidence, root caries, or cervical caries and who might fit into one or more of the following groups:
- High consumption of carbonated beverages (pH, 3.2-3.5) or citric fruits (e.g., lemons, limes)
- Bulimic patients (higher incidence in adolescent females than males)

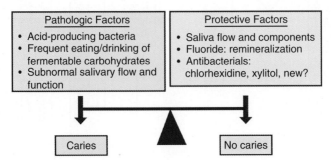

Fig. 8-15. The caries balance. (Adapted from Featherstone JDB: The caries balance: Contributing factors and early detection, J Calif Dent Assoc 31:129–133, 2003.)

- Geriatric and/or adults who live in residential care facilities
- Gastric reflux patients
- Chemotherapy and head and neck radiation–treated patients
- Individuals with medically related xerostomia or diagnosed with Sjögren syndrome

48. **What is tooth attrition?**
Attrition is the physiologic wear of tooth structure resulting from normal tooth to tooth contact over time.

49. **What is erosion? What are its possible causes?**
Erosion is the loss of tooth structure by a chemical process that does not involve bacterial action. It is generally caused by the consumption of foods that contain phosphoric or citric acid, such as fruits, fruit juices, and carbonated or acidic beverages. Excessive exposure to gastric acids because of vomiting is also a contributing factor.

50. **What is the theory of tooth abfraction?**
Abfraction is defined as the pathologic loss of tooth substance caused by biomechanical loading forces. The loss of structure is usually seen as wedge-shaped cervical lesions at the cementoenamel junction (CEJ) that may not be carious. This theory is used as an alternative explanation for areas that historically were attributed to toothbrush abrasion. They are also referred to as noncarious cervical lesions (NCCLs).

51. **List generally accepted principles for cavity preparation.**
   1. Cavity preparations should be governed by tooth anatomy, tooth position in the dental arch, extent of the carious lesion, and physical properties of the filling material.
   2. Gingival margins should be ended on enamel whenever possible.
   3. Cavity preparation margins should be supragingival whenever possible.
   4. Margins of posterior cavity preparations should not end directly in occlusal contact areas. Contact areas should be composed of one material to allow even wear. Uneven wear results if two materials meet at the contact area, thereby producing open margins.
   5. Weakened and unsupported tooth structures should be removed.
   6. Maintaining a dry work field with the use of a rubber dam always enhances the consistent quality of restorations.

52. **Describe the principles of cavity preparation for composite resins and amalgam alloy.**
The classic cavity preparations, according to Black's principles, are generally not needed for contemporary bonded retained composite and amalgam restorations. Dovetails, retention grooves, and extension into uninvolved occlusal grooves are generally not needed. Maximizing tooth structure dominates design, with sealants replacing groove extensions.

53. **How do the basic principles of operative microdentistry differ from those of traditional operative dentistry, as advocated by Black?**
The Black approach to operative dentistry tends toward the destruction of healthy tooth structure to remove smaller amounts of unhealthy tooth structure (extension for prevention). The concept of microdentistry seeks to diagnose unsound tooth structure that is a threat to the tooth and remove that threat, with minimal encroachment on the surrounding healthy tooth structure.

54. **What is a fissurotomy procedure? What are its applications?**
A fissurotomy involves the conservative preparation of occlusal pits and fissures using air abrasion or special burs designed for this purpose; This procedure is used to treat pits and fissures with incipient decay. Preparations are typically narrow, long, and irregularly deep, so they are often restored with flowable composites. Hybrid composites, although stronger and more wear-resistant than flowables, may be clinically more difficult to place into such preparations without the incorporation of voids.

55. **What are the advantages of the fissurotomy procedure over pit and fissure sealants?**
It is often difficult to determine caries activity in pits and fissures, particularly with conventional means. Concerns arise about the placement of sealants over undiagnosed caries. Questionable occlusal grooves covered with a sealant, particularly in fluoridated communities, may mask more extensive subsurface caries activity. The fissurotomy offers better access and is a conservative technique for maximizing the retention of healthy tooth structure while ensuring certain removal of all decay.

56. **Describe the "tunnel preparation."**
The tunnel preparation is a conservative approach to restoring class II caries in teeth with relatively small interproximal lesions. It conserves the proximal marginal enamel by using only occlusal, buccal, or lingual access and then angulating mesially or distally until the external tooth enamel is perforated. Usually, application of a matrix band beforehand protects the adjacent tooth wall. The tooth cavity is then packed from the access dimension.

57. **What is a slot preparation?**
Any narrow access to reach interproximal caries can be called a slot preparation. The access may be buccal or lingual, as in a class III lesion, or from the occlusal aspect. The ideal is to conserve tooth structure by removing only caries and a minimal amount of tooth structure.

58. **Define micro air abrasion. When is it used?**
This technique uses pressurized delivery of an abrasive powder (e.g., aluminum oxide) to prepare teeth for restoration. The claimed advantages are less trauma and a less invasive, heatless procedure, often not requiring local anesthesia. It is ideally suited for pit and fissure sealant preparations and conservative class I and V preparations using flowable composites. Disadvantages include the need for special high-speed evacuation equipment and high cost of the units.

59. **Describe the principle behind air abrasion for cavity preparation.**
Air abrasion is based on kinetic energy. Abrasive particles, typically 27- to 50-μm aluminum oxide, are propelled at high velocity to remove tooth structure. By varying the speed of the particles, the length of time to remove tooth structure and often the level of sensitivity can be controlled.

60. **What are the various sources of propellant for air abrasion units?**
Depending on the type of unit and manufacturer, the propellant can range from compressed air or nitrogen to operatory-compressed air lines or units with built-in air compressors.

61. **What dental procedures are well suited for the use of air abrasion? Are any procedures contraindicated?**
All classes of cavity preparation may be performed with air abrasion. Some operators may use a high-speed handpiece to gain initial access to deep grooves, pits, marginal ridges, and hard-to-reach areas. Although air abrasion units have the ability to remove dental amalgam, some questions remain about the amount of mercury released by air abrasion versus removal with conventional, high-speed handpieces.

62. **Why is air abrasion considered well suited to the application of microdentistry?**
Treatment goals of microdentistry include preservation of sound occlusal enamel with minimally invasive occlusal preparations and the use of tunnel or slot preparations to treat primary interproximal caries. Air abrasion is much more selective in the structure it cuts, thereby removing very little sound tooth structure relative to the use of high-speed handpieces. Additionally, the vibration from high-speed handpieces can cause enamel fractures that air abrasion cannot.

DENTAL ADHESIVES

63. **What are dental adhesives?**
Dental adhesives are products that allow the predictable adhesion of restorative material to dentin and enamel. They are based on using a number of agents to prepare the surface, bond to the tooth surface, and act as a substrate to which the restorative material bonds. In general, they are technique-sensitive and constantly evolving in the marketplace.

64. **What are the goals of dental bonding?**
- Eliminate or minimize the contraction gap of composite polymerization.
- Sustain thermal expansion and contraction cycles.
- Create 20- to 30-MPa bond strengths to enamel and dentin.
- Eliminate microleakage.

65. **What are signs of microleakage?**
They are stains, sensitivity and pulpal symptoms, recurrent caries, and bond failures.

66. **What are the components of adhesive systems?**
Most current systems are combinations of components. Some are multicomponent, depending on whether they are self-cure, light-cure, or both, whereas others have a single component. Unlike early-generation systems, all the new bonding agents are hydrophilic to allow compatibility with dentin bonding. The basic components are an acid etchant solution, hydrophilic primer, and resin.

67. **What types of adhesive systems are available?**
Type 1. Etchant applied, washed off to remove smear layer; primer and adhesive resin applied separately as two solutions. Type 1 systems are all-purpose types. They generally bond to light-, dual-, and self-cured composites.
Type 2. Etchant applied and washed off to remove smear layer; primer and adhesive applied as a single solution. Type 2 systems have almost all-purpose capability.
Type 3. Self-etching primer (SEP) is applied to dissolve smear layer and not washed off; adhesive is applied separately.
Type 4. Self-etching primer and adhesive are applied as a single solution to dissolve and treat the smear layer simultaneously.

68. **What types of adhesive systems are currently used in clinical practice?**
Many variables, including timing, rinsing, drying, rewetting dentin, and maintaining a controlled operative field are important in the placement of dental adhesives. Over time, manufacturers focused research efforts on the

development of simplifying these systems to reduce the potential for inconsistencies in treatment by reducing the number of steps required for application. Classification systems became confusing as generational models advanced. Bonding systems that required phosphoric acid etching with rinsing were referred to as total etch whereas those that did not require the additional step were called self-etch. The sixth- and seventh-generation systems were self-etching models. In current practice, adhesives can be classified as total etch (TE) and self-etch.

69. **What is the hybrid layer?**
The hybrid layer is a multilayered zone of composite resin, and dentin and collagen. After removing the organic and inorganic debris of the smear layer by etching and reducing some hydroxyapatite from the intertubular dentin down to 2 to 5 μm, a plate of moist collagen remains on the dentin floor. Priming agents penetrate this moist collagen substrate and migrate into the tubules, lateral canals, and all areas of peritubular dentin. This becomes the hybridization process as the dentin, both collagen and hydroxyapatite crystals, become totally impregnated with bonding resin. The resin further penetrates the dentin tubules. Light curing produces a mechanically and chemically bonded surface that can polymerize to composite restoratives.

70. **What is essential for successful hybrid layer formation?**
Supersaturating the dentin substrate with primer or wetting agent is essential. If the etchant time is 15 seconds, the wash should be at least as long. The water is then dispersed to leave the dentin moist. Multiple coats of priming agent are applied to achieve a glossy surface on air dispersion. Resin is then applied and cured.

71. **How is enamel bonding achieved?**
Bonding to enamel is micromechanical; a low-viscosity resin penetrates the microporosity created by acid etching on the enamel surface. Once the resin is cured, it strongly adheres to the enamel and forms the suitable substrate for composite bonding. Although previously done under dry conditions, contemporary adhesive systems use a wet bond to enamel. If one is bonding only to enamel, it is necessary to use only an unfilled resin without the primer application.

72. **How is bonding to dentin achieved?**
Dentin is largely composed of organic materials, mostly collagen and water. (Enamel is 86% mineralized, whereas dentin is 45%.) Bonding to dentin can require removal of preparation debris **(smear layer)** and demineralization of the dentin surface by acid etchant. This leaves a lattice of unsupported collagen as long as the surface stays moist. Hydrophilic primers and resins (applied in solvents of acetone or alcohol) can then penetrate this matrix, infusing a micromechanical lock similar to enamel. When cured, this resin-reinforced dentin complex forms the **hybrid layer,** and is a suitable substrate for composite bonding. With newer self-etch primer adhesives (SEPs), the etchant and primer are applied and not washed off; the smear layer remains. An adhesive is applied separately. The dentin with these latter systems is never denuded, and there may be less technique sensitivity because the process of leaving dentin to damp-dry is eliminated.

73. **How long should you etch?**
Etching dentin demineralizes its surface to a depth of 1 to 10 μm. If you etch too long, you may create a depth of demineralized collagen that is too deep for adhesives to penetrate, thus weakening the bond or denaturing the remaining collagen. The total etch of a tooth preparation with 32% to 40% phosphoric acid gels should be a **maximum of 15 seconds,** which also works for enamel.

74. **Why must the dentin surface be kept wet?**
When using types 1 and 2 adhesive systems, the etching step leaves the dentin collagen lattice largely unsupported. If this layer dehydrates, it will collapse, and the applied adhesives will not be able to infuse through the collagen. The surface should be left moist by only the slightest application of air to eliminate puddles of water—or, even better, blotted with a sponge or gauze. Some adhesive systems rehydrate the demineralized zone, even if it is overdried.

75. **What potential problem may cause an incomplete seal of dentin tubules?**
Incomplete placement of the bonding reagents may result in an increase in postoperative pulpal sensitivity. There may be incomplete wetting on application of the primer agent or incomplete curing of the bonding agent. One must be sure to place incremental layers of wetting agent until a glossy appearance is observed on gentle air dispersion, and a well-calibrated curing light must be used for sufficient exposure times.

76. **What factors contribute to increased pulpal sensitivity, even with proper technique?**
If the dentin is dried too completely, air emboli may enter the dentin tubules and the dentin bonding layer may overseal the layer of air. There is thus a potential for mechanical masticatory stresses and a resultant sensitivity on biting on the tooth restoration unit. To avoid this problem, leave the dentin moist by gentle air dispersion. Then the hydrophilic primers will follow fluid down the tubules and fill intertubular dentin and tubules with resin.

77. **How long should you apply the adhesive?**
The adhesive must penetrate through the demineralized dentin to form the hybrid layer for maximal bond strength. Some systems are faster than others; thus, following the manufacturer's instructions is important. In

general, after applying the adhesive, 15 to 20 seconds should be allowed for penetration. Air evaporation of the solvent (acetone or alcohol) is followed by curing (generally, visible light-cured). This should leave a shiny dentin surface. If this goal is not achieved, reapplication of the adhesive should be performed until a shiny layer appears.

78. Describe the composition of contemporary primers in adhesive systems.
Primers are bifunctional molecules. One end is hydrophobic to bind to the adhesive, and the other end is hydrophilic. The hydrophilic end permeates conditioned dentin and chases the water of the moist surface, assisted by solvents (acetone or alcohol). After this penetration, the solvents need to be evaporated by air drying. Examples of primers are HEMA (2-hydroxyethyl methacrylate), 4-META (4-methacryloyloxyethyl trimellitate anhydride), and PENTA (dipentaerythritol penta-acrylate monophosphate). Generally, they do not have any light-curing capabilities.

79. Describe the bonding resin adhesive.
Bonding resins are unfilled bis-GMA (bisphenol A glycidyl methacrylate) or UDMA (urethane dimethacrylate). They may be visible light-cured (VLC), autocured, or dual-cured. The later generation of adhesive systems consolidated the primer and adhesive into premixed applications, which leads to time savings. There has been a trend to add fillers to the adhesive bonding agents to enhance their physical properties.

80. What enhancement do fillers contribute to newer adhesive bonding resins?
- Increase the bond strength at the hybrid layer
- Improve stress absorption at the tooth restoration interface, enabling better retention
- Have a lower modulus of elasticity to impart added flexibility and thus relieve contraction stress caused by polymerization shrinkage; adhesive absorbs within itself some of the contraction stress
- Help adhesive cover the dentin in one application rather than multiple applications

81. What are the seventh-generation adhesive systems?
The latest systems combine applications of conditioning, priming, and adhesive resin all in one bottle. They are referred to as "single-component, one-step, self-etch adhesives" or "all-in-one adhesives."

82. Can you use any adhesive with any composite?
Generally, any light-cured composite should bond to any light-cured adhesive. However, self-cured composites such as core pastes are not compatible with most single-component adhesives. Dual-component or self-cure adhesives must be used with self-cure composites.

83. Outline the adhesive procedures for bonding composites and amalgam to tooth structure.
1. For composite materials:
   To enamel: Clean surface with pumice, wash, etch 15 seconds, wash, air-dry, and apply unfilled VLC resin only.
   To dentin and enamel: Clean surface, etch 15 seconds, wash, leave moist, use VLC adhesive components in layers before composite, and consider filled adhesives.
2. For amalgam (bonding to dentin only):
   Clean surface, etch 15 seconds, wash, use VLC primer to seal tubules, self-cure resin adhesive (two-component system), and pack amalgam before resin sets.

COMPOSITES

84. What are the components of composite resins?
- Monomers: Bis-GMA, UDMA
- Diluent monomers: TEGDMA (tetraethyleneglycol dimethacrylate), MMA (methyl methacrylate)
- Inorganic fillers: quartz, glass, zirconium
- Organic fillers: silica
- Coupling agents: silane
- Initiators: tertiary amines, camphorquinone (CMP), phenyl propanedione (PPD), benzoyl peroxide
- Inhibitors: ether of hydroquinone
- Ultraviolet absorbers: benzophenone

85. Describe the function of each monomer component.
Principal monomers are high-molecular-weight compounds that can undergo free radical addition polymerization to create rigid, cross-linked polymers. The most common monomer is Bis-GMA (an aromatic dimethacrylate that is the addition product of bisphenol A and glycidal methacrylate [GMA]). An alternative monomer is urethane dimethacrylate.

   Diluent monomers are low-molecular-weight compounds used to reduce the viscosity of the unpolymerized resins to improve physical properties and handling. There are two types, monofunctional (MMA) and difunctional (ethylene glycol dimethacrylate or triethylene glycol). The latter are used most often because they form harder and stronger cross-linked composite structures because of a lower coefficient of thermal expansion. They also have less polymerization shrinkage, are less volatile, and have less water absorption.

86. **What are filler particles?**

Inorganic filler particles used in composite resins include quartz, glass, and colloidal silica, along with additions of lithium, barium, or strontium to enhance optical properties. These fillers are coated with a silane coupling agent (organosilane) to bond adhesively to the organic resin matrix. Silane bonds to the quartz, glass, and silica particles, whereas the organic end bonds to the resin matrix.

87. **Describe the mechanism of silane coupling.**

During free radical polymerization of the organic Bis-GMA, covalent bonds are formed between this polymer matrix and the silane coupling agent, commonly gamma-methacryloxypropyltrimethoxy silane. The coupling agent that coats the filler particles at the silane end thus holds the inorganic and organic phases together, which prevents further water absorption.

88. **What is the mechanism of polymerization in composite resin systems?**

Benzoyl peroxide and aromatic tertiary amines are used to initiate polymerization reactions by supplying free radicals. This process is induced by photoactivation with visible light in the 420- to 470-nm range using alpha diketones and a reducing agent, often a tertiary aliphatic amine. The diketone absorbs light to form an excited triplet state, which together with the amine produces ion radicals to initiate polymerization.

89. **Describe the function of polymerization inhibitors.**

Inhibitors are necessary to provide shelf life and delay the polymerization reaction, thus allowing clinical placement of composite materials. The dimethyl acrylate monomers spontaneously polymerize in the presence of atmospheric oxygen. To this end, monomethyl ethers of hydroquinone are used as inhibitors.

90. **What are radiation absorbers?**

Ultraviolet absorbers provide color stability to composite resins and thus limit discoloration.

91. **How are composites classified?**

There are a number of classification systems, generally based on filler particle size and how the fillers are distributed.
- Large-particle (conventional) composites: 20 to 50 μm in diameter
- Intermediate: 1 to 5 μm
- Hybrids or blends: 0.8 to 1.0 μm
- Fine particle and minifilled: 0.1 to 0.5 μm
- Microfilled: 0.05 to 0.1 μm
- Nanofilled: 5 to 75 nm
- Homogenous microfilled: organic matrix and directly admixed microfiller particles
- Heterogeneous microfilled: organic matrix, directly admixed microfiller particles, and microfiller-based complexes

92. **Which are the most commonly used composite materials?**

The microfilled, hybrid, and nanofilled composites.

93. **List major characteristics of hybrid composites.**
- Most universal in application, anterior and posterior usage
- Combine strength and polishability
- Easier to use than thin microfills and more closely match the refractive index of tooth structure
- Composed of several filler particles, a glass in the 1- to 3-μm range plus silica, 0.04 μm
- Hybrids get darker when cured; match shade with cured sample
- Fillers are 75% to 80% by weight:
  1. First-generation hybrid composite, with smaller filler size (1-2 μm) and high filler content (70%-75% by weight).
  2. Second-generation hybrid composite with high filler content (70%-75% by weight) and uniform cut (1 μm) glass and submicron particles.

94. **What are microhybrid composites?**

Microhybrid composites evolved from hybrid composites in efforts to decrease the size of the largest particles. Typically, the largest size particle found in today's microhybrid is <1 μm. They maintain the strength of hybrid composites with improved handling and esthetics.

95. **What are the major properties of microfill composites?**
- Allow the most esthetic polishability and mimic porcelain in result
- Used in class III, IV, and V restorations; diastema closure; hand-sculpted facial veneers
- Resist wear: more elastic than hybrids and may be better suited for abraction lesions
- Particle size 0.01 to 0.1 μm
- Color gets lighter when cured; match shade with cured sample
- Fillers are 40% to 50% by weight

96. **What are nanofilled composites?**

The application of nanotechnology to composites is one of the greatest advancements in this field. Microfilled composites were the precursor material for nanofilled formulations that contain filler particles, ranging from 5 to 100 nm, and nanoclusters. Nanoclusters are 0.6- to 1.4-μm agglomerates of primary zirconia-silica nanoparticles, 5 to 20 nm in size, fused together at contact points. The remainder of the porous structure is infiltrated with silane. Overall, nanofilled composites have similar mechanical and physical properties as microhybrids but provide superior polish and sustained gloss. They are highly esthetic, with favorable handling properties, and have demonstrated excellent strength and wear. Thus far, they are commercially successful, suggesting more clinical acceptance.

Another category, nanohybrid composites, includes a combination of glass particles and nanofillers.

97. **How are hybrids, microfilled, and nanofilled composites used together for maximizing strength and esthetics, the so-called sandwich technique?**

1. A sandwich technique is a layering of materials to create the maximum of desirable properties in a restoration. In a class IV anterior restoration of an incisal angle, for example, using a hybrid composite first to build up the body of the underlying dentin provides strength and dentin-like opacity. Then, overlaying the final tooth structure with a microfilled composite provides incisal translucency, desired reflective characteristics, and high polishability of a microfill.
2. A layer of hybrid, together with opaquers, may block out undesirable colors prior to using a microfill.
3. All posterior restorations, as well as porcelain repairs and periodontal splinting, benefit from the superior strength of a hybrid.
4. Nanofilled composites can be used for the entire restoration and are stronger than microfills. They can be finished as smooth as microfills, but the process may be more technique-sensitive and time-consuming.

98. **What are packable composites?**

Packable composites have a consistency that more closely resembles that of amalgam than conventional composites. They are most commonly used in class I and II restorations. However, they cannot be condensed, but are more packable than hybrids. Because they are much stiffer in consistency, there is some ability to sculpt the restoration before curing. Bulk curing, however, is 2 to 3 mm at best.

99. **What are low-shrinkage composites?**

Most current microhybrid and nanohybrid composites have a 2% to 3.5% polymerization shrinkage. Minimizing shrinkage is the goal of composite resin manufacturers.

100. **What are self-adhesive composites?**

Self-etching bonding agents set the stage for the self-adhesive composites that contain the bonding agent within the restorative material. These restorative products bond and seal without the need for etchants or adhesives.

101. **What are composite opaquers or tints? How may they be used?**

Opaquers and tints are light-cured, low-viscosity, highly shaded composites used to add esthetic characteristics to restorations. They often match commonly used shade guides and can be brushed on in layers to create lifelike matches to natural teeth. They may be applied on a bonded tooth, between layers of the sandwich buildup, or even on the surface to characterize the restoration.

102. **What is a compomer?**

A compomer is a polyacid-modified composite that incorporates the properties of resin ionomers and composites. Compomers are self-adhesive to dentin due to an acid-base reaction when light cured and they release fluoride. They still require a primer-adhesive and may not require etching first for dentin bonding, but etching increases bond strength to enamel. They may be used in carious class V lesions, as a flow application in the gingival wall of a proximal box in class II preparations, and to block out undercuts in inlay-only crown preparations. They are also suitable for all restorations in primary teeth.

103. **Define composite sealant.**

Composite sealants are unfilled resins applied to seal microcracks that may be left after finishing and polishing of composite or bonded restorations. They are very thin-filmed and have a minimal air-inhibited layer. Application is done after a 20-second etch, wash, and then allow a 20-second light cure.

104. **What are flowable composites?**

Flowable composites are low-viscosity, VLC, radiopaque hybrid composite resins, often containing fluoride and dispensed by syringe directly into cavity preparations. They have 37% to 53% filler by volume (compared with 60% for conventional composites). They are claimed to be easy to deliver via a narrow syringe tip, offer flexibility for class V preparations, and are able to access small areas. They may be used as a base material under class I and II restorations. Although long-term performance is not known, they seem well suited for the long channels of air abrasion preparations, cementing veneers, dental sealants, margin repairs of all types, inner layer in sandwich techniques, porcelain repairs, and sealing the head of implants.

105. How are flowable composites used?

Class V defects: Use for abfraction, erosions, and sealing marginal defects.

Minimal class I restorations: Use like a thick sealant for pit and fissure restorations prepared with air abrasion or fissurotomy burs.

Gingival wall of class II restorations: Use in the gingival wall of a proximal box has been shown to reduce leakage at this margin in composite restorations.

Blocking out small undercuts: This eliminates removing sound tooth structure and is a fast and simple application.

106. What are the advantages of all-purpose composite resins?

These multipurpose products are small-particle composites, release fluoride, are self- or dual-curing, and have high compressive strengths and low viscosity. They have applications as cements, bases and liners, or pediatric restoratives. They bond to dentin, enamel porcelain, amalgam, precious and semiprecious metals, and moist surfaces. They function as luting materials for crowns (with dentin-bonding systems) and are suitable for Maryland bridge bonding.

107. What is an ormocer?

Ormocer is an acronym for *or*ganically *mo*dified *cer*amic. Ormocers are a class of restorative material that links glasslike inorganic components with organic polymer components to make them almost as hard as glass but similar to polymer materials in behavior. The prepolymerized filler particles in ormocers are large and tightly packed, which leads to less shrinkage on curing. The technique for placement is direct and similar to that for traditional composites.

108. What is a ceromer?

Ceromer is an acronym for *cer*amic *o*ptimized poly*mer*. The formulations of these materials give them many of the ideal properties found in composites and porcelain, but with a much higher level of fluoride release. These materials have high strength because of their low modulus of elasticity, as well as high flexural strength and fracture toughness. Also, their surface hardness is similar to that of enamel, giving them low wear and excellent polishability. These materials can be used for inlays, onlays, veneers, and crowns, using the direct-indirect or indirect techniques.

109. What are "smart" composites?

Smart composites have an ion-releasing composite formulation that releases fluoride, hydroxyl, and calcium ions in response to a decrease in the pH in the area adjacent to the material. What makes these composites "smart" is that the greater the decrease in pH, which results from plaque, the greater the release of active ions. The effect is a reduction in secondary caries formation by inhibiting bacterial growth and reducing demineralization. The fluoride release from this material is not as high as from glass ionomer but is much higher than from other aesthetic materials.

110. With all these products, how does the clinician know the best to use?

It depends on physical and mechanical properties, esthetic appeal, ease of use and, most importantly, personal preference.

111. Define direct resin, indirect resin, and indirect-direct resin restorations.

- **Direct resin** restorations are the placement of composite resins into class 1, 2, 3, 4, and 5 preparations directly at chairside. They are the most commonly performed.
- **Indirect resin** procedures involve tooth preparation, impressions, and temporization at a first visit. Laboratory fabricated onlays or inlays of resin or ceramic restorations are cemented on a second visit.
- **Indirect-direct resin** restorations are a single-visit technique using fast-setting die stones to allow preparation, impression taking, chairside fabrication of the restoration, and delivery of the final inlay or onlay.

112. What are the characteristics of indirect composite resin systems?

These composite resin systems are fabricated in the laboratory from impressions of prepared teeth. They are referred to as prosthetic composites or laboratory composites. They may be fiber-reinforced for crowns and bridges. By treating with heat, high-intensity light, vacuum, nitrogen, and/or pressure, the restoration's physical properties are greatly advanced. They exhibit reduced polymerization shrinkage, increased flexural and tensile strength, resistance to abrasion and fracture, and improved color stability.

113. What criteria are used to choose direct placement composite resins in class II restorations?

1. The best use is in narrow slot-type restorations and smaller restorations of one-fourth to one-third of the intercuspal distance.
2. If used in larger restorations, more than one-third of the intercuspal distance, weak cusps must be covered, and longevity is not considered long term.
3. Persons with known metal allergies or patients who wish to avoid metal restorations should use these.

4. Use is contraindicated in bruxers or clenchers or when extensive tooth loss aligns the resin margin in occlusal contact.

114. **Discuss the challenges of the class II composite restoration.**
    1. Most current resins wear significantly more than amalgam, gold, or porcelain. To minimize wear, sufficient light curing is suggested (30- to 40-second cures on facial, occlusal, and lingual surfaces, with a calibrated light source).
    2. They are generally time- and technique-sensitive restorations. Contact areas are harder to establish, and finishing is time consuming. Use magnification to view; also use thin, dead, soft matrix bands or sectional matrices, well burnished against the proximal tooth, and held tightly. Finish with sharp 12-bladed burs and a light touch.
    3. Sufficiently light-cure the primer and bonding agents before placing composite to avoid postoperative tooth sensitivity. Apply composite in 2-mm increments.

115. **Compare indirect resins with porcelain.**
    Indirect resin inlays tend to fit better, are easier to adjust/polish intraorally, can be repaired with similar materials in the mouth and, most importantly, are not as hard or abrasive to the opposing teeth as porcelain. Porcelain restorations may be better for onlays or when restoring multiple cusp and occlusal schemes, but the wear to opposing teeth is significant and the need to adjust occlusion and polish intraorally after cementation requires time and is more difficult.

116. **Summarize guidelines for indirect resin and full-coverage ceramic crown preparations.**
    1 Indirect resin preparations
      • 1.5-mm reduction on occlusal aspect
      • 1.5- to 2.0-mm reduction on cusps
      • Rounded internal line angles
      • No bevel margins
      • Butt joint or deep chamfer margins
      • Divergent walls
    2 Specialized ceramics full crowns
      • 2.0-mm occlusal reduction
      • 1.5-mm chamfer margin or butt joint margin
      • 1.5 to 2.0 facial reduction

117. **Outline the step-by-step procedure for the direct posterior resin restoration.**
    1. Apply rubber dam or isolation system.
    2. Remove the defective tooth structure or restoration.
    3. Use a caries indicator if desired.
    4. Prepare the tooth for the restoration.
    5. Place a matrix system (sectional matrix or full-band); wedge.
    6. Wash and clean preparation; you may use an antibacterial, if desired.
    7. Use total etch time of 15 seconds for enamel and a maximum of 10 to 15 seconds for dentin with phosphoric acid. Do not over-etch dentin.
    8. Rinse etchant off well, and lightly air-dry or blot excessive water; leave surface moist.
    9. Apply multiple layers of primer-adhesive to enamel and dentin, leaving for 20 seconds to allow penetration and hybrid layer formation.
    10. Air-disperse to evaporate the solvent.
    11. Light-cure for 10 to 20 seconds.
    12. Apply a layer (<2-mm increments) of flowable composite to the pulpal floor in the proximal box, cure per manufacturer's guidelines.
    13. Build up with composite (e.g., hybrid, packable, reinforced microfill).
    14. Sculpt, shape, and cure per the manufacturer's guidelines.
    15. Perform gross occlusal adjustment.
    16. Remove rubber dam or equivalent isolation system and adjust occlusion further.
    17. Apply occlusal resin stains, if desired.
    18. Polish with points, cups, discs, and wheels.

118. **What methods are used to provisionalize indirect resin restorations?**
    Take a preoperative polyvinyl matrix in a triple tray, fill with an acrylic or provisional composite resin and cement with a temporary cement. Light-cure, and trim.

119. **Outline the cementation technique for resin-bonded inlays and onlays.**
    1. Remove provisional restoration.
    2. Apply rubber dam or isolation system.
    3. Clean preparation, rinse, dry; try restoration, checking margins, interproximal contacts, and overall fit.

4. Remove restoration, clean with etch, and rinse; place a silane coupling agent on the internal surface for 1 minute.
5. Etch tooth enamel and dentin for 15 seconds, rinse, and lightly air-disperse moisture.
6. Apply multiple layers of single-component adhesive; air-disperse to evaporate solvent; leave for 20 seconds.
7. Light-cure 20 seconds.
8. Apply thin layer of adhesive to internal surface of restoration.
9. Mix dual-cure resin cement and apply into preparation; seat restoration.
10. While holding restoration, remove as much cement as possible with brush or rubber tip.
11. Spot cure into place 10 seconds from buccal and lingual aspects.
12. Apply floss through contacts.
13. Light cure finally for 30 seconds on each surface; remove rubber dam or equivalent isolation system and adjust occlusion; finish and polish.

120. **Describe the direct-indirect technique for posterior resin restorations.**
This combination technique involves taking an elastomeric impression of the prepared teeth and pouring up a die in a fast-setting material, such as an ultrafast-setting gypsum product. The clinician then generates the restoration in the office laboratory, light-cures it, and cements it in the same visit.

121. **List the advantages and disadvantages of the direct-indirect technique over the indirect, laboratory-processed, resin restorative technique.**
1. Major advantages
   • Decreased chair time
   • Decreased laboratory expenses
   • No need for temporization
2. Major disadvantages
   • Possible deformation of the restoration, especially if a flexible die material is used
   • Restorative material formulations available in the dental laboratory provide better strength and wear resistance
   • Processes available in the dental laboratory provide a better cure of the resin polymer material

122. **Give examples of laboratory-processed resin restorative materials. How are they cured compared with in-office resins?**
Most laboratory-processed resins are cured by a combination of light of varying intensities, pressure, and heat. Alternatively, other materials in this category are processed in a nitrogen environment under heat and pressure. The nitrogen removes any oxygen-inhibiting air from the resin and improves the cure.

123. **What cementing materials should be used with indirect resin restorations?**
All three of the polymer resin systems mentioned above should be luted with resin cements. Only resin cements possess the ability to bond adequately to tooth structure and the internal surface of the restoration. All other types of cements are strictly contraindicated. Hybrid-type resin cements are best suited for onlay and full-coverage restorations because of their higher strength. Microfill resin cements are preferred for inlays because they possess greater wear resistance to occlusal masticatory forces.

124. **Why are the polymer resin restorative materials well suited for restoring the occlusal surfaces of implant-supported restorations as opposed to conventional porcelains?**
Because porcelain has poor shock-absorbing ability, masticatory energy in implant restorations is transferred almost totally to the interfacial region between the implant and osseous tissue that supports the fixture. In contrast, polymer resins are much more energy-absorbent while still providing excellent resistance to wear on occlusal surfaces.

125. **What considerations shall be kept in mind for repair of older composite restorations?**
As composites age, it is harder to bond to the surface chemically. There are fewer reactive sites on the resin surface, and impregnated proteins and debris limit the bonding capacity. It is necessary to remove the outer surface with a bur to remove contaminants and increase the surface area. Pumice, followed by etching, proceeds as usual. Coating with silane allows better bonding to the silica particles. Final application of unfilled resin and curing before placement of the composite should result in predictable bonding.

126. **How is a fractured porcelain restoration repaired?**
The first step is to determine the cause. Is it a structural weakness or perhaps an occlusal stress-related fracture? Try to resolve any causative factors first. The next step is to create some mechanical hold wherever possible. Roughen and bevel around the defect because the restorative cannot bond to a glazed surface. Microetch when possible with an air abrasion microetcher, or use a porcelain acid etchant such as 10% to 12% hydrofluoric acid gel. Then silanate and apply bonding resin, opaquers, and finally the appropriate color of composite restorative.

127. **What is the function of a curing light?**
Primarily curing lights apply a visible light spectrum (400-700 nm) to photo imitators such as camphorquinone (450-525 nm) and PPD (430 nm) that allow polymerization on demand of a vast array of dental materials. Output should be at least 300 mW/cm^2, and built-in radiometers are advantageous.

128. List the current basic light types.
    - Quartz halogen bulb
    - Most common, least expensive, reliable
    - Wide-spectrum bandwidth, 400 to 510 nm
    - Cures all materials
    - Plasma arc curing (PAC)
    - Very fast, expensive, larger than halogen
    - May not cure all materials
    - Argon laser
    - Fast, expensive, larger than halogen
    - May not cure all materials
    - Light-emitting diode (LED)
    - Cordless, lightweight, small, long battery life
    - May not cure all materials
    - High-powered LED
    - Reduced curing times
    - More efficient curing
    - Caution pulp temperature
    - Lightweight, portable, long lifespan

129. Why and how should lights be tested and maintained?
    The power output of a light is critical to proper curing of a restoration. Any decrease is likely to give inadequate polymerization. The power output should be tested with a radiometer (built into many newer lights) when new and weekly thereafter. Any decrease should be checked. Usually, a deterioration in bulb strength (change the bulb), a dirty wand tip (clean regularly), or a worn light filter or optical guide (replace as needed) can decrease output. When all these steps fail, return the light to the manufacturer.

130. What constitutes an ideal cure?
    - Pack and cure materials incrementally to a 2-mm maximal thickness.
    - Keep light at right angles to the cure material.
    - Use infection control barriers with excellent transparency, that will stay in place when the light is in use.
    - Keep distance from tip to material less than 6 mm, the further from the restoration you are the lower the output delivered.
    - Use a proper diameter tip for the curing objective.
    - Darker shades and thicker layers need more time.
    - There is apparently no difference in ramped, stepped, or pulsed delivery of light and final cure results.
        Check manufacturer's recommendations for cure time based on type of composite and light source used, as cure times can vary based on combination of products used.

131. When in doubt, should you just cure for longer time?
    No! It is always best to understand the requirements of the material and equipment you are using. Depending on your light source, you can overheat the tissue unnecessarily, causing damage to the tooth and surrounding gingiva.

CEMENTS

132. What are resin cements?
    They are modified, low-viscosity composites used to bond ceramic and indirect resin restorations.

133. Summarize the types of resin cements and the indications for each.
    1. Light-cured
        Metal-free restorations <1.5 mm in thickness
        Metal-free orthodontic retainers
        Metal-free periodontal splints
    2. Dual-cured
        Metal-free inlays, onlays, crowns, and bridges
        Any application where a curing light may not reach
    3. Self-cure
        Metal-based inlays, onlays
        Ceramometal crown and bridges
        Full metal crowns and bridges
        Endodontic posts
        Bonded amalgams

134. What are the advantages of glass ionomer restorative materials?
    They bond to tooth structure, have an almost ideal expansion-to-contraction ratio and low microleakage, and release fluoride. Glass ionomers tolerate moisture and adhere directly to tooth structure with a solid marginal

seal. The light-cured materials are the easiest to work with because they provide extended working times, have rapid on-demand set, and are less technique-sensitive on mixing. The chairside experience is quicker and easier for the patient and dentist.

135. What are metal-reinforced GICs?

Metallic silver particles of up to 40% by weight are added to GICs to increase the strength and to speed up the setting time. Metal-reinforced GICs may be used for the following: (1) core buildups when at least 50% of tooth structure remains (GICs alone do not have the strength to be a total core); (2) as a temporary filling material; and (3) as a filler, base, or liner for undercuts in any cavity preparation. They provide excellent thermal and electrical insulation and are radiopaque.

136. What are resin-modified glass ionomers?

The addition of methacrylate monomer in aqueous polyalkenoic acid solution with monomer containing free radical double bonds in a fluoroaluminosilicate-containing component improved the strength of traditional glass ionomers. The monomer sets via VLC polymerization and cross-links, but the acid-base setting reaction is undisturbed. The initial self-setting is accelerated and light curing offers final control. The latest products do not require any etching, priming, or bonding, and the dual cure provides longer working times and shorter setting times. A variety of aesthetic shades are available.

137. What are glass ionomer resin (GIR) cements?

These resin-modified glass ionomers improve the properties of glass ionomers significantly.
1. They are easy to mix and place.
2. They are equal or higher in fluoride release.
3. They have higher retention, higher strength, lower solubility, and lower postoperative sensitivity than glass ionomer or zinc phosphate cements.

TECHNIQUE TIPS

138. What is considered the most important requisite for successful adhesive dentistry?

The formation of maximal-strength bonding requires a clean operating field, free of debris and contamination. Whenever possible, this goal is best accomplished with a rubber dam or isolation system.

139. What is the function of a matrix band? What types are currently available?

Matrix bands establish the foundation for a missing proximal wall of a tooth preparation. They may be metal or plastic and usually have a retainer to keep their form against the axial tooth walls and support tight contacts. The use of a wedge adapts the band fully at the gingival margin, but the wedge should not be placed under too much pressure to avoid unwanted effects on the gingival papilla. The traditional metal band retainers have been replaced by **sectional types,** which are used to form predictable proximal contacts when posterior direct resins are placed. They require an individual matrix for each proximal box (two are used for mesial-occlusal-distal boxes). The concaved metal or transparent form is placed interproximally and gently wedged. Then, using a rubber dam or dedicated forceps, the retaining ring is grasped, expanded, and positioned over the proximal line angles. When released, the ring tines grab the matrix and hold it against the tooth. The result is close adaptation of band to tooth to minimize excessive composite at the line angles but also to exert pressure on the band against the adjacent tooth to ensure a tight contact.

140. How can one achieve a tight interproximal contact in direct class II posterior composite restorations?

1. Use a thin burnished band, well-adapted and wedged, or a prefabricated sectional matrix system.
2. Apply a proximally applied force with an instrument to the band while curing the composite. This technique keeps the restoration tightly against the band and provides optimal contact.

141. What are clinical procedures that may cause injury to pulps of teeth?

1. Dull burs and diamonds can result in increased heat production.
2. Noncentric hand pieces traumatize teeth like mini-jackhammers.
3. Inadequate water delivery causes heat and dehydration.
4. Overdrying tooth preparations dehydrates the pulp, causing sensitivity.
5. The acidity of astringent materials can injure if left in dentin or root contact. Use only minimally on packing cord or in the gingival sulcus.
6. Temporary resin exothermic reactions for provisional restorations may be harmful. Cool with water often during exothermal period.
7. Poor-fitting temporary restorations can result in leakage that injures pulps. Margins should fit well.
8. Overcontoured restorations can result in trauma from occlusion. Carefully adjust occlusion and check in all excursions.

142. Describe the symptoms generally associated with cracked tooth syndrome

Patients who have cracked tooth syndrome (CTS) typically present with pain on chewing, particularly with hard foods and at the correct contact angle on the offending tooth. Additionally, there may be some sensitivity to cold and sweets, depending on the extent and nature of the fracture. Symptoms that include lingering temperature sensitivity may indicate that the pulp has undergone irreversible damage as a result of the fracture.

143. **What diagnostic tools and methods may be used to determine the location of the fracture in a patient with CTS?**
   In addition to the customary methods of locating dental pathology, the use of a bite stick enables you to isolate cusps to see whether pain can be elicited by occlusal stress on a potential offending cusp. The offending cusp often elicits a response on release of the bite on the stick. Intraoral cameras, magnification, and light refraction are also helpful in determining the location and extent of fractures.

144. **What types of restorations should be considered for teeth with CTS?**
   Generally speaking, restorations that bond and/or provide cuspal reinforcement should be used on CTS teeth. Fractures that have minimal dentin involvement may be restored with direct or indirect resins. Fractures involving significant amounts of dentin or involving one or more cusps should be restored with ceramic or gold onlays and crowns.

145. **Describe the clinical relationship among bruxism, tooth wear, and the incidence of CTS.**
   Bruxism and tooth wear often lead to loss of cuspid guidance, resulting in more of a group function occlusal scheme. This leaves the posterior teeth, especially those that are more heavily restored, prone to fracture.

146. **Describe the use of diagnostic restoration removal in the treatment of coronal fracture syndrome.**
   Diagnostic restoration removal is the removal of an existing filling material to inspect the pulpal floor visually and evaluate the integrity of the dentin at the base of the cusps. This procedure is performed when a hairline crack is visible externally but its extent and disposition are unclear.

147. **If a patient presents with tooth sensitivity to biting and cold in a clinically normal-appearing molar with a MOD amalgam, what are the possible differential diagnoses? What is the suggested treatment?**
   First, to confirm the specific tooth, attempt to duplicate the symptoms with a cold spray and when biting on a wet cotton roll. Take a radiograph to rule out recurrent decay, periapical pathology, or periodontal involvement. If there are no positive radiographic findings, consider a cracked tooth or a pulp that is hyperemic and may or may not be approaching irreversible change.

   The best initial treatment is to remove all old amalgam and explore the tooth for cracks or decay. Placing a bonded nonmetallic restoration allows one to see whether the pulp can resolve. If symptoms subside within 3 to 6 weeks, a permanent restoration (full-coverage crown or onlay) may be placed. If symptoms persist or worsen at any time, endodontic treatment should begin. If endodontic treatment does not resolve the pain, it may be concluded that the fracture proceeds subgingivally or through the furcation. At this time, extraction must be considered.

   Advanced imaging, such as with a cone beam CT could be considered. They may be able to determine signs of the fracture, such as a vertical bone defect, but typically are unable to detect fine cracks in the root definitively.

148. **What is the biologic width? Explain its relationship to restorative dentistry.**
   The biologic width is an area that ideally is approximately 3 mm wide from the crest of bone to the gingival margin. It consists of approximately 1 mm of connective tissue, 1 mm of epithelial attachment, and 1 mm of sulcus. As it relates to restorative dentistry, if a restorative procedure violates this zone, there is a higher likelihood that periodontal inflammation will ensue, causing the attachment apparatus to move apically.

149. **When it becomes necessary for restorative reasons to impinge on the biologic width, what steps can be taken before final restoration to create a maintainable periodontal environment?**
   Crown lengthening and orthodontic extrusion are the two most common ways to deal with this problem. Crown lengthening exposes more tooth structure surgically and is, in effect, surgical repositioning of the biologic width. Orthodontic extrusion is done when crown lengthening would unduly compromise the periodontal health of the adjacent teeth or create an unfavorable aesthetic situation, as can often occur in the anterior maxilla.

150. **What techniques can be used to achieve marginal exposure and to control hemorrhage in a class V cavity preparation?**
   If the preparation is less than 2 mm below the gingival sulcus, an impregnated retraction cord with a gingival retraction rubber dam clamp may be effective. If the defect approaches 3 mm or more, the hemostasis and margin exposure often require surgical exposure (crown lengthening) or excision via electrosurgery.

151. **Describe the options for treatment of root surface sensitivity.**
   Root sensitivity is a common problem and can be adequately resolved in many cases by modifying the patient's tooth-brushing technique and having her or him use desensitizing toothpaste or a fluoride gel. Other desensitizing agents use oxalate precipitates or a glutaraldehyde-hydroxyethyl methacrylate formula to occlude and seal the dentin tubules. Dentin-bonding systems also work well to reduce sensitivity.

152. **Should composite resins be placed to cover exposed root surfaces in a patient with gingival recession?**

In the absence of caries, the placement of composite to cover exposed root surfaces should generally be performed after careful consideration. Composites bond only marginally well to cementum and, like all restorative materials, can further promote gingival recession. In addition, if surgical root coverage is performed, success depends on the establishment of a biologic attachment between the grafted tissue and cementum. Grafts do not attach to composites. Root surface coverage may be considered in cases of protracted and extreme root sensitivity or when it is of significant aesthetic concern to the patient.

153. **Should direct placement composites be placed in bulk or in increments to the cavity preparation?**

Opinions vary about the optimal method of composite placement. Some manufacturers and clinicians advocate bulk placement, but most recommend the layering and curing of material in approximately 2.0-mm increments to allow more thorough curing. Incremental placement also allows the layering of materials of different shades, opacities, and viscosities to achieve a better aesthetic result.

154. **What is the relationship between the size and location of the restoration and the potential for failure when direct resins are used on posterior teeth?**

The more posterior the composite resin is placed, the greater the occlusal force. This force greatly increases the possibility of fracture, especially when there is an occlusal stop on the resin. Additionally, the larger the restoration, the greater the likelihood that polymerization shrinkage will compromise the integrity of the margins, leading to postoperative sensitivity and failure.

155. **Describe the ideal clinical situation for placement of a class II direct resin restoration.**

Ideally, a class II resin should be fairly conservative, with minimal exposure of dentin, all margins should be in enamel for optimal seal and marginal integrity, and there should be no occlusal stops on the restoration to minimize the likelihood of resin fracture.

156. **What are helpful aids in shade matching for anterior teeth?**

Choose the shade with color-corrected or natural light. Match teeth that are moist. Liquid coatings (saliva) alter reflected light. Place a cotton roll behind adjacent teeth to study changes in color, and note incisal shade changes that occur with light and dark backgrounds. Place a small amount of composite on the facial aspect of a tooth and light-cure. Hybrid composites turn darker and microfills lighter on curing.

157. **Describe recent technologic advances in chairside shade taking for porcelain restorations.**

In the past, shade taking involved manual shade tabs and the subjective viewpoint of the practitioner. Today, digital shade-taking systems allow dentists to digitally map teeth with all their variations of hue, value, and chroma. This information can be sent to the laboratory electronically. The software then calculates the shades of porcelain to be layered to achieve the proper match.

158. **List uses of the stainless steel crown in adult dentition.**

1. Extensive decay in the dentition of young adults may leave a vital tooth with limited structure that requires a crown. If a permanent cast or ceramic restoration is not feasible, one may use the stainless steel crown (SSC) in conjunction with a core buildup to stabilize the tooth until a permanent crown is constructed. A typical restoration involves the following steps: (1) complete excavation; (2) application of a glass ionomer liner or dentin bonding; (3) beveling of the cervical enamel or dentin margin; (4) trial fitting of the stainless steel crown (SSC) with careful adaptation of the cervical margins and checking for occlusal clearance; (5) etching of the preparation; (6) application of a self-cure bonding resin; (7) filling of a well-adapted SSC with self-curing composite core material; and (8) seating of the crown. Removal of excessive and expressed composite leaves a well-sealed restoration that may serve for many years. When it is time to prepare the tooth for the permanent crown, slitting the SSC leaves the core buildup ready for final preparation.
2. SSCs may be used to stabilize rampant decay at any age.
3. SSCs may be used as a substitute for the copper band to stabilize a tooth before endodontic treatment. The SSC is more hygienic and kinder to the periodontium when it has been well adapted. Traditional access is through the occlusal dimension.
4. The SSC may be used as a temporary crown when lined with acrylic.

159. **Outline design criteria for closing spaces in the anterior dentition.**

1. Usually, composite bonding and/or porcelain veneers may close the maxillary central diastema. Careful space analysis with calipers allows the most aesthetic result. The width of each central incisor is measured, along with the diastema space. Half the dimension of the diastema space is normally added to each crown, unless the central incisors are unequal. Then adjustment is made to create equal central incisors.
2. If the central incisors appear too wide aesthetically, one can reduce the distal incisal to narrow the tooth and bond it over to seal any exposed dentin. One then adds to the mesial incisal of the lateral incisor to effect closure of space.
3. Peg laterals may similarly be transformed by bonding and/or porcelain veneers.

160. **List the indications for the porcelain veneer restoration.**
   1. Stained teeth or teeth in which color changes are desired and available bleaching options have been unsuccessful
   2. Enamel defects
   3. Malposed teeth where orthodontic movement is not an option
   4. Malformed teeth
   5. Replacement for multi-surfaced composite restoration when adequate tooth structure remains (at least 30%)
       Each patient must be evaluated on an individual basis. A general requirement is excellent periodontal health and good hygiene practices.

161. **Describe the basic tooth preparation for the porcelain veneer restoration on anterior teeth.**
   1. **Vital bleaching.** This is optional, but preferable first step to determine if patient's desired outcome can be achieved without more invasive procedures.
   2. **Preparation.** Consider wax-up of final contours as well as fabrication of reduction guide. Preparation of tooth includes enamel reduction of at least 0.5 mm, which may extend to 0.7 mm at the cervical line angles, is necessary to avoid overcontouring. The only exception may be a tooth with a very flat labial contour and slight linguoversion. Chamfer-type labial preparations can be achieved with bullet-type diamonds, and the use of self-limiting 0.3-, 0.5-, or 0.7-mm diamond burs is essential for consistent depth of preparation. The gingival cavosurface margin should be level with the free gingival crest. The mesial and distal proximal margins are immediately labial to the proximal contact area. The contacts are not broken but may be relaxed with fine specialty strips of 15- to 120-μm thickness. This allows placement of smooth metal matrix strips at the time of placement. The incisal margin is placed at the crest of the incisal ridge. Placing retraction cord into the gingival sulcus prior to preparing the gingival cavosurface margin helps in the atraumatic completion of the preparation.
   3. **Impressions.** Standard impression techniques use vinyl polysiloxane materials.
   4. **Temporization.** If at all possible, this should be limited in use; it may be time-consuming and add to the expense of the procedure. One should use **fine** discs on the labial enamel surface for polishing the rough surface of the diamond-cut preparation to limit the accumulation of stain and debris. If it is necessary to temporize, preconstructed laboratory composite veneers or chairside direct temporization may be used. The techniques are similar. Spot-etch two or three internal enamel areas on the labial preparation. Apply unfilled resin and tack-bond the veneer, or place some light-cured composite on the tooth and spread it with a gloved finger dipped in unfilled resin to a smooth finish. The preparation should be light-cured, and one should be able to lift it off relatively easily at the unetched areas and polish down the etched spots.

162. **Describe the technique for insertion of porcelain veneers.**
   1. After isolation, pumicing, and washing, the fragile porcelain veneers are tried on the chamfer-prepared tooth. First, the inside surface of the veneer is wetted with water to increase the adhesion. Margins are then carefully evaluated.
   2. Try-in pastes are used to determine the correct color matching. Water-soluble pastes are the easiest to use. The try-in pastes closely match the final resin cements but are not light-activated.
   3. The porcelain veneers are prepared for bonding. Apply a 30-second phosphoric acid etchant for cleaning. Wash and dry. Apply a silane coupling agent, and air-dry. Apply the unfilled light-cured bonding resin, and cure for 20 seconds.
   4. To bond the porcelain veneer to the tooth, first clear interproximal areas with fine strips. Pumice and wash thoroughly. Place strips of thin interproximal matrix, and etch the enamel for 30 seconds. Wash for 60 seconds and dry. Apply the bonding resin. Any known dentin areas should be primed (with dentin primer materials) before applying the bonding resin. Any opaquers or shade tints may now be applied. The light-cured resin luting cement is then applied to tooth and veneer. The veneer is carefully placed into position, and gross excessive composite is removed. Precure at the incisal edge for 10 seconds, and remove any partially polymerized material gingivally and proximally. Light-cure fully for 30 to 60 seconds. Finish the margins with strips, discs, and finishing burst. Check for protrusive excursions. Apply the central incisors first and then the laterals and the cuspids.

163. **What are the "no-prep" veneers?**
   "No-prep" veneers are made of ultrathin, highly translucent porcelain (0.2-0.3 mm) and are used to close diastemas and cover stained, discolored, crowded, or chipped teeth in the anterior region. Little to no reduction in tooth structure is necessary for placement, so the use of local anesthesia, provisionals, and postoperative sensitivity may be eliminated. The downside of nonpreparation veneering techniques includes poor marginal adaptation and poor aesthetics. If the palatal or functional side remains uncorrected, maintenance and restoration may be challenging.

164. **What are CAD-CAM restorations?**
   CAD-CAM stands for computer-aided design–computer-aided manufacturing. It is a digital technology from which the practitioner or laboratory technician can design, plan, and fabricate a crown, onlay/inlay, or denture using 3D image obtained from an impression or intraoral scan.

165. Describe the process whereby the CAD-CAM unit fabricates a restoration.

The intraoral camera is placed over the tooth preparation, and a 3D image of the preparation is generated. The operator then delineates the margins on the computer screen, and the system calculates and proposes the other morphologic contours, which the operator accepts or modifies. Once the design is accepted, the software directs the modular milling unit to fabricate the restoration from a preselected block of restorative material. When completed, the restoration can be adjusted chairside, if necessary, and stained internally and externally to modify the shade.

166. What are the classifications for dental casting gold alloys?

Dental gold casting alloys are classified as types I to IV according to their composition as it affects surface hardness and strength as measured by their Vickers hardness number (VHN).

Type I   (soft): VHN 50 to 90
Type II   (medium): VHN 90 to 120
Type III   (hard): VHN 120 to 150
Type IV   (extra hard): VHN 150+

Table 8-1. Type, Vickers Hardness Number (VHN), Composition, Properties and Suggested Uses of Gold Alloys

TYPE	STRENGTH	VHN	AU %	AG %	CU %	PT/PD %	ZN %	SUGGESTED USES
I	Low	50-90	85	11	3	-	1	Inlays
II	Medium	90-120	75	12	10	2	1	Inlays and onlays
III	Hard	120-150	70	14	10	5	1	Onlays, pontics, full crowns
IV	Extra hard	150+	65	9	15	10	1	Bridges, bars, frameworks

167. What are the benefits of cast gold inlays and onlays?

It is generally accepted that cast gold is the standard against which all other restorative materials are judged. The gold onlay provides cuspal protection, as well as the following benefits:
1. Low restoration wear
2. Low wear of opposing teeth
3. Lack of breakage
4. Burnishable and malleable
5. Proven long-term service
6. Bonded cast gold restorations offer improvement in their main weakness, the cementing media

168. What are the advantages of cast gold onlays over other materials for restoring posterior teeth?

It is generally accepted that cast gold is the standard against which all other restorative materials are judged. Cast gold onlays afford cuspal protection to prevent fracture, have excellent marginal integrity and, unlike porcelain, are kind to the opposing dentition.

TOOTH WHITENING

169. What are the most common methods to lighten vital teeth?

Generally, most tooth whitening is done with home bleaching kits using custom tray fabrication. In-office techniques are suitable for some patients based on the type and intensity of stain and temperament and wishes of the patient. Home treatment requires compliance and patience, whereas chairside techniques are faster, but often more costly.

Direct composite or laboratory porcelain veneers are the next most conservative approach and may be used when bleaching does not produce satisfactory results. Veneers are also useful when the shape, size, or arrangement of teeth is aesthetically unacceptable.

Finally, full-coverage porcelain and porcelain fused to metal crowns are the most invasive methods; these may be used when there is a need to replace damaged or missing tooth structure.

170. What factors influence tooth discoloration?

Extrinsic agents either consumed or not subject to removal by proper hygiene can stain and darken teeth. Intrinsic discoloration may be caused commonly by aging (increased yellowing), disease, injury, or certain exposures, such as to tetracycline.

171. For intrinsic stains, what agent has proved most effective for general use?

Intrinsic stains respond favorably to the chemical oxidation actions of peroxides. Vital tooth whitening is a popular dental service, and the in-office and at-home markets continue to grow. It is important that the patient is in good oral health prior to proceeding with any whitening program to minimize potential side effects and unexpected outcomes. Patients should be encouraged to have an evaluation with their dentist first to discuss which option is best for them.

172. What are the peripheral benefits of tooth whitening?

Often, patients describe increased self-esteem, improved oral hygiene practices, and increased interest and involvement in dentistry.

173. List appropriate expectations of present bleaching techniques.

1. Natural teeth generally darken with age. Patients older than 50 years accumulate brown, orange, or yellow stains that are decreased by bleaching. Light yellow or brown shades lighten better than gray shades. External stains respond better than deeper internal stains, such as those from tetracycline staining or staining related to endodontic events.
2. Teeth lighten visibly regardless of the system used (in-office or home methods).
3. The degree of lightening is a function of the concentration of active ingredient and time of contact. In-office techniques use higher concentrations applied for up to 1 hour on isolated teeth, whereas home methods use lower concentrations applied over several weeks in custom-molded trays constructed with or without reservoirs on the facial surfaces.
4. Generally, few side effects are reported, and they tend to be transient.
5. Bleached teeth retain color for up to several years, although some patients request touchups at 6- to 12-month intervals. Patients with high consumption of coffee, tea, cola, or red wine, and tobacco users may require more frequent applications.
6. All current tooth-lightening products are generally similar when adjusted for contact time and concentration of reagent. Changes of two to six or more shades on the Vita scale are common.

174. How are bleaching procedures currently performed?

1. **Professionally administered chairside.** After tooth isolation with a paint on dam, a peroxide gel is coated on teeth and usually activated via high-energy light to shorten the treatment interval. Higher concentrations of peroxide gels in the form of up to 35% carbamide peroxide are used in 1- to 2-hour treatment sessions.
2. **Professionally dispensed systems.** These use custom-fabricated trays to deliver 10% to 20% carbamide peroxide solution in-home procedures. Trays are worn according to manufacturer guidance, approximately for 2 hours for a period of 2 to 3 weeks. Favorable results have been reported, even with tetracycline staining, with prolonged applications of up to 3 to 6 months.
3. **Self-administered, over-the-counter, and professionally dispensed whitening strips.** Whitening strips containing 5% to 6.5 % hydrogen peroxide (equivalent to 10% carbamide peroxide) that are adherent to the teeth and worn for one to two 30-minute intervals daily for up to 2 weeks take about half the time of tray-delivered systems.

175. What are the active ingredients in bleaching systems?

Hydrogen peroxide (H_2O_2) is the active ingredient in all bleaching systems. In carbamide peroxide formulations, the H_2O_2 is stabilized by urea and appears to be more stable than H_2O_2 alone and produces fewer side effects. A 10% carbamide peroxide solution contains 7% urea and 3% H_2O_2. Presently available formulations contain 3% to 50% H_2O_2. Formulations are based in viscous gels to avoid side effects and maximize the retention to teeth. They are buffered to a near-neutral pH.

176. Describe the mechanism of action of hydrogen peroxide in lightening teeth.

Hydrogen peroxide oxidizes and removes interprismatic organic matter within the tooth to lighten the shade.

177. Describe "energized" in-office methods to speed the lightening of teeth.

The application of a curing light or laser has been claimed by manufacturers to shorten the lightening process; generally, less than 1 to 2 hours in the office will equal 2 weeks at home. This is because much higher peroxide concentrations are delivered on properly isolated teeth; it does not seem to be based on the method of energizing. Higher in-office concentrations require tooth isolation by paint on rubber dam material or a traditional dam.

178. Which method of bleaching produces the best results?

Split arch comparisons seem to indicate that no discernable differences in lightening are achieved by any properly performed home or energized method; the effect is a function only of concentration and time.

179. What are the two major complications of vital tooth bleaching?

Tooth sensitivity and gingival irritation may affect up to two-thirds of patients during the course of treatment. Tooth sensitivity is often mild and self-limiting and usually involves increased response to cold. Gingival irritation is often attributed to peroxide contact with tissues or poorly contoured trays that irritate the marginal tissues. There are no structural or functional effects on teeth.

180. What is thought to be the cause of bleach-induced tooth sensitivity?

Pulpal penetration of peroxide, dehydration, and tray-related tooth movements have been implicated. This sensitivity is transient and generally dissipates within a short time.

181. If a patient reports tooth sensitivity during the initial phase of treatment, what strategies may be implemented?

Decreasing the contact intervals may be a start—using 1-hour instead of 2-hour contact times or even every other day. Decreasing the concentration of the product chosen, 10% or less carbamide peroxide rather than higher levels, is a second choice. It has been reported that not prebrushing the teeth decreases sensitivity without undue impairment in bleaching result. Dentifrices contain detergents (e.g., sodium lauryl sulfate) that may readily denature proteins on contact, which allows greater penetration of peroxide into the tooth and increases transient irritation. A prescription-strength fluoride dentifrice can be used to resolve persistent cases. Soft tissue irritation can occur with in-office methods unless proper isolation is used. Home bleaching trays must be well adapted and properly contoured to prevent prolonged soft tissue contact. Patients should be instructed not to overfill their trays to avoid swallowing excessive bleach material on insertion.

182. What contributes to the safety of peroxide as an oral bleaching agent?

Natural tissue peroxidases available on tooth and tissue surfaces limit the penetration of peroxide and degrade it readily. These enzymes are thought to play a role in the efficacy and tolerability of vital bleaching.

183. All methods of tooth whitening improve tooth color to some degree, provided there is what?

There needs to be a sufficient degree of peroxide diffusion into the tooth surface.

184. Is bleaching safe for children?

Studies in those in the 11- to 18-year-old group have shown no ill effects greater than those seen in the general population. The use of whitening strips is well accepted because of the shortened application intervals required, however at the parent's discretion.

185. What concentrations of bleaching gel are used for home bleaching?

Available products for home bleaching come in concentrations ranging from 10% to 30%. A higher concentration allows shorter exposure times within the trays, which may decrease the effects of dehydration and lessen the chances of sensitivity. When using a higher concentration, bleaching trays must be especially well adapted and trimmed to prevent soft tissue exposure.

186. Can tetracycline-stained teeth be successfully treated with home bleaching?

Depending on the nature and severity of the discoloration, significant aesthetic improvement of tetracycline-stained teeth can be achieved with home bleaching. Tetracycline stain exists primarily in the dentin of teeth; discoloration in the incisal two-thirds responds more favorably than that in the gingival third. Deeper and more pronounced stain is the most resistant to extensive color change.

187. How would you modify the home bleaching regimen for patients with tetracycline-stained teeth?

If only certain teeth exhibit stain, bleaching may be selectively limited. Treatment times often must be extended to between 2 and 6 months.

188. When is the optimal time to bleach in the treatment-planning sequence?

In general, the optimal time is before beginning the final restorative phase. Bleaching lightens tooth color. Subsequent shades of crowns and composites need to be matched to the final tooth color. This is necessary because composite and porcelain restorations do not change color and will be mismatched if subsequent bleaching is performed.

189. Describe the technique of enamel microabrasion.

Microabrasion is the controlled removal of discolored enamel using a rubber cup and a paste composed of medium pumice and an acid, usually 20% hydrochloric acid. This technique is effective for treating superficial enamel discolorations (white or brown spots) often seen postorthodontically and in cases of fluorosis.

190. How can microabrasion be used as an adjunct to vital bleaching procedures?

Although vital bleaching is extremely effective in many aesthetic cases, it tends to make areas of decalcification (white spots) even whiter in contrast to the surrounding tooth. Additionally, stains common with fluorosis are usually minimally affected by bleaching. Microabrasion is an effective technique for removing such lesions if they are superficial in nature.

191. What are the limitations of the microabrasion technique?

Microabrasion is useful only for the removal of enamel lesions in the outer few hundred microns (100-200 μm) of the tooth. Lesions that penetrate deeper into enamel or into dentin must be restored with restorative materials. Teeth with deeper intrinsic staining, such as that caused by tetracycline, cannot be treated effectively with microabrasion.

192. Should you wait to do bonded restorations on recently bleached teeth?

Alterations in the surface microstructure from peroxide treatments can reduce bond strength. It is advised to wait 3 weeks or longer before doing bonded restorations.

193. Describe a logical sequence for whitening an anterior dentition with older class III and IV composite restorations.

Usually, older restorations are replaced after whitening because they will not match the new enamel shade. Before gel application, these older restorations should be carefully disked back to uncover all facial enamel. This process allows full bleach coverage of exposed enamel and leaves a more uniformly colored surface to replace and match the composite restorations.

194. Are reservoirs necessary in prefabricated bleaching trays?

It was thought that leaving a space on the facial surface of models before making a custom tray allows more of the gel to stay in contact with the teeth. There is generally no difference reported with or without tray reservoirs; they may not be necessary.

195. How effective are whitening toothpastes?

Generally, given their low concentration of bleaching agent and short tooth contact time, whitening toothpastes have a minimal effect on actual tooth color but may prolong the effect of direct bleaching.

196. How are endodontically treated teeth bleached?

Most discoloration of pulpal degeneration is internal and/or from remnants of endodontic paste fillers. Such teeth generally require bleaching from the access cavity. The sooner the bleaching is started after the endodontic event, the more successful is the lightening. Often, the pulp chamber is packed with a mixture of hydrogen peroxide and sodium perborate, so-called walking bleach. This mixture is changed as needed until the result is satisfactory. Care must be taken not to allow the bleach mixture to leach into the pulp canal, especially if there is any doubt about the integrity of the pulpal seal.

AMALGAM

197. What is the difference between an alloy and an amalgam?

An **alloy** is a mixture of metals; an **amalgam** is an alloy containing mercury.

198. What is the composition of dental amalgam?

Dental amalgam is an alloy composed of silver, tin, copper, and mercury. The basic setting reaction involves the mixing of the alloy complex of silver (Ag) and tin (Sn) with mercury (Hg) to form the so-called gamma phase alloy (original silver and tin) surrounded by secondary phases called gamma-1 (silver and mercury) and gamma-2 (tin and mercury). The weakest component is the gamma-2 phase, which is less resistant to corrosion.

$$\underset{\text{gamma}}{Ag_2Sn} + Hg \longrightarrow Ag_3Sn + \underset{\text{gamma-1}}{Ag_2Hg_3} + \underset{\text{gamma-2}}{Sn_3Hg}$$

Alloys are manufactured as filings or spherical particles; dispersed alloys are mixtures of both. Smaller particle size results in higher strength, lower flow, and better carvability. Spherical amalgams high in copper usually have the best tensile and compressive characteristics.

199. What is the function of each component?

- Silver increases strength, hardness, and reactivity while decreasing creep.
- Tin increases reactivity and corrosion but decreases strength and hardness.
- Copper increases strength, expansion, and hardness while decreasing creep.
- Zinc increases plasticity, strength, and the mercury-to-alloy ratio; it also decreases creep and causes secondary expansion.
- Mercury wets alloy particles, but decreases strength in excessive amounts.

200. How can one tell when an amalgam is properly triturated?

A properly triturated amalgam mix appears smooth and homogeneous. No granular appearance or porosity should be evident. An over-triturated mix is preferable to an undermixed preparation.

201. What types of amalgam alloys are commonly used today?

Alloys are supplied in different particle shapes and sizes to influence the handling and setting properties. The blended alloy is a mixture of fine-cut and spherical particles, whereas all-spherical alloys are composed of spherical particles. Because spherical alloys are very fast-setting, they are particularly suitable for core buildups and impression taking in one visit.

202. What are the indications for the various amalgam product types?

- All class I preparations: spherical or spheroidal
- Class II preparations: admixed or spheroidal
- Around pins and for internal retention: spherical
    It is not advisable to combine spherical and admixed types.

203. List current principles for amalgam tooth preparations.

Basically, a conservative preparation that salvages the maximal amount of tooth structure while removing carious material is advocated:
- Use of the 330 and 245 burs allows slot and tunnel preparations.
- Prepare rounded internal line angles, 90-degree cavosurface margins, with removal of unsupported enamel during excavation of all caries past the DEJ.
- Use a caries detector solution when necessary.
- Create mechanical retention by undercuts, channels, and grooves or bonding.
- Place band and properly wedge; create tight interproximal contacts.
- Seal dentin tubules with adhesive liners.
- Provide enough amalgam bulk for strength.

204. List six common causes of amalgam failure.

1. Inadequate retention
2. Insufficient bulk for strength
3. Insufficient removal of unsupported enamel
4. Incomplete caries removal
5. Inadequate condensation
6. Recurrent caries caused by microleakage

205. What is the purpose of finishing and polishing amalgam restorations?

Amalgam restorations should be finished and polished for three main reasons: (1) to reduce marginal discrepancies and create a more hygienic restoration; (2) to reduce marginal breakdown and recurrent decay; and (3) to prevent tarnishing and increase the quality of appearance of the restoration. Polishing is often a neglected part of treatment because of lack of opportunity for recall visits or from the consideration of not being compensated for the added service. However, polishing one or two restorations at each recall may be a cost effective means to provide this valuable service.

206. Describe the sequence for polishing amalgams.

Begin gross contouring with multifluted finishing burs, usually at least 1 day after insertion. Burs come in a variety of round, pear, flame, and bullet-nosed shapes and allow anatomic contouring. Amalgam polishing points can be used to create a high luster. Final pumicing with rubber cups can complete the finishing.

207. What additional means may be used to retain alloy restorations?

Optimal retention warrants the use of pins, grooves, channels, or holes placed in sound tooth areas. Although bonding has replaced much of pin usage, it arguably still provides the best possible retention.

208. List guidelines for the use of pins to retain dental restorative material.

1. Pins should extend 2 mm into tooth structure and then backed off a half-turn to reduce stress.
2. Pins should be placed fully in dentin. If they are too close to the DEJ, the enamel may fracture from the tooth. In general, they should be placed at the line angles where the root mass is the greatest and at least 0.5 mm from the DEJ.
3. Pins should extend 2 mm into amalgam; further extension only weakens the tensile and shear strength of the amalgam.
4. Pins should be aligned parallel to the radicular emergence profile or parallel to the nearest external enamel wall. Additional angulations may be used when there is no danger of pulpal or periodontal ligament perforation.
5. If the tooth structure is flat, the use of small retentive channels that are cut into the tooth structure prevents potential torsional and lateral stress.

209. What are the major complications to the use of pins to retain restorations?

Pin placement can result in pulpal exposure, perforation through the periodontal ligament, and fracture of a tooth. Additionally, pins may weaken an amalgam if they extend more than 2 mm into the mass. The use of a dentin-bonded resin liner can help seal any potential fracture lines, but placement requires skill and expert technique.

210. What should be done if accidental exposure of the pulp or perforation of the periodontal ligament occurs during pin placement?

If the pulp is exposed by the pinhole, allow the bleeding to stop, dry with a sterile paper point, and place calcium hydroxide in the hole. Bond over with an adhesive glass ionomer resin. Do not place a pin in the hole. Usually, the pulp will heal. If penetration of the gingival sulcus or periodontal ligament space occurs, clean, dry, and place the pin to the measured depth of the external tooth surface to seal the opening.

211. Discuss current concepts of pulpal protection.

Formerly, a thermal liner or base under amalgam restorations was advocated. If 1 to 3 mm of dentin remains under the cavity preparation, sufficient thermal protection is present. Sealing dentin tubules is considered important to minimize postoperative pulpal sensitivity and prevent bacterial contamination by microleakage.

Microleakage can wash out liners such as calcium hydroxide. Sealing dentin tubules by bonding protects the pulp from postoperative sensitivity and offers long-term protection against bacterial contamination from microleakage.

212. **Discuss the classic role of calcium hydroxide.**
Calcium hydroxide compounds have a long tradition of providing pulpal protection as a liner under restorative materials. Calcium hydroxide is known to serve as an insulator, stimulator of repair dentin via bridge formation, and bactericidal agent because of its high pH. However, it does not bond to dentin, does not seal tubules, and is prone to wash out if microleakage occurs. If calcium hydroxide is used, it should be sealed by using some type of bonded resin system.

213. **What compounds stimulate dentin bridging?**
    - Calcium hydroxide
    - Zinc phosphate cements
    - Resin composite systems
      Eugenol and amalgam compounds do *not* show bridge formation.

214. **Summarize the recommended treatment for a direct vital pulp exposure.**
    1. Control hemorrhage using irrigation with saline or sodium hypochlorite.
    2. Apply a calcium hydroxide capping agent.
    3. Cover with a layer of glass ionomer cement.
    4. Etch, bond, and restore.
    5. Alternatively, some advocate direct etching, priming, and bonding after hemorrhage control as a direct cap procedure.

215. **What is a cavity liner? What are the indications for its use?**
A cavity liner is a relatively thin coating over exposed dentin. It may be self-hardening or light-cured, and it is usually nonirritating to pulpal tissues. The purpose is to create a barrier between dentin and pulpally irritating agents or stimulate the formation of reparative secondary dentin. Calcium hydroxide has traditionally been placed on dentin, with a thickness of 0.5 mm, as a pulpal protective agent. Contemporary practice uses newer dentin bonding agents for liner materials. They not only provide a barrier to pulpally toxic agents but also seal the dentin tubules against bacterial microleakage and provide a bondable surface to increase the retention of the restoration. Glass ionomer cements and dentin bonding systems have become the standard liner materials in restorative dentistry.

216. **What is a base? What are the indications for use?**
Generally, cements thicker than 2 to 4 mm are termed *bases* and, as such, function to replace lost dentin structure beneath restorations. A base may be used to provide thermal protection under metallic restorations, increase the resistance to forces of condensation of amalgam, or block out undercuts in taking impressions for cast restorations. A base should not be used unnecessarily. Pulpal thermal protection requires a thickness of at least 1 mm, but covering the entire dentin floor with a base is not thought to be necessary. Generally, the following guidelines may be used:
    1. For deep caries with frank or near exposures or with less than 0.5 mm of dentin, apply calcium hydroxide.
    2. Under a metal restoration, a hard base may be applied (over the calcium hydroxide) up to 2.0 mm in thickness to increase resistance to forces of condensation.
    3. If more than 2 mm of dentin is present, usually no base is needed under amalgam; a liner may be used under the composite.
    4. Use of a dentin bonding agent that seals the dentin tubules and bonds to the restorative material is desirable.

POSTS AND CORES

217. **What is the purpose of placing a post in an endodontically treated tooth?**
Posts are needed only to retain coronal buildup when the remaining coronal tooth structure to support a build-up by itself. Although the cast post had been the standard for years, it is insufficient, requires additional time and expense, and has been replaced by alternatives. The use of titanium posts and metal-free, fiber-reinforced posts for better aesthetics in anterior teeth has become popular. Retention of posts is usually by micro (sand blasting) or macro (channel undercuts) mechanical methods. Furthermore, posts are now bonded into place by self-cured or dual-cured resin cements.

218. **Does a post strengthen endodontically treated teeth?**
Contrary to what was formerly thought, posts do not reinforce teeth and may weaken some root structures. Widening a canal space for a larger post can weaken a root. Long posts are more retentive, but too much length may perforate a root or compromise the apical seal. A good guide is to make the length about half of the bone-supported root length, allow at least 1 mm of dentin lateral to the apical end of the post, and leave at least 3 to 5 mm of apical gutta percha filling.

219. **Which canals are generally chosen for post space?**
Generally, the largest canal is chosen—in maxillary molars, it is the palatal canal and in mandibular molars, it is the distal canal. Two-rooted bicuspids with minimal tooth structure may require one post in each canal.

220. **How may vertical fractures develop in roots from a post?**
- Wedged or tight-fitting posts may cause fractures.
- Overpreparation of the internal canal space may weaken a root and cause fractures.

221. **When are posts indicated? When are they not needed?**
1. Indicated
   - If more than half the coronal tooth structure is missing, place a post to attach the core material to the root structure.
   - If all the coronal tooth structure is missing, place a post to attach the core material to the root structure.
2. Not needed
   - If minimal coronal tooth structure is missing, as when an access cavity is made centrally with no caries on proximal walls, no post is required. Placement of a bonded filling material to the level of the pulpal floor adequately restores the endodontic access preparation.
   - If up to half of the coronal tooth structure is missing, a post may not be needed, except for teeth with high lateral stresses (e.g., cuspids with a cuspid rise occlusion). Place a bonded crown buildup.

222. **How are antirotational features created?**
1. Cast cores can be placed in anterior teeth with recessed boxes to limit rotation.
2. Small cut boxes or channels 1 to 1.5 mm deep and about the width of a 330 bur may be placed into the remaining tooth structure.
3. An accessory pin may be placed nonparallel to the posts.

223. **When a crown preparation is made, where should the finish line be placed?**
The gingival margin should be 1 to 1.5 mm apical to the core buildup material and on the root surface for optimal retention and antirotational resistance. If there is a ferrule post and core, the crown margin may be placed on the core material.

224. **List the characteristics of ideal posts.**
- The post space must provide adequate retention and support for the core, and the core must provide adequate support for the fixed restoration.
- Passive-fitting posts are best.
- Resin-bonded posts transmit less force to the root and increase the structural integrity by bonding the post to the root.

225. **What are the indications for a cast post?**
For buildup of a single-rooted tooth with little supragingival structure or thin-walled roots, a cast post or core with an inset lock preparation and ferrule design may strengthen the root and prevent rotation. The casting is air-abraded or microetched and bonded into the root.

226. **Of what materials are prefabricated posts constructed?**
Fiber-reinforced resin, stainless steel, and titanium alloys.

227. **Outline the clinical steps in resin-bonding a cast or prefabricated posts.**
1. Prepare the canal space by removing gutta percha to a depth of half the bone-supported root length, or as dictated by root shape.
2. Refine the canal preparation.
3. Cleanse the canal of debris with hydrogen peroxide using a syringe.
4. Treat with 37% phosphoric acid etchant for 15 seconds or with 17% EDTA for 1 minute to remove the smear layer.
5. Rinse well with water and lightly dry.
6. Microetch the post with air abrasion.
7. Apply resin cement primers and resins to the post and canal according to product directions.
8. Mix the resin cement and inject into the canal quickly, seating the post.
9. Wipe the excessive cement with a brush dipped in resin while holding the post until the cement has set.

228. **Summarize the guidelines for fillers, buildups, and post and cores.**
For full-crown preparations, all old restorative material should be removed after preliminary tooth preparation. Small areas or missing teeth can be replaced with a bonded filler; larger sections of missing teeth should be replaced with a buildup; and an endodontically treated tooth with more than half its coronal structure missing should have a post with a composite core buildup.

229. **What materials are used to rebuild tooth core structure?**
These are gold, amalgam, composites, and glass ionomers.

230. **List advantages of using composite materials for core buildups.**
- Composite materials can bond to tooth structure.

- Usually, they achieve adequate strength in 5 to 10 minutes so that preparation of the core may be done at the same appointment as placement.
- They may be tooth-colored to avoid shade-matching problems with the final restoration.
- They may also be shaded to differentiate core structure from tooth when placing finish lines.
- They can be prepared easily and placed into a matrix or core form or placed freehand.

231. What current types of core composite materials are available?

Light cure. These use traditional large-particle materials that are made to cure deeply. Any hybrid composite also may be used.

Dual cure. These materials have the advantage that the surface may be light-cured immediately, whereas deeper layers can be chemically cured, allowing preparation to take place soon after placement.

Self-cure. In areas in which light penetration cannot be achieved, such as around posts and in deep recesses, these materials may be the best choice.

   NOTE: Some self-cure or dual-cure materials will not bond to light-cured adhesives. It is important to use a self-cure adhesive system and read the manufacturer's instructions carefully.

AMALGAM, MERCURY, AND HEALTH ISSUES

232. Summarize the current status of the use of amalgam.

Dental amalgam continues to be a popular material for the restoration of carious teeth worldwide due to its durability, cost, and ease of placement. As newer materials evolve, it is likely that mercury-containing restorations will be phased out. Until then, it is the opinion of world health agencies, medical and dental societies, and the scientific community at large that amalgam is a safe, easy, durable, bacteriostatic, and cost-effective restorative material. The choice of using a particular material should be left to an informed patient, with adequate scientific information supplied by a knowledgeable professional.

233. What three forms of mercury are found in the environment and may result in human exposure?

1. **Elemental mercury** is a small contributor to the total human body burden. It is very short-lived because of rapid oxidation. It is the common form found in dentistry; it is lipid-soluble and adsorbed in the lungs. Elemental mercury is the least toxic form.
2. **Inorganic mercury** is formed by the oxidation of elemental mercury and has limited solubility. It is sequestered in the kidney and excreted slowly in urine, with a half-life of about 60 days. It is of moderate toxicity.
3. **Organic mercury** is usually in the methyl mercury form. It is only found in nondental sources. Organic mercury forms in the gut of fish from bacterial action on mercury and accumulates in red blood cells; it is sequestered in the central nervous system and liver and has high lipid solubility. It is not found in urine but is secreted in feces, and 90% is absorbed in the gut. Organic mercury is the most toxic form.

234. What should a dentist know to be prepared to respond to a patient's inquiry about amalgam restorations and safety?

The clinician must know all the facts about amalgam, health-related sensitivities, ethics of replacements, and alternative restorative choices. Informed consent brochures and written consent for amalgam restorations are required in several US states.

235. What consideration should be given to a patient's concern about sensitivity to dental alloys?

A real allergy or hypersensitivity (as differentiated from toxicity or poisoning) to dental alloys and metals is not uncommon. Approximately 3% of the population has some type of metal sensitivity. Health questionnaires should ask about skin reactions to jewelry and/or known metal sensitivities. Allergy testing can confirm these sensitivities.

   It is important to determine the type of inquiry:

1. Patients who have aesthetic concerns and do not wish to have non–tooth-colored restorations
2. Patients who have phobias about the alleged toxicity of dental materials
3. Patients who have chronic diseases, such as multiple sclerosis, and are looking for some causative agent
   Each group of patients requires appropriate information from dental and medical sources to help them make informed choices about dental health.

236. What dental materials are reported to be the most allergenic? What are the manifestations of these exposures?

Allergic reactions have been reported to chromium, cobalt, copper, nickel (the most common), palladium, tin, zinc, silver, and gold and platinum (least allergenic). The symptoms may range from localized chronic inflammation around restorations and crowns to more generalized oral lichen planus, geographic glossitis, angular cheilitis, and plicated tongue.

237. Are certain people hypersensitive to mercury?

Yes. However, according to the North American Contact Dermatitis Group, true sensitivity to mercury in subtoxic doses is rare. Studies have shown that 3% of people respond to a 1% mercury patch test. Of these, less than

0.6% have any clinical manifestations of mercury sensitivity allergy. It is important to note that these testing levels are extreme in relation to the exposure possible from dental amalgam restorations.

238. **Are there any known harmful effects from the mercury content of dental amalgam?**
As a restorative material, silver amalgam has been used in dentistry for more than 200 years. Its safety has been studied throughout this long period, and in nonallergic patients, no epidemiologic evidence has associated general health problems with this amalgam. Furthermore, no recovery or remission from any chronic disease after removal of amalgams has been scientifically demonstrated.

The FDA issued its final rule on encapsulated dental amalgam in July 2009, classifying it and its component parts as a class II medical device. This places amalgam in the same class as other restorative materials, such as gold and composite resin.

239. **Discuss the relative safety of composite resins as restorative materials.**
Although they appear safe, health concerns have been raised about the use of composite resins. Composite materials contain many components that are potentially hazardous and possibly carcinogenic during the polymerization reaction or later because of degradation of the material. To consider these materials a "nontoxic" alternative to dental amalgam is premature and surely warrants further study.

240. **By what physical pathways can mercury enter the body?**
Elemental mercury is abundant in the earth's environment. It exists in the soil, oceans, and air. The burning of fossil fuels and even volcanic eruptions have contributed to the widespread decimation of this element. The use of mercury in manufacturing through the centuries has led to much of the environmental contamination. Furthermore, in high enough doses, mercury is neurotoxic. The questions of exposure to mercury from dental amalgams require some clinical elucidation.

Dental amalgam fillings contain up to 50% mercury and elements of silver, tin, and copper, bound into a metallic complex from which the mercury is not free. Small amounts of mercury vaporize from the surface with function, pass into the air, and are exhaled. This amount, which is absorbed into the body as a function of the number of surfaces of amalgam, is largely excreted by the kidneys into the urine. The smaller amount, which may accumulate in other organs, has raised concern. Mercury accumulates in organs such as the brain, lungs, liver, and gastrointestinal tract, but this accumulation represents exposure from all environmental sources. The ultimate question is the percentage of the dental amalgam component compared with total mercury exposure from all sources.

The daily intake of mercury attributable to dental amalgams, as measured by urine levels of mercury, is reported to be only one-seventh (14%) of that measured from eating one seafood meal per week. The total daily intake from 8 to 12 amalgam surfaces is about 1 to 3 µg. This is again seven times lower than the intake from one seafood meal per week and only about 10% to 20% of the average total exposure (9 µg/day) from all environmental sources. Clearly, the general environmental exposure is much more of a concern.

By comparison, the maximal limit of elemental mercury inhalation exposure for industrial workers was found to be urine levels of 82 µg/L. People without amalgam fillings have urine levels of 5 to 10 µg/L, and dentists have urine levels of less than 10 µg/L. It may easily be seen that the ambient environmental exposure to mercury is the significant exposure.

There should be an overall effort to lower environmental mercury, and there appears to be no dispute on this issue. It is therefore predicted that as newer substitutes for silver amalgam are developed that prove to be as durable, simple to use, and cost-effective, we may see the gradual phasing out of its use. Many dental practices are now amalgam-free.

241. **What are the ethical issues related to removing a patient's amalgams?**
According to the ADA's Principles of Ethics and Code of Professional Conduct with official advisory opinions, revised in 2012: "Based on current scientific data, the ADA has determined that the removal of amalgam restorations from the non–allergic patient for the alleged purpose of removing toxic substances from the body, when such treatment is performed solely at the recommendation of the dentist, is improper and unethical."

If a dentist represents that such dental treatment has the capability to cure or alleviate systemic disease, when there is no scientific evidence or knowledge of this, this action is considered unethical. However, a dentist may remove amalgams at a patient's request, as long as no inference is made to improving the patient's health and the risk and benefits are discussed. A dentist may also ethically decline to remove the amalgam if there is no sound medical reason.

242. **How can one maintain mercury hygiene in the dental office?**
- Use capsulated amalgam.
- Calibrate amalgam triturators.
- Use rubber dam, high-volume suction, and amalgam traps in-office procedures.
- Dispose of amalgam waste by certified collectors.

ACKNOWLEDGMENT

The authors gratefully acknowledge the contributions of previous chapter authors.

BIBLIOGRAPHY

Atlanta GA. *Centers for Disease Control and Prevention.* US Dept of Health and Human Services; 2019. https://www.cdc.gov/oralhealth/publications/OHSR-2019-index.html.

Bellinger DC, Trachtenberg F, Barregard L, et al. Neuropsychological and renal effects of dental amalgam in children: A randomized clinical trial. *JAMA.* 2006;295:1775–1783.

Centers for Disease Control and Prevention. Vital signs: dental sealant use and untreated tooth decay among US school-aged children. *MMWR.* 2016;65(41):1141–1145.

Centers for Disease Control and Prevention: *Oral Health Surveillance Report: Trends in Dental Caries and Sealants,* Tooth Retention, and Edentulism, United States, 1999–2004 to 2011–2016.

Clarkson BH. Introduction to cariology. *Dent Clin North Am.* 1999;43:569–578.

Clarkson TW, Magos L, Myers GJ. The toxicology of mercury—current exposures and clinical manifestations. *N Engl J Med.* 2003;349:1731–1737.

Clinical Research Associates. CRA Newsletter. Enamel-Dentin Adhesives. *Self-Etching Primers (SEP).* 2000;24(11). www.CliniciansReport.org.

Cury JA, Rebelo MA, Del Bel Cury AA, et al. Biochemical composition and cariogenicity of dental plaque formed in the presence of sucrose or glucose and fructose. *Caries Res.* 2000;34:491–497.

Darby ML, Walsh M. *Dental Hygiene: Theory and Practice.* 4th ed. St. Louis: Mosby; 2015.

de Camargo EJ, Moreschi E, Baseggio W, Cury JA, Pascotto RC. Composite depth of cure using four polymerization techniques. *J Appl Oral Sci.* 2009;17(5):446–450.

Dental Board of California. *Dental Materials Fact Sheet;* 2001. http://c1-preview.prosites.com/42675/wy/docs/dentalmaterialsfactsheet.pdf.

Freedman G, Goldstep F, Seif T. Ultraconservative resin restorations. *Dentistry Today.* 2000;19:66–73.

Garcia-Godoy F. Restorative dentistry. Preface. *Dent Clin North Am.* 2002;46:xi–xii.

Gill T, Pollard AJ, Baker J, Tredwin C. Cracked tooth syndrome: assessment, prognosis and predictable management strategies. *Eur J Prosthodont Restor Dent.* 2021;29(4):209–217.

Hedge T, Mason E, Hale T. Selecting the most appropriate milling block for use with the Cerec system. *Contemp Esthet Restor Pract.* 2002;6:24–34.

Horst JA, Ellenikiotis H, Milgrom PL. UCSF Protocol for caries arrest using silver diamine fluoride: rationale, indications and consent. *J Calif Dent Assoc.* 2016;44(1):16–28.

Huckabee T. Combining microabrasion with tooth whitening to treat enamel defects. *Dentistry Today.* 2001;20:98–101.

Kidd EAM, Joyston-Bechal S. *Essentials of Dental Caries.* London: Oxford Medical; 1998.

Kugel G, Garcia-Godoy F. Direct esthetic adhesive restorative materials: A review. *Contemp Esthet Restor Pract.* 2000;4:6–10.

Knosp H, Holliday R, Corti C. Gold in dentistry: alloys, uses and performance. *Gold Bulletin.* 2003;36:93–102.

Leinfelder K, Kurdziolek S. Indirect resin restorative systems. *Contemp Esthet Restor Pract.* 2000;4:14–18.

Lussi A, Imwinkerleid S, Pitts N, et al. Performance and reproducibility of a laser fluorescence system for detection of occlusal caries in vitro. *Caries Res.* 1999;33:261–266.

Milicich G. The use of air abrasion and glass ionomer cements in microdentistry. *Compend Contin Educ Dentistry.* 2001;22:1026–1039.

NIH Consensus Statement. *Diagnosis and management of dental caries throughout life;* 2001. http://consensus.nih.gov/2001/2001DentalCaries115PDF.pdf.

Ozer F, Blatz MB. Self-etch and etch-and-rinse adhesive systems in clinical dentistry. *Compend Contin Educ Dent.* 2013;34:12–14. 16, 18.

Paes Leme AF, Koo H, Bellato CM, et al. The role of sucrose in cariogenic dental biofilm formation—new insight. *J Dent Res.* 2006;85:878–887.

Price RBT. Light curing in dentistry. *Dent Clin North Am.* 2017;61(4):751–778.

Radz GM. Direct composite resins. *Inside Dentistry.* 2011;7:76.

Rainey JT. Understanding the applications of microdentistry. *Compend Contin Educ Dentistry.* 2001;22:1018–1025.

Reality 2005, Vol. 19, p 816 http://www.realityesthetics.com/protected/book/2005/Packable_Composites.pdf

Rechmann P, Rechmann BM, Featherstone JD. Caries detection using light-based diagnostic tools. *Compend Contin Educ Dent.* 2012;33:582–584. 586.

Ross S. One visit makeovers. *Contemp Esthet Restor Pract.* 2001;5:42–53.

Shafer WG, Hine MK, Levy BM. *Textbook of Oral Pathology.* Philadelphia: WB Saunders; 1963.

Small BW. The esthetic use of cast and direct gold in 2001. *Contemp Esthet Restor Pract.* 2001;5:16–24.

Small BW. Direct resin composites for 2002 and beyond. *Gen Dentistry.* 2002;50:30–33.

Sun Y, Shi W, Yang JY, et al. Flagellin-PAc fusion protein is a high-efficacy anti-caries mucosal vaccine. *J Dent Res.* 2012;91:941–947.

U.S. Department of Health and Human Services. *Oral Health in America: A Report of the Surgeon General, Executive Summary.* Rockville: National Institutes of Health, National Institute of Dental and Craniofacial Research; 2000.

U.S. Department of Health and Human Services. *Oral Health in America: Advances and Challenges Executive Summary.* Rockville: National Institutes of Health, National Institute of Dental and Craniofacial Research; 2021.

van Meerbeek B, De Munck J, Yoshida Y, et al. Buonocore memorial lecture. Adhesion to enamel and dentin: current status and future challenges. *Oper Dent.* 2003;28:215–235.

Young DA, Kutsch V, Whitehouse J. A clinician's guide to CAMBRA: A simple approach. *Compend Contin Educ Dent.* 2009;30:92–94. 96, 98.

CHAPTER 9

PROSTHODONTICS

Jennifer L. Frustino, Amanda C. Colebeck

FIXED PROSTHODONTICS

1. **What is the definition of *fit* for a full-crown restoration? What is the clinical acceptance of the fit of a full-crown restoration?**
   The fit of a full-crown restoration is normally measured in relationship to two reference areas, (1) the occlusal seat and (2) the marginal seal. The two areas are interrelated and affect each other. The ideal fit of a full crown (marginal discrepancy) is related to the film thickness of the cementing medium (normally, 10-30 μm). The clinical acceptance of marginal discrepancy is approximately 80 μm (Fig. 9-1).

2. **What is the best marginal tooth preparation?**
   There is no ideal marginal tooth preparation. The selection of the marginal design depends on many factors, including:
   1. The material used in construction of the full crown:
      - All-ceramic restoration—shoulder or deep chamfer
      - Metal-ceramic with porcelain extended to marginal edge—shoulder or deep chamfer
      - Metal-ceramic with metal collar—shoulder with bevel or chamfer
      - Full gold crown—feathered edge, bevel, or chamfer
   2. The amount of retention needed. A beveled or feathered edge affords the most retention.
   3. Seating resistance. Shoulder preparation affords the least resistance.
   4. Sealing capability. A beveled or feathered edge affords the best seal.
   5. Pulpal consideration. More tooth reduction is necessary with a shoulder preparation than with a chamfer; the feathered edge requires the least reduction.

3. **How does one determine the number of abutments to be used?**
   There is no rigid rule. Determining factors include:
   1. The greater the number of pontics, the greater the increase in loading forces on the abutments.
   2. The position of the pontics affects the loading forces of the abutments; the more posterior the pontics, the greater the loading forces on the abutments.
   3. The crown-to-root ratio of the abutments (bone support); a periodontally compromised mouth increases the abutment-to-pontic ratio.
      Roots of the abutments that are parallel to each other distribute the loading forces down the long axis of the teeth. When the loading forces do not fall within the long axis of the tooth, the lateral forces on the abutments are increased. This situation necessitates the use of additional abutments.

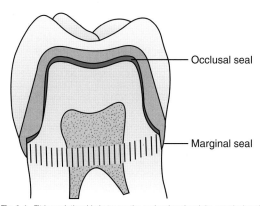

Fig. 9-1. Fit is a relationship between the occlusal seal and the marginal seal.

4. **In periodontally compromised patients, is splinting the entire dental arch with a one-piece, roundhouse fixed bridge the treatment of choice?**
Splinting an entire dental arch with a roundhouse fixed bridge is not an ideal treatment because it is fraught with potential problems, including the following:
1. All tooth preparations must be parallel to each other.
2. Impression taking and die construction are extremely difficult.
3. Accuracy of fit for the one-piece unit is extremely difficult.
4. Premature setting of the cement is a major risk because total seating of the fixed bridge onto the abutments is made extremely difficult by the mobility of the existing teeth.
5. If one of the abutments fails, it may be necessary to replace the entire prosthesis.
6. Difficult for patient to clean and maintain adequate dental hygiene.
   It is better to split up the prosthesis in some fashion than to construct a one-piece unit.

5. **Is the cantilever fixed bridge a sound treatment?**
A cantilever fixed bridge places more torquing forces on terminal abutments than desirable. Certain guidelines should be followed if a cantilever is used:
1. Cantilever pontics are limited to one per fixed bridge.
2. If the cantilever is replacing a molar, the size of the pontic should be the same as for a bicuspid, and at least one more abutment unit should be incorporated than in a conventional bridge. In addition, there should be no lateral occlusal contact on the pontic, and the bridge should be cemented with a rigid medium.
3. If the cantilever pontic is anterior to the abutments, the mesial aspect of the pontic should be designed to allow some interlocking effect.

6. **Can a three-quarter crown be used as an abutment for a fixed bridge?**
A three-quarter crown can be used successfully as an abutment for a fixed bridge if certain guidelines are followed:
1. Because there is less tooth reduction than with a full crown, retention may be compromised. Internal modifications, such as grooves or pins, must be used to compensate for potential loss of retention.
2. Proper tooth coverage is necessary for a three-quarter crown abutment:
   • Anterior—linguoincisal
   • Posterior, upper—linguo-occlusal
   • Posterior, lower—linguo-occlusal plus coverage over the buccal cusp tips
3. A three-quarter crown on a fixed bridge should be made only of metal; therefore, aesthetics may be compromised.

7. **Must a post and core be constructed for an endodontically treated tooth that is to be used in a fixed bridge?**
An endodontically treated tooth is generally more brittle than a vital tooth. The need for a post is based on the retention required to retain the core. If the access cavity is small and sufficient tooth structure remains after tooth preparation, a post is not necessary. In this case, the coronal chamber should be filled, preferably with a bonded material.

8. **What is the proper length for the post? Should a post be made for each canal in a multirooted tooth?**
In general, the length of a post should be such that the fulcrum point, determined from measuring the height of the core to the apex of the tooth, is in bone. This guideline normally places the post approximately two-thirds into the root length. Improper length allows a potential for root fracture. It is not necessary to construct a post for each canal in a multirooted tooth, provided that the dominant root (i.e., palatal root of maxillary molar) is used and proper length has been established. If proper length cannot be obtained, it is necessary to place posts in at least one of the other remaining roots.

9. **Can one use the preformed single-step post and core in place of the two-step cast post and core?**
There is no conclusive evidence favoring cast post and cores over direct post-and-core restorations. The traditional cast post-and-core technique is more time consuming and frequently involves greater laboratory and material costs. Direct core restorations can reduce both time and financial burdens on the patient without compromising outcome.

10. **Where should a crown margin be placed in relationship to the gingiva—supragingivally, equigingivally, or subgingivally?**
It is better for gingival health to place a crown margin supragingivally, 1 to 2 mm above the gingival crest or equigingivally at the gingival crest. Such positioning is often not possible because of aesthetic or caries considerations. Subsequently, the margin must be placed subgingivally. The question then becomes whether the subgingival margin ends slightly below the gingival crest, in the middle of the sulcular depth, or at the base of the sulcus. In preparing a subgingival margin, the major concern is not to extend the preparation into the attachment

apparatus. If the margin of the subsequent crown is extended into the attachment apparatus, there is potential for a chronic gingival irritant. Therefore, for clinical simplicity, when a margin is to be placed subgingivally, it is desirable to end the tooth preparation slightly below the gingival crest (Fig. 9-2).

MATERIALS

11. **What materials are used in the construction of a full crown?**

- Gold alloy
- Nongold alloy
- Acrylic resin
- Acrylic resin with a metal alloy
- Composite resin
- Composite resin with a metal alloy
- Ceramic with a metal alloy
- All ceramic

12. **Are the same materials used in the construction of a fixed bridge?**
All of these materials can be used for the construction of a fixed bridge, however, for longevity and strength, only metal, porcelain fused to metal, or high-strength ceramics such as zirconia and lithium disilicate are recommended for fixed bridges. Porcelain fused to metal was the most common material used for bridge fabrication historically due to the need for metal support for strength and ceramic for esthetics. However, newer ceramic materials, including lithium disilicate and zirconia, have increased strength and in most cases can be used to eliminate the metal substructure.

13. **What are the major advantages and disadvantages of the metal-ceramic crown?**
In general, the metal-ceramic crown combines certain favorable properties of metal in its substructure and of ceramic in its veneer coating.
     Advantages
1. The metal substructure gives high strength, which allows the materials to be used in fixed bridgework and for splinting teeth.
2. The fit of a metal casting can also be achieved with the metal-ceramic crown.
3. Aesthetics can be achieved by the proper application of the ceramic veneer.
     Disadvantages
1. To allow enough space for the metal-ceramic materials, adequate tooth reduction is necessary (≥1.5 mm). The marginal tooth preparation is critical in relation to the design of the metal with the ceramic.
2. The fabrication technique is complex. The longer the span of bridgework, the greater the potential for metal distortion and/or porcelain problems.
3. Esthetics are typically inferior to crowns fabricated without metal substrate that allow for more translucency such as lithium disilicate.

14. **What tooth preparation is necessary for the metal-ceramic crown?**
The amount of tooth reduction necessary for the metal-ceramic crown depends on the metal and ceramic thickness. The necessary thickness of the metal is 0.5 mm, whereas the minimal ceramic thickness is 1.0 to

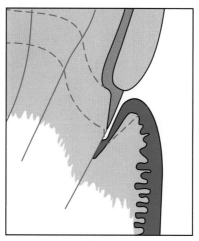

Fig. 9-2. The subgingival margin should not impinge into the attachment apparatus.

1.5 mm. Therefore, the tooth reduction is approximately 1.5 to 2.0 mm. With this porcelain-metal sandwich, a shoulder preparation is generally necessary for adequate tooth reduction.

15. **What tooth preparation is necessary for the all-ceramic crown?**
The amount of tooth reduction necessary for monolithic (solid) lithium disilicate crowns is 1.0 mm for fracture resistance in occlusal areas. In contrast, zirconia has such high fracture resistance that the amount of tooth reduction for monolithic zirconia crowns can be a minimum of 0.5 mm. If porcelain layering is desired for either ceramic material, an additional 1.0 to 1.5 mm reduction should be made to allow for this restorative space.

16. **What happens if tooth preparation or reduction is inadequate in the marginal area of a tooth that is planned for a PFM restoration?**
If the tooth reduction is less than 1.5 mm at the marginal area, only metal can be present in that area. If porcelain is applied on metal that has been reduced in thickness because of lack of space, marginal metal distortion is likely during the firing cycle. If the porcelain thickness is reduced to compensate for the reduced space, the opaque porcelain layer is likely to be exposed or to dominate, leading to an unaesthetic result. If both the porcelain and metal have adequate thickness, then the crown is over-contoured (Fig. 9-3).

17. **Can the marginal area of a metal-ceramic crown be constructed in porcelain without metal?**
Yes. There are many techniques to construct a porcelain margin with optimal aesthetics, proper fit, and correct contour (emergence profile) but adequate finish line reduction has to be present for the strength of the porcelain (ideally a shoulder preparation of 1.0 mm or more).

18. **If the tooth preparation is sufficient to accept the porcelain edge of the metal without distortion, why is it necessary to construct a margin in porcelain solely for aesthetic reasons?**
It is possible to cover the metal correctly with porcelain in the marginal area, but most often the aesthetic results fall short of expectation in the most critical area. Incident light that transmits through the porcelain and reflects from the metal often creates a shadowing effect. If porcelain is present only at this marginal area, light transmission and reflection through the porcelain and the tooth create the proper blend between the marginal aspect of the crown and the tooth.

19. **For a successful porcelain marginal construction, how far should the metal extend in relation to the shoulder?**
Originally, the metal was finished slightly shy of the edge of the shoulder, with porcelain extending to the edge. Another technique finished the metal at the axiocaval line angle of the preparation, creating a porcelain margin that totally covered the horizontal shoulder. With both techniques, however, shadowing was still present. To create

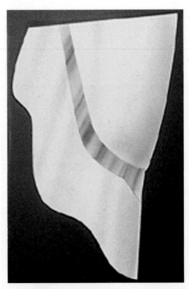

Fig. 9-3. Margin tooth reduction (1.0-1.5 mm) is necessary for acceptance of the porcelain to cover metal.

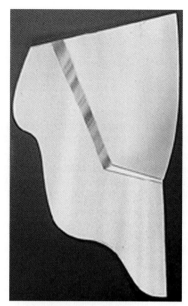

Fig. 9-4. Diagram of porcelain margin.

proper light transmission and reflection of the porcelain-tooth interface, the metal should be finished to about I to 2 mm above the axiocaval line angle of the shoulder (Fig. 9-4).

20. **What are noble alloys?**
Noble alloys in general do not oxidize on casting. This feature is important in a metal substrate so that oxidation at the metal-porcelain interface can be controlled by the addition of trace oxidizing elements. If oxidation cannot be controlled on repeated firings, porcelain color may be contaminated, and the bond strength may be weakened. Noble alloys are gold, platinum, and palladium. A silver alloy that oxidizes is considered semiprecious.

21. **What is a base metal alloy? Can it be used in the construction of a metal-ceramic crown?**
The base metal or nonprecious alloys most often used in the construction of a metal-ceramic crown are nickel and chromium. Because these alloys readily oxidize at elevated temperatures, they create porcelain-to-metal interface problems. The oxidation must be controlled by a metal-coating treatment, which is somewhat unpredictable. Casting and fitting are also difficult. A noble alloy is preferable.

22. **What are the criteria for selecting a specific alloy?**
    1. Compatibility of the coefficient of thermal expansion with the selected porcelains
    2. Controllability of oxidation at interface
    3. Ease in casting and fabrication
    4. Fit potential
    5. High yield of strength
    6. High modulus of elasticity (stiffness) to avoid stress in the porcelain

23. **How does porcelain bond to the alloy?**
Ceramic adheres to metal primarily by chemical bond. A covalent bond is established by sharing O_2 in the elements in the porcelain and the metal alloy. These elements include silicon dioxide (SiO_2) in the porcelain and oxidizing elements such as silicon, indium, and iridium in the metal alloy.

24. **How is a porcelain selected?**
The criteria for selecting a specific porcelain include:
    1. Compatibility with the metal used in regard to their respective coefficients of thermal expansion (of prime importance)
    2. Stability of controlled shrinkage with multiple firings
    3. Color stability with multiple firings
    4. Capability of matching shade selection with various thicknesses of porcelain
    5. Ease of handling (technique-sensitive)
    6. Full range of shades and modifiers

25. How many layers or different porcelains can be applied in the buildup of a metal-ceramic crown?

   1. Shoulder
   2. Opaque
   3. Opacious dentin
   4. Body
   5. Incisal
   6. Translucent
   7. Modifiers in every layer
   8. External colorants

26. What is the function of the opaque layer?
   The elements in the opaque layer create the chemical bond of the porcelain to the metal substrate. The opaque layer masks the color of the metal and is the core color in determining the final shade of the crown.

27. What is opacious dentin?
   Opacious dentin is an intermediary modifying porcelain that affords better light transmission than the opaque layer, in part because of its optical properties. Opacious dentin is less opaque than the opaque layer but less translucent than the body (dentin) porcelain. It is also used for color shifts or effect properties.

28. What differentiates shoulder porcelain from dentin (body) porcelain?
   The principal difference between shoulder and body porcelain is the firing temperature. Because the shoulder porcelain is established before the general buildup, its color and dimension must remain stable during subsequent firings. Therefore, the shoulder porcelain matures at a higher temperature than the subsequent body porcelain firings.

29. What is segmental buildup in the construction of the metal-ceramic crown?
   Segmental buildup refers to the method of applying the porcelain powders in incremental portions horizontally. Each increment differs from the others in opacity and translucency or hue, value, or chroma. This technique is used to construct a crown that attempts to mimic the optical properties of a natural tooth (Fig. 9-5).

30. What is the coefficient of thermal expansion? What is its importance in prosthodontics?
   The coefficient of thermal expansion is the exponential expansion of a material as it is subjected to heat. The coefficient is extremely important during joint firing of two dissimilar materials. For example, the coefficient of thermal expansion should be slightly higher (rather than the same) for the metal substrate than for the porcelain coating. This slight difference results in compression of the fired porcelain coating, which gives it greater strength.

31. What is the proper coping design for the metal-ceramic restoration?
   The purpose of the metal coping is to ensure the fit of the crown and maximize the strength of the porcelain veneer. The metal must have the proper thickness so as not to distort during the firing. The coping should be reinforced in load-bearing areas, such as the interproximal space and can be strengthened in areas in which metal exists alone, such as the lingual collar. To maximize the strength potential of the porcelain, uniform thickness should be attempted in the final restoration. This thickness can be obtained by designing the wax-up of the framework to accommodate the porcelain layer.

32. How does the marginal tooth preparation affect the design of the metal-ceramic crown?
   The marginal tooth preparation determines the marginal configuration of the metal-ceramic crown. The three options are:
   1. Beveled or feathered edge—the preparation is covered only in metal.
   2. Chamfer—if the depth of the chamfer is at least 1 mm, the porcelain can extend over the metal and a supported porcelain margin can be constructed.
   3. Shoulder—the preparation must be 1 mm for the porcelain to cover the metal.

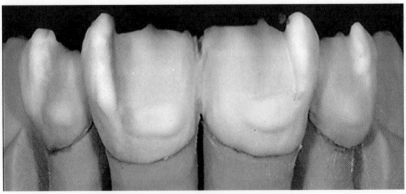

Fig. 9-5. Segmental buildup to construct a porcelain crown.

33. **Is the design of the metal framework of a fixed bridge different from the design of a single unit?**
The design of the metal framework must incorporate four basic interrelationships—strength, aesthetics, contour, and occlusion. In fixed bridgework, however, strength of the substrate plays the dominant role. Therefore, greater attention must be paid to reinforcement of the framework than of a single unit.

34. **How do design problems of the metal framework influence the function of the metal-ceramic restorations?**
    1. The color of the porcelain is compromised between abutments and pontics if the thickness of the porcelain varies.
    2. If the porcelain veneer is too thick (>2 mm) because of improper framework design, much of the strength of the interface bond is lost.
    3. If the porcelain veneer is too thin (≤0.75 mm), the aesthetic effect is compromised.
    4. The metal framework is designed to resist deformation. If strut-type connector design is not used in the fixed bridgework, the bridge may flex and result in porcelain fracture.

35. **What is metamerism? How does it affect the metal-ceramic restoration?**
Metamerism is the optical property whereby two objects with the same color but different spectral reflectance curves do not match. This property is important in matching the shade of the metal-ceramic restoration to the natural tooth. Even if the colors are the same, different reflectance curves can create a barely noticeable difference.

36. **What is the importance of fluorescence in porcelain?**
Fluorescence is the optical property whereby a material reflects ultraviolet radiation; it reflects different hues. Natural teeth can fluoresce yellow-white to blue-white hues. Fluorescence in porcelain is important to minimize metamerism of porcelain to natural teeth in varying light conditions.

37. **What are hue, value, and chroma? What is their importance in dentistry?**
Color consists of three properties:
    1. *Hue* refers to color families (e.g., red, green).
    2. *Value* refers to lightness or darkness as related to a scale from black to white.
    3. *Chroma* refers to the saturation of a color at any given value level.
       The properties have a practical use in ordering color.

38. **What is opalescence?**
Opalescence is the optical property seen in an opal during light transmission and light reflection. During transmission, the opal takes on an orange-white hue, whereas during reflection it takes on a bluish-white hue. This phenomenon also occurs in the natural tooth as a result of light scattering through the crystalline structure of the opal. The structure size is in the submicron range (0.2-0.5 μm). A porcelain restoration can demonstrate the opal effect by incorporating submicron particles of porcelain into the enamel (incisal) layer.

39. **How do you select a shade to match the natural teeth?**
There is no truly scientific method to analyze the shade of a natural tooth and apply this information to the selection of porcelain and fabrication of the crown. Attempts to establish such a technique have met with limited success. At present, shade determination is designed to match natural teeth with a synthetic replication (shade guide) that results in a range of acceptability rather than an absolute match. The most widely used guide is the VITA Classical Shade Guide by Vident.

40. **What improvements have been made in selecting a shade in more recent years?**
The **3D guide** was developed based on the three dimensions of hue, chroma, and value. The VITA® 3D-Master Shade Guide® (Vident) improves accuracy in selection based on a value numbering system of 0 to 5, with 0 being the brightest and 5 the darkest shade. Chroma is also categorized from 1 to 3, with 1 being the lowest and 3 being the highest. Hue is categorized as left, middle, or right (orange to red).
    Digital photography for shade analysis has also been used. Digital photography with Adobe Photoshop has been used in shade selection. Images of the compared tooth and the shade guide are taken in the same vertical plane in a RAW file format. The images are then opened in Photoshop and the background area is turned to black. A duplicate image is made and turned to gray scale. The "HSB" color model is selected in the "INFO" palette, and when the cursor is placed on the shade guide or the compared tooth, the hue will be given by an "H" number, chroma by the "S" number, and the value by the "B" number. The difference in these parameters can be measured between the tooth and the guide. The ceramist can use this information to choose the most appropriate porcelains to match the tooth structure.
    Computerized digital shade technology and software are used in conjunction with visual shade guides and digital photography. Instruments store data for various shade guides and use fiberoptics along with spectrometers to aid dentists in determining the tooth shade and color zones. Light waves are sent through the tooth and refracted or reflected back to the receiver in the spectrometer. The digital spectrophotometers determine the shade, hue, chroma, and value. VITA Easyshade V® by Vident and Crystaleye® by Olympus are two product examples.

41. **Can you change a shade with external stains?**
External stains or colorants are frequently used to minimize the differences between natural and ceramic teeth. They should be used rationally rather than empirically. An understanding of the color phenomenon is necessary in all aspects of shade control and is essential if extrinsic colorants are to be used correctly. Extrinsic colorants follow the physical laws of subtractive color.

42. **What guidelines derived from the color phenomenon apply to the use of external colorants?**
The understanding of hue, value, and chroma and their effect on external staining of a crown are essential. The major guidelines are as follows:

   Hue: Drastic change of the shade of the ceramic restoration by use of external colorants is often impossible. Slight changes in shade may be accomplished (e.g., orange to orange-brown).
   Value: External colorants can be used to lower the value of the ceramic. The complementary color of the shade to be altered may have a darkening effect. It is almost impossible to increase the value or shade of the ceramic.
   Chroma: Chroma can be successfully increased by external colorants, usually in the gingival or interproximal areas.

43. **What effects can be created with surface stains?**
   1. Separation and individualization with interproximal staining
   2. Coloration of a cervical area to emulate root surface and produce the illusion of change of form
   3. Coloration of hypocalcified areas
   4. Coloration of check lines
   5. Coloration of stain lines
   6. Neutralization of hue for increase of apparent translucency (usually violet)
   7. Highlighting and shadowing
   8. Incisal edge modification—emulated opacities, high chrome areas, stain areas
   9. Synthetic restorations
   10. Aging

44. **Are external colorants stable in the oral cavity?**
External colorants are metallic oxides that fuse to the ceramic unit during a predetermined firing cycle. Although stable in an air environment, they are susceptible to corrosion when subjected to certain oral environments. Depending on the stain and pH of the oral fluids, external colorants may be lost from the ceramic unit over a long period of time.

45. **What is the most important factor in determining the strength of a ceramic?**
The most important factor in the strength of a ceramic material is control of small flaws or microcracks, which often are present at the surface and internally. In most cases, the strength of the ceramic depends on surface flaws rather than porosity in the normal range.

46. **Should porcelain be used on the occlusal surface of a metal-ceramic, zirconia, or lithium-disilicate crown?**
In general, the surface hardness of dental porcelains is greater than that of tooth structure, metal alloys, and all other restorative materials. This may lead to excessive wear of the opposing dentition if certain occlusal guidelines are not followed. In the best scenario, the opposing material is porcelain, but results are good if the occlusal loads have good force distribution. Porcelain is contraindicated in patients who engage in bruxism or parafunctional activities. This is because porcelain is strongest under compressive stress (chewing forces) but weak in tensile and shear stresses (excursive forces) and likely to chip or break in these patients.

47. **Can a porcelain fracture of a metal-ceramic restoration be repaired?**
It is now possible to bond composite or ceramic materials to a fractured restoration. The bond, which may occur on porcelain or on the metal substrate, is sufficiently strong to be resistant in a non- or low-stress-bearing area. However, if the fracture occurs in a stress-bearing area, the probability of a successful repair is low.

48. **On what basis do you choose between an all-ceramic and metal-ceramic crown?**
The terminology for all-ceramic crowns includes a wide range of materials including high-strength ceramics like lithium disilicate and zirconia, as well as low-strength layered porcelain jacket crowns. For the most part, anytime that a metal-ceramic crown is considered, a zirconia crown can be an option as well. Limitations to lithium disilicate come from its lower strength compared to the other two materials, and it is contraindicated in regions of very high occlusal load such as second or third molars, and bridges replacing molars or requiring multiple pontics. The material is best suited for anterior teeth and premolars where esthetics are most important and functional stress is lower. Unlike the metal-ceramic crown, which is hindered by the metal substrate, the all-ceramic crown can mimic the optical properties of the natural tooth.

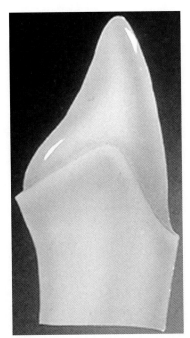

Fig. 9-6. Tooth preparation for an all-ceramic crown.

49. **Is tooth preparation the same for an all-ceramic crown and metal-ceramic restoration?**
    The same amount of overall tooth reduction is needed for a metal-ceramic restoration as for an all-ceramic crown (1.0-1.5 mm labially, lingually, and interproximally). However, unlike the metal-ceramic restoration, which will accept any marginal design, marginal tooth preparation for the weaker strength all-ceramic crowns should be a shoulder or deep chamfer (minimum of 1.0 mm tooth reduction) (Fig. 9-6).

50. **What tooth preparation is necessary for solid zirconia crowns?**
    Monolithic zirconia restorative material is used for crowns, bridges, screw-retained implant crowns, inlays, or onlays with no porcelain overlay. The material was originally designed to provide a more durable and aesthetic alternative to posterior metal occlusal PFMs (porcelain fused to metal crowns) and cast gold restorations for demanding situations such as bruxers or restorations with limited occlusal space. These restorations are milled through CAD-CAM (computer-aided design–computer-aided manufacturing) technology and are meant to be fracture- and chip-resistant. Marginal preparation can be feather-edged and a shoulder is not necessary. A conservative preparation is indicated, similar to a full-cast gold crown, so any preparation with at least 0.5 mm of occlusal reduction is acceptable. Occlusal reduction of 1.0 mm is ideal. Labial, lingual, and interproximal reduction is 1.0 mm. Tooth preparation for a monolithic Zirconia crown is shown in Fig. 9-7.

51. **Can the newer all-ceramic materials with high strength values be used in place of metal-ceramic restorations?**
    In terms of strength and esthetics, zirconia crowns can be used in place of metal-ceramic restorations. Lithium disilicate, while still being considered a high-strength ceramic, is considerably lower in strength compared to the other two materials, and it is contraindicated in regions of very high occlusal load. It is advisable to use the all-ceramic crown in the anterior segment, in which aesthetics is the dominant factor (Fig. 9-8).

52. **What are the different types of all-ceramic crowns?**
    All-ceramic crowns may be categorized by composition and method of fabrication:
    Composition
    1. Feldspathic porcelain, such as a conventional porcelain jacket crown
    2. Aluminous porcelain: Vitadur, HyCeram, Cerestore, Procera, InCeram
    3. Mica glass: Dicor, Cerapearl
    4. Crystalline-reinforced glass: Optec, IPS Empress, IPS e.max
    5. Zirconia: BruxZir, Prismatik, Lava, ZirCAD
    6. Lithium silicate: Obsidian

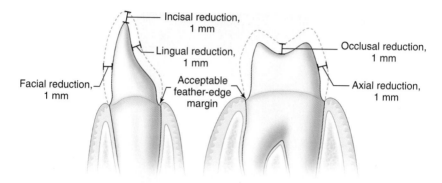

Fig. 9-7. Requirements for the preparation of a monolithic zirconia crown consist of using a feather edge, a shoulder preparation is not necessary, and a minimum 0.5 mm occlusal reduction. A 1 mm occlusal reduction is ideal, though.

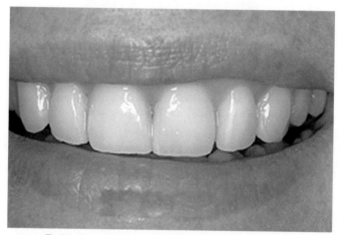

Fig. 9-8. All-ceramic crowns on maxillary anterior segment (teeth #6-11).

Method of fabrication
1. Refractory die technique: Optec, Mirage, HyCeram, InCeram
2. Casting: Dicor
3. Press technique: Cerestore, Procera, Empress, IPS e.Max
4. CAD-CAM or milled technique: IPS e.Max CAD, Prettau, Izir, BruxZir

53. **What is crystalline-reinforced glass?**

A crystalline-reinforced glass is a glass in which a crystalline substance such as leucite is dispersed. This composition is used in the Optec and Empress systems. Strength is derived from the crystalline microstructure within the glass matrix. The higher concentration of leucite crystals in the matrix limits the progress of microcracks within the ceramic.

54. **What is the importance of alumina in an all-ceramic restoration?**

Alumina (Al_2O_3) is a truly crystalline ceramic, the hardest and probably the strongest oxide known. Alumina is used to reinforce glass (as in HyCeram). The strength is determined by the amount of alumina reinforcement. Alumina is also used in total crystalline compositions (Cerestore, Procera, InCeram), which may serve as the substructure, much like metal coping. With this technique, the ceramic has high strength.

55. **Is the cementing of an all-ceramic crown different from the cementing of a metal-ceramic crown?**

The major difference is that a trial cement is not recommended for the all-ceramic crown, which obtains much of its strength from the underlying support of the tooth. If the cement washes out, the unsupported crown is susceptible to fracture. In general, all-rigid cements can be used, but a bonded resin cement is highly recommended to maximize the underlying support.

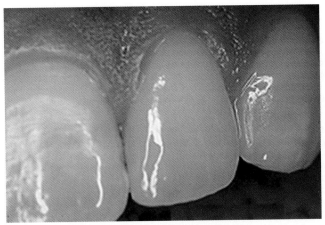

Fig. 9-9. Ceramic veneer (tooth #10) bonded to tooth.

56. **Can all-ceramic materials be bonded to the tooth preparation?**
It is important that the ceramic material be chemically etched for bonding to a tooth. If the ceramic material cannot be properly etched, alumina is used in the substrate (Fig. 9-9).

57. **What is the significance of the refractory die?**
A refractory die is used in many techniques for the construction of different types of all-ceramic crowns and veneers. Basically, it is a secondary die obtained by duplicating the master die. The ceramic material is applied on the refractory die for the firing cycles. Once the cycles have been completed, the refractory die is removed, and the ceramic piece is returned to the master die. Refractory die material must have the following properties:
    1. Compatibility with impression materials
    2. Dimensional stability for measurements
    3. Tolerance of high-heat firing cycles
    4. Compatible coefficient of thermal expansion with the ceramic material used
    5. Easy removal from the ceramic piece

58. **What determines the design of the pontic?**
The design of the pontic is dictated by the special boundaries of the following: (1) edentulous ridge; (2) opposing occlusal surface; and (3) musculature of tongue, cheeks, or lips. The task is to design a tooth substitute within these boundaries that favorably compares in form, function, and appearance with the tooth it replaces. The tooth substitute must provide comfort and support to the adjacent musculature, conformity to the food flow pattern, convenient contours for hygiene, and cosmetic value, if indicated.

59. **How should the contact area of the pontic on the edentulous ridge be designed?**
Three concepts in pontic design are popular:
    1. The sanitary pontic design leaves space between the pontic and ridge.
    2. The saddle pontic design covers the ridge labiolingually. Total coronal width is usually concave.
    3. The modified ridge design uses a ridge lap for minimal ridge contact. Labial contact is usually to the height of the ridge contour (straight emergence profile).
        The selection of the design depends on the following factors:
    1. Spatial boundaries
    2. Shape of edentulous ridge (normal, blunted, or excessive resorption)
    3. Maxillary or mandibular posterior arch
        In contrast to the mandibular posterior pontic, the maxillary edentulous ridge is usually broad and blunted and has superior cosmetic effects.
    4. Anterior pontic
        The overriding cosmetic requirement is that form and shape reproduce the facial characteristics of the natural tooth.

60. **What is the emergence profile? What is its importance?**
The emergence profile is the shape of the marginal aspect of a tooth or a restoration and relates to the angulation of the tooth or restoration as it emerges from the gingiva. This gingival contour is extremely important for tissue health after placement of a crown.
    The most obvious error of the emergence profile of a crown is overcontouring, which creates abnormal pressure of the gingival cuff and leads to inflammation in the presence of bacteria. Overcontouring and a poor

emergence profile are caused primarily by the following: (1) inadequate tooth preparation, (2) improper handling of materials, and/or (3) inadequate communication between the dentist and technician.

61. After periodontal therapy, when can the dentist complete the marginal tooth preparation?
A certain waiting time is necessary between completion of periodontal therapy and completion of the marginal tooth preparation so as to establish and stabilize the attachment apparatus on the root surface. If this waiting time is not observed, impingement of the restoration into the attachment apparatus frequently occurs. The result is an iatrogenic gingival inflammation. The amount of waiting time necessary depends on the aggressiveness of the gingival procedure. A reasonable guideline, however, is to wait at least 6 weeks for tissue resolution.

62. What is a biologically compatible material?
A biologically compatible material elicits no adverse response in the tissue or systemically. Adverse tissue response may be the result of any of the following:
1. Allergic reaction
2. Toxic response
3. Mechanical irritation
4. Promotion of bacterial colonization
   In general, highly polished noble alloys and highly glazed porcelains are the most biologically compatible materials.

63. Is any material used to construct crowns suspected of biologic incompatibility?
In general, most materials used in the construction of crowns are biologically compatible. Adverse reactions have occurred with some materials, primarily because of unpolished metal or unglazed porcelain surfaces. However, literature reports have indicated that nickel-chrome alloys used in castings may be biologically incompatible. An allergic response may occur in 10% of women and 5% of men.

REMOVABLE PARTIAL DENTURES

64. What is the most important factor in determining the success of a bilateral, free-end mandibular removable partial denture (RPD)?
The most important factor in determining success is proper coverage over the residual ridge. Coverage should extend over the retromolar pad to create stability of the RPD and minimize the torquing forces on the abutment teeth.

65. When clasps are to be used on the abutment teeth, what important factors must be considered?
When clasps are used, it is important to design the prosthesis so that the path of insertion is parallel to the abutment teeth. This factor is important in eliminating torquing forces on the abutment teeth during insertion and removal of the partial denture. If the planes are not parallel, the abutment teeth must be adjusted. The abutment teeth must also be evaluated for placement of the retentive clasps and reciprocal bracing arm. The abutment teeth are then shaped to accept the clasps. The proper positioning of occlusal rests on the abutment teeth is extremely important, and the teeth are prepared to optimize positioning.

66. What are the advantages and disadvantages of the cingulum bar as a connector?
Advantages
1. Space problems for bar placement seldom exist unless anterior teeth have been worn down by attrition.
2. No pressure is exerted on the gingival tissues with movement of the RPD.
3. The major connector forms a single unit with the anterior teeth, thus contributing to comfort of the RPD.
4. Indirect retention is provided.
5. Repair of the RPD is simple when natural anterior teeth are lost.
Disadvantages
1. The metal bar situated on the lingual surface of the anterior teeth is relatively bulky, especially if crowding is present.
2. Aesthetics is compromised if spacing exists.
3. Marked lingual inclination of the anterior teeth precludes use of the bar.

67. What laboratory requirements should be implemented when a cingulum bar is used?
1. For sufficient rigidity, a minimal height of 4 mm and thickness of 2.5 mm are necessary. These dimensions should be increased when the cingulum bar traverses more natural teeth.
2. No notches should be made in the metal to stimulate tooth contour because they weaken the bar. In the presence of reduced height, the bar is placed more gingivally and made thicker to provide rigidity.
3. The junction of the bar to the denture base must be sufficiently strong. The bar can cover the lingual surfaces of premolars, if present. The contour of the teeth should be adapted to the path of insertion of the RPD.

68. Are indirect retainers necessary in the construction of an RPD? If so, where should they be placed?

The function of an indirect retainer is to prevent dislodgment of the RPD toward the occlusal plane. In a total tooth-bearing RPD, it is unnecessary to include indirect retainers. However, when the RPD has a free-end saddle portion, it is advisable to include indirect retention to prevent vertical dislodgement.

The ideal positioning of the indirect retainer is at the furthest point from the distal border of the free-end saddle. For example, if the free-end saddle is on the lower right quadrant, the indirect retainer is placed on the lower left canine.

69. Is it advantageous to place stress-breaking attachments adjacent to a free-end saddle in an RPD?

The advantage of constructing a stress-breaking attachment next to a free-end saddle is to relieve torquing forces on abutment teeth that have been periodontally compromised. However, further displacement of the free-end saddle toward the underlying ridge may cause an acceleration of resorption of the residual ridge. It is preferable, therefore, to compensate for torquing forces on the abutment teeth by the proper extension of the saddle area.

70. Is it necessary to use clasps around abutment teeth in an RPD?

Clasps may be eliminated around abutment teeth if the teeth are restored with a partial or full crown containing some form of attachment that replaces the functions of the clasps. These functions include the following:
1. Guide planes for the RPD
2. Prevention of vertical displacement toward the ridge by the occlusal and cingular rest
3. Retentive function from the retentive arm
4. Bracing function from the reciprocal arm
      Depending on the type of attachment, all or part of these functions may be replaced. With partial replacement, the remaining functions are incorporated into the RPD.

71. What is the difference between a precision and semiprecision attachment?

A **precision attachment** is preconstructed with male and female portions that fit together in a precise fashion, with little tolerance. Normally, there is no stress, and retention can be adjusted within the attachment. The attachment parts, constructed of a metal that can be placed into the crown and RPD, normally are joined by solder. In general, no other clasps are necessary.

A **semiprecision attachment** is cast into the crown and RPD. The female portion is normally made of preformed plastic that is positioned into the wax form and then cast. The male portion is cast with the RPD framework. The female and male parts fit together with much more tolerance than in the precision attachment, resulting in less retention. Secondary retentive clasping is necessary. Less torque is induced on the abutments with a semiprecision than with a precision attachment.

72. What is the difference between an intracoronal and extracoronal attachment?

An intracoronal attachment is placed within the body of the crown, whereas the extracoronal attachment is attached to the outer portion. The selection of one over the other depends on many factors; if designed properly, both types can be used successfully.

73. What are the advantages and disadvantages of an intracoronal attachment?

Advantages
1. Placement of torquing forces near the long access of the tooth, thus minimizing these forces
2. Elimination of clasps
3. Parallel guide planes for proper RPD insertion
4. Capability to establish proper contour at the abutment-RPD interface
Disadvantages
1. More tooth reduction
2. Need for adequate coronal length
3. Lack of stress-bearing capability
4. Difficulty in performing repairs

74. What are the advantages and disadvantages of an extracoronal attachment?

Advantages
1. Same amount of reduction of the abutment tooth and conventional restoration
2. Elimination of clasps
3. Incorporation of stress breaking into attachment
4. Ease of replacing parts
5. Improved aesthetics
Disadvantages
1. The attachment is positioned away from the long axis of the tooth, creating a potential for torquing forces on the abutment tooth.
2. Adequate vertical space is necessary for placement of the attachment.
3. Interproximal contour at the crown-attachment interface is difficult to establish correctly.

75. **What are other options to increase partial denture retention that avoid the use of clasps?**
It has become common practice to place osseointegrated implants in edentulous ridges with overdenture stud attachments for the retention of partial dentures. In these cases, unesthetic clasps can typically be avoided as the implant attachment provides significant retention.

76. **Is the unilateral RPD an acceptable treatment modality?**
In general, a unilateral RPD is not an ideal treatment modality because cross-arch stabilization is necessary for success. A unilateral RPD may be used, however, when a single tooth is replaced and abutment teeth are on either side of the replacement tooth (Nesbitt appliance).

COMPLETE DENTURES

77. **What is the best material for taking a complete-denture impression?**
In taking a complete-denture impression, it is important to understand that the topography of an edentulous arch includes soft displaceable tissue with undercut areas. An impression material must not distort the tissues. Therefore, the material must be low in viscosity and elastomeric so that it can rebound in the undercut areas.

78. **Is border molding necessary for a complete lower denture?**
Unlike a complete upper denture, a lower denture does not rely on a peripheral seal for retention. Thus one may assume that border molding is an unnecessary procedure during impression taking. This assumption is incorrect because inadvertent overextension can greatly reduce denture stability as well as irritate tissue. Underextension of the peripheral border decreases tissue-bearing surfaces, thereby affecting denture stability.

79. **What is the importance of the posterior palatal seal? How is its position determined?**
The posterior palatal seal is an important component because it completes the entire peripheral sealing aspect of a maxillary denture. Anatomically, the seal is located at the juncture of the hard and soft palates and joins the right and left hamular notches. If the seal is positioned more posteriorly, tissue irritation, gagging reflex, and decreased retention can result. If the seal is positioned more anteriorly, tissue irritation and decreased retention can result. Manual palpation and phonetics (the "ah" sound) are the best ways to determine the anatomic position for the palatal seal. Indelible ink can be used to transfer the vibrating line from the mouth to the record base to the master cast to determine the posterior border.

80. **What are the critical areas in the border-molding procedure of taking impressions for a maxillary arch?**
The most critical area to capture in an impression is the mucogingival fold above the maxillary tuberosity area. Proper three-dimensional extension of the final prosthesis is extremely important for maximal retention. Other critical areas are the labial frena in the midline and the frena in the bicuspid area. Overextension in these areas often leads to decreased retention and tissue irritation.

81. **Should an impression be taken under functional load or passively at one static moment?**
The answer to this question has been debated for years. Soft tissue constantly changes, and a static impression captures the tissue at one point in time. On the other hand, a functional impression is taken with abnormal masticatory loads. Therefore, there is no absolute method of taking the impression. Denture stability with occlusal forces and periodic tissue evaluation, however, are critical with both methods.

82. **What are the critical areas to capture in an impression of a mandibular arch?**
Mandibular dentures do not rely on suction from a peripheral seal for retention but rather on denture stability in covering as much basal bone as possible, without impinging on the muscle attachments. Movement of the tongue, lips, and cheeks greatly affects the amount of the tissue-bearing area. Therefore, apart from identifying and covering the retromolar areas, the active border molding performed by the lip, cheeks, and tongue determines the peripheral areas of a mandibular arch, thus establishing maximal basal bone coverage.

83. **How do you determine the peripheral extent of a denture?**
For a peripheral border impression, a moldable material should be used around a well-fitting tray. The material should have moderate or low viscosity so as not to displace tissue and should be set in a short period of time. The lips, cheeks, and tongue dictate the extent of the peripheral impression. The impression is captured by exaggerated movements of the anatomic structures made by the patient or manipulated by the dentist.

84. **How is vertical dimension established in a totally edentulous mouth?**
Vertical dimension is established with the aid of bite rims. The most important aspect of vertical dimension is to establish the freeway space. The minimal opening in freeway space, which is determined phonetically (the "s" sound), is normally 1 to 2 mm.

85. **How are overlap and overjet established?**
Overlap and overjet are established by the maxillary bite rim, which also establishes the occlusal plane. The bite rim is adjusted by its position relative to the lip and cheek.

86. **Is the bite registration taken in the centric relation or centric occlusion position?**
This controversy has been argued for years and remains unresolved. However, certain principles are generally accepted:
1. A centric relation position may be duplicated.
2. A centric relation is the same position in various openings of the vertical dimension.
3. A centric relation should be an unstrained position.
4. Centric occlusion may be used if the bite registration is done without increasing the vertical dimension.

87. **What does the tooth try-in appointment accomplish?**
The try-in appointment is important in order to visualize the aesthetics of the final teeth in regard to lip line, overbite and overjet, shape, and arrangement. The try-in appointment can also determine the fullness of the labial flanges in relationship to the cheeks and lips. The occlusal relationship can be checked and verified, and a new bite registration can be performed. Above all, the try-in appointment affords the dentist and patient a preview of the final completed denture.

88. **How is posterior occlusion selected with regard to tooth morphology?**
Posterior occlusion can range from monoplane (flat plane) to steep anatomic occlusal cusps. In general, the more anatomic the occlusion, the more efficient its function. However, it is more difficult to establish balanced occlusion with a steep anatomic denture, and lack of balance leads to denture instability. It is therefore easier to establish occlusal harmony with monoplane teeth. Overbite and overjet of the anterior teeth also affect the selection of the posterior teeth.

89. **How do overbite and overjet affect the selection of cuspid inclines of the posterior teeth?**
Overbite and overjet of the anterior teeth affect the selection of the cuspid inclines of the posterior teeth when balanced occlusion is to be achieved in lateral and protrusive movements:

Steep overbite—steep cuspal incline
Small overbite—monoplane
Wide overjet—monoplane
Narrow overjet—steep cuspal incline

90. **Of what materials are denture teeth composed? How are they selected?**
Denture teeth are made from basically three materials—porcelain, acrylic, and composite-filled resin. All three materials afford excellent aesthetic capabilities.
    Porcelain teeth afford the greatest degree of hardness and best withstand wear. However, they are brittle and difficult to change or adjust; they also have a low mechanical bond strength to the resin base.
    Acrylic teeth, on the other hand, are the softest of the materials and therefore the least resistant to wear. They are, however, easy to use, can be easily changed or adjusted, and have the best bond strength to the denture base.
    Composite-filled resin teeth have hardness and strength values between those of porcelain and acrylic; they bond well to the denture base and can be adjusted easily.

91. **What procedure should be followed for insertion of a complete maxillary and complete mandibular denture?**
During the processing of the denture base, the probability of dimensional change is high. Dimensional change affects the adaptation of the base to the tissue-bearing area and also affects the occlusion. It is advisable, therefore, to verify the adaptation of the dentures to the tissue-bearing areas. This procedure can be accomplished by placing some type of pressure-indicating material inside the denture. The extension of the peripheral borders, especially in the frenum area, should be evaluated. Once the individual bases are adjusted, the occlusal balance should be carefully checked and adjusted. A remount procedure is recommended for this equilibration.

92. **When the treatment plan calls for an immediate (transitional) denture, what are the expectations?**
If the anterior teeth are to be extracted at the time of denture insertion, the patient should be informed that the denture teeth can be placed in the same position as the existing teeth. However, the patient's facial appearance will change because of the presence of the labial flange, which affects the fullness of the lip. The patient also should be made aware of the necessary process of adaptation to the palate and of the increase in salivary flow that will become normal over time. Finally, the patient should be told that most people adapt well to such oral changes.

93. **Is the impression procedure the same for a transitional denture as for a conventional denture?**
The impression procedure is approximately the same for establishing the peripheral border. The major concern in taking an impression around existing teeth and exaggerated undercut area is to select a material that has the lowest viscosity and is nonrigid after setting. These properties are important to avoid damaging existing teeth during the removal of the impression.

94. **How is vertical dimension established in the construction of a transitional denture?**
It is important to use the existing teeth to establish the centric occlusal position, regardless of the amount and position of the teeth. At the bite registration phase, a bite rim is constructed in the edentulous space adjacent to the existing teeth, and the teeth with the wax rims are used to capture the occlusal relationship.

95. **If the master casts are altered in a transitional denture procedure (e.g., elimination of gross tissue undercuts), how is the surgical procedure altered?**
It is necessary during the surgical procedure to know exactly how the master cast has been altered. This information is critical for successful insertion of the transitional denture. It is advisable to construct a second denture base that is transparent. This surgical stent is placed over the ridge after the teeth are extracted. Pressure points and undercuts are readily visible, and surgical ridge correction can be performed.

96. **When a transitional denture is inserted, what procedures should be followed?**
It is always beneficial to have a surgical stent available to ascertain the fit of the denture base. Because many soft tissue undercut areas may be present, it is critical to establish a single path of insertion of the denture. Gross removal of areas inside the dentures may lead to poor adaptation of the denture base and instability. In this situation, immediate use of a soft lining material is indicated.

97. **During the healing phase, what procedures should be followed?**
The patient should be instructed not to remove the denture and return after 24 hours. At that time, tissue irritation and occlusion are checked, and the denture is adjusted. Then the patient is instructed about insertion and removal of the denture and told that as the ridges heal, resorption will occur. Each case varies, but in general resorption leads to a loosening of the denture. Therefore, transitional soft lining procedures should be performed throughout the healing phase, on approximately a monthly basis. The final healing may take from 3 to 6 months, at which time a permanent lining in the existing denture or a new denture is constructed.

98. **Is a face-bow transfer necessary in jaw registration in the complete-denture construction?**
It is advisable to take a face-bow transfer in the construction of a complete denture. The purpose of the registration is to relate the maxillary bite rims to the temporomandibular joint and facial planes. This registration aids in determining not only aesthetic factors, but also the type of occlusal plane.

99. **Is it necessary to take eccentric bite registrations in the construction of complete dentures?**
Although eccentric bite registrations are not essential, they aid in establishing a balanced occlusion. A stable occlusion is important for the retention and stability of dentures and for functional efficiency.

100. **What are digital dentures?**
Computer-aided technology has recently emerged as a mechanism for fabricating complete dentures. Digital dentures can be fabricated in as few as two appointments, as opposed to the traditional four or five patient visits. The first clinical appointment is for impressions, jaw records, and tooth selection. Impressions and jaw records are scanned, and digital files are created and merged. Virtual digital dentures are designed, the denture bases are milled from highly compressed biohygienic base material, and standard denture teeth are added. At the second appointment, the denture is inserted and adjusted. The digital record is maintained and, if the denture is ever lost or broken, an identical model can be refabricated and sent to the dentist, without patient involvement. The application of CAD-CAM complete dentures has considerable potential for patient care but prospective clinical trials are necessary to validate this new technology.

101. **What is the neutral zone? How does it relate to the alveolar ridge?**
The neutral zone is the potential space between the lips and cheeks on one side and the tongue on the other. Natural or artificial teeth in this zone are subject to equal and opposite forces from the surrounding musculature. The alveolar ridge, which normally dictates the position of the denture teeth, may conflict with the neutral zone. Therefore, the neutral position zone also should be considered when denture teeth are positioned.

102. **Are there any advantages to retaining roots under a denture apart from retention properties?**
Retention is a critical aspect in root-retained dentures. Of equal importance, however, is that retained roots help prevent resorption of the residual ridges. Retained roots also afford the patient some proprioceptive sense of "naturalness" in the function of the dentures.

103. **What is the ideal type of attachment in a root-retained denture?**
The ideal type of attachment affords maximal retentive forces for the denture, with minimal torquing forces to the roots. Because these ideal properties cannot be totally attained, a compromise is necessary. Many factors determine how much retention a tooth can withstand without subjection to harmful forces, including the following:
1. The amount of supportive bone around the retained roots
2. The number of existing roots
3. The type and amount of occlusal forces

4. The type of attachment (e.g., intra- or extraradicular, rigid, or stress-bearing attachment)
5. Splinting or nonsplinting of roots

104. **In a root-retained denture, which is better—an intraradicular or extraradicular attachment?**
Both attachments can be equally retentive, but the intraradicular attachment places the fulcrum forces more deeply into the bone than an extraradicular attachment and thus helps withstand deleterious torquing forces. The intraradicular attachments, however, are more difficult to implement because of the following: (1) length of existing root; (2) width of existing root; (3) paralleling to other roots; (4) inability to splint; and (5) difficulty in hygiene.

105. **Is splinting a preferred treatment in a root-retained denture?**
The main purpose of splinting roots in a tooth-borne denture is to dissipate the forces, thus minimizing the torque on the existing roots. Splinting does not necessarily result in increased denture retention, but it creates a more difficult construction procedure. Splinting should be attempted after certain aspects are evaluated, such as paralleling, amount of freeway space, placement of the bar to the ridge, and type of bar.

106. **What is the difference between a rigid and stress-breaking attachment?**
In a **rigid attachment,** the male and female components join in a precise fashion, allowing almost no movement between the two parts. This creates a rigid nonflexible attachment that affords the greatest amount of retention but also produces the greatest amount of torque on the retained roots. A rigid attachment is not recommended for periodontically compromised teeth.
A **stress-bearing attachment** affords movement between the male and female components, thereby relieving torque. In most cases, a stress-bearing attachment is recommended.

107. **How many roots must be retained to construct a root-retained denture?**
There is no fixed rule. A root-retained denture can be constructed with only one root. The fewer the roots, the less the retentive force that should be applied to them. The ideal distribution of retained roots would be cuspid regions and bilateral molar regions.

108. **Is it necessary to place attachments or cover the roots of a root-retained denture?**
It is not always necessary to cover a root beneath an overdenture. Retention is not the only goal of this treatment modality. Equally important is preservation of the residual ridge by retaining the roots. However, if a root is not covered, the exposed surfaces are highly susceptible to decay. Oral hygiene must be stringently maintained.

109. **Are the principles the same for a maxillary as for a mandibular overdenture?**
Yes. The majority of the principles for root-retained dentures are the same for the maxillary arch as for the mandible. One aspect that may differ is related to morphologic differences of the residual ridges. The maxillary arch has a greater probability of undercut areas in the anterior region above the roots. This difference is apparent in the canine area. It is necessary to design the path of insertion to take the undercuts into consideration. Therefore, attachment selection may have to be altered, and the peripheral border of the denture may have to be reduced or eliminated.

110. **Can the palate be eliminated in a root-retained maxillary denture?**
If retention is adequate from the retained roots with their attachments, it is possible to eliminate the palate. It must be remembered that the palatal area affords the denture the greatest bearing area and also creates cross-arch stabilization.

111. **What are the causes of denture stomatitis? How can it be treated?**
Denture stomatitis is caused by trauma from poorly fitting dentures, by poor oral and denture hygiene, and by the oral fungus *Candida albicans.* Denture stomatitis can be treated by using resilient denture liners that stabilize ill-fitting dentures, thereby treating the inflamed tissue. Some liners may also inhibit fungal growth.

IMPLANTS

112. **What types of implants are most commonly used for prosthetic replacement of the tooth?**
1. **Endosteal implants:** Blades, screws, or cylinders are implanted into the maxilla or mandible. These implants support the dental prosthesis.
2. **Subperiosteal implants:** A metal framework is inserted on top of the maxillary or mandibular bone. Vertical posts attached to the framework protrude from the soft tissue and support the dental prosthesis.

113. **What is an osseointegrated implant?**
An osseointegrated implant is a cylinder or screw constructed of a biocompatible material that is precisely embedded into the ridge of the maxilla or mandible (Fig. 9-10). The fixture is allowed to integrate with the bone without any loading forces for a certain period. Histologically, the bone cells grow tightly around this anchor, with no membrane attachment at the interface (unlike the natural tooth-bone interface).

114. **What are mini–dental implants?**
These are implants fabricated of the same biocompatible materials as conventional implants but with smaller dimensions (diameter $\cong$ 1.8-2.9 mm). They are generally one piece, with a fused implant-abutment complex designed to support or retain prosthetics. They are typically placed by a surgical approach that does not require

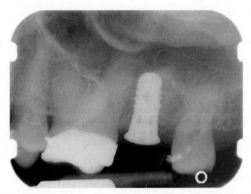

Fig. 9-10. Osseointegrated implant. (From Spitz SD: Lasers in prosthodontics: clinical realities of a dental laser in a prosthodontic practice. Alpha Omegan 101:188–194, 2008.)

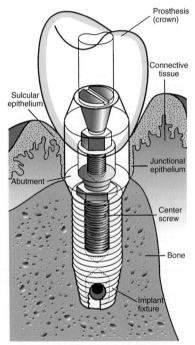

Fig. 9-11. Components of an implant. (From Perry DA, Beemsterboer PL: Periodontology for the Dental Hygienist, ed 3, St. Louis, Saunders, 2007.)

a flap or bone augmentation. They can be immediately loaded and therefore offer instant patient satisfaction. Also, they typically cost significantly less than conventional implants. Historically, mini-implants were used for interim or transitional fixed and removable prosthetics or orthodontic treatments. Some practitioners advocate for their use for the long term or permanently, but the evidence is still unclear.

115. Describe the components of an implant and the clinical procedures used with each.
The technique and biocompatible materials used in the osseointegrated implant were developed by Per-Ingvar Brånemark, an orthopedic surgeon, more than 50 years ago. Brånemark identified the biocompatible material, titanium, and described the following components (Fig. 9-11):
1. **Fixture**—the anchor embedded into the edentulous ridge. It is constructed of titanium and may be coated with a biocompatible bone regeneration material, such as hydroxyapatite. The fixture is carefully embedded into precision-drilled holes and allowed to integrate with the bone undisturbed for 3 to 6 months.

2. **Abutment**—the transitional piece that connects the fixture to the prosthesis. The abutment is normally attached to the fixture after a second surgical procedure.
3. **Dental prosthesis**—the dental prosthesis can then be constructed and attached to the abutment. This stage may begin a few weeks after the second surgery.

116. What is the success rate of an osseointegrated implant prosthesis?
Many factors affect the success rate of an implant prosthesis; however, studies for long-term predictability have demonstrated a success rate of more than 90%.

117. What factors affect the success rate of the implant?

- Careful patient selection
- Exacting diagnostic records
- Integrated treatment planning
- Precise clinical procedures

118. What are the important factors in patient selection?
1. Patient's general health
   - Medical considerations
   - Medications
   - Psychiatric considerations
2. Intraoral factors
   - Bone tissue site of fixture installation free from pathologic conditions (e.g., cysts)
   - Site free from unerupted or impacted teeth, root remnants, or any other foreign bodies
   - No open communication between the bone and oral cavity
   - Healthy mucosa, free from ulceration
   - Anatomic factors

119. What type of bone is important to osseointegration?
Good bone consists of a thick layer of compact bone surrounding a core of dense trabecular bone of favorable strength. Poor bone consists of a thin layer of cortical bone surrounding a core of low-density trabecular bone.

120. What anatomic factors are important to consider for implant replacement?
- Transverse shape of the jaw bone
- Degree of resorption
- Maxilla—location of sinuses, nasal cavity, and incisive canal
- Mandible—mental foramen, inferior alveolar nerve, and blood vessels

121. How is the intraoral condition evaluated?
The intraoral condition is determined through radiographic evaluation:
- Intraoral radiograph of proposed site
- General view of the jaws (a panoramic radiograph reveals any pathologic processes)
- Lateral cephalometric radiograph (to show relationship between jaws)
- Cone-beam computed tomography (CBCT) records (provides valuable information about the width of the alveolar crest and location of important anatomic structures)

122. How do you plan for the proper treatment modality?
Planning the actual course of therapy is essential to success. Before the surgery, an evaluation should be made of the desired prosthetic results. This evaluation dictates the following:
- Type of prosthetic replacement
- Number of implants
- Placement of fixtures
- Models of the jaw mounted on an articulator, if necessary
  The setup of teeth on these models determines the prosthesis and helps the dentist performing the surgery to visualize the proposed prosthesis. The surgeon also may be guided for implant placement by the use of a surgical template.

123. What are radiographic and surgical stents?
Radiographic and surgical stents are templates constructed on the diagnostic models that aid in the position and placement of the implants. A stent with metal markers over the proposed fixture sites should be used to aid in the evaluation of radiographs. A surgical stent is also useful when the fixtures are implanted. The optimal position from a prosthetic point of view can be visualized.

124. What are the treatment modalities for a totally edentulous jaw?
- Overdenture supported by implants
- Fixed, high-water prosthesis
- Conventional fixed crown and bridges using implants

125. **Describe the concept of implant-supported overdenture.**
An implant-supported overdenture is supported by the implants and edentulous ridge covered by resilient mucosa. The surgeon must accommodate for this resiliency in the attachments of the implants to permit small rotational movements.

126. **What are the indications for the overdenture treatment?**
This treatment modality is a comparatively simple procedure with relatively low cost and meets the demands imposed by many patients. The most common indications are the following:
- Retention of denture
- Compromised hygiene skills (i.e., reduced dexterity, as with some older individuals)
- Interarch positions (difficulty in placing proper interdental relationships with fixed restorations)
- Phonetics and aesthetics (especially in the maxilla)
   An overdenture may improve aesthetic and/or phonetic results compared with an implant-supported fixed prosthesis.

127. **How many implants are necessary to support the overdenture?**
The number of implants ranges from a minimum of two fixtures to an ideal of four. It is also important to consider the loading forces on the implant.

128. **What is the effect of loading forces on implant-supported overdentures?**
The loading forces are important to fixture survival because overloading can lead to implant failure. To reduce improper loading conditions, the following points should be considered:
1. The implants should be positioned as perpendicular to the occlusal plane as possible.
2. Shear loads and bending movements are reduced if leverages are shortened by using short abutments and low attachments.
3. Resilient attachments reduce bending movements. Occlusal forces are shared between fixtures and overdenture-bearing mucosa.
4. Extension bars represent a potential risk of overloading.

129. **What is the fixed high-water prosthesis on an edentulous arch?**
The fixed prosthesis supported by implants on an edentulous arch was first developed and investigated by Brånemark in the 1960s (Fig. 9-12):
- Placement of fixtures with transmucosal abutments as parallel as possible to each other
- Cast metal frameworks that fit precisely on the abutments and support the prosthesis
- Denture teeth and processed denture material on the metal framework

130. **What does *high water* mean?**
High water refers to the design of an implant-supported prosthesis. The implants support the prostheses without the aid of the mucosal edentulous ridge, which is used in the implant-supported overdenture. Space between the prosthesis and mucosa is necessary for proper hygiene, thus leading to the descriptive term *high water.*

131. **What happens when the fixtures are not parallel in a fixed prosthesis?**
A precise prosthesis fit is necessary for osseointegrated rigid fixtures; therefore, relative paralleling is required. Lack of paralleling, however, can be compensated with proper abutment selection. The divergence of axial fixtures can differ by up to 40 degrees.

132. **How many fixtures are necessary to support a high-water fixed prosthesis?**
Many factors determine the number of fixtures necessary to support a fixed prosthesis, including quality of bone, placement and length of fixture, and loading of fixtures. In general, however, four to six fixtures are sufficient to support a fixed high-water prosthesis.

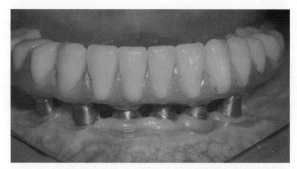

Fig. 9-12. High-water prosthesis. (From Babbush CA, Hahn JA, Krauser JT, et al.: Dental Implants: The Art and Science, ed 2, St. Louis, Saunders, 2011.)

133. **Can conventional fixed bridgework be used over implants to restore a totally edentulous arch?**
Conventional fixed bridgework rather than the high-water prosthesis can be used with implants to restore a totally edentulous arch. However, fixture positioning, loading forces, and aesthetic and phonetic considerations are more critical. In addition, more fixtures are necessary to support the prosthesis (minimum of six).

134. **Should an implant prosthesis be considered in partially edentulous patients?**
The partially fixed implant-supported prosthesis is a viable treatment and should be considered as the treatment of choice when the alternatives are a removable partial denture or fixed bridge attached to previously untouched teeth, or if the proposed abutments are periodontally compromised. Conventional bridgework may be the appropriate treatment of choice when the proposed abutment teeth are periodontally sound but need extensive restorative work (Fig. 9-13).

135. **What factors should be considered when selecting implant treatment for partially edentulous patients?**
    1. Implant placement is limited and defined by existing edentulous space; therefore, fixture placement may be near sensitive structures such as nerves and blood vessels.
    2. Good aesthetic results may be difficult to achieve.
    3. Greater horizontal loading forces place high demands on the anchorage of the fixture.
    4. Topographic conditions of the existing bone and its relationship to the remaining teeth must be considered.
    5. Occlusal considerations are essential—that is, when canines and premolar teeth are replaced in a cuspid-protected articulator with a deep overbite.
    6. Periodontal disease on remaining teeth creates a pathologic condition that may contraindicate implantation.

136. **What factors influence abutment selection?**
The abutment selection is an important prosthodontic phase of treatment because it may determine the final prosthesis design. Factors for abutment selection should include the following:
    1. Articulated casts with a diagnostic wax-up of the proposed prosthesis aid in determining the size and angulation of the abutment.
    2. The type of abutment depends on whether the prosthesis is to be screwed to the implant or cement-retained.
    3. Transmucosal space should be determined because it affects the height selection of the abutment.
    4. Aesthetic and phonetic considerations also affect the selection of abutment.

137. **What diagnostic procedure may be used for abutment selection?**
To determine the proper abutment angulation height, aesthetic factors, and occlusal considerations, it is necessary to know the position of the fixture to the bone in relation to the gingival mucosa and interarch space between the fixture and opposing dentition. Fixture angulation and transmucosal height can be measured intraorally with diagnostic gauges. However, the following is a more precise method:
    1. Obtain an impression of the arch with the fixtures.
    2. Construct a cast that contains replicas of the fixtures with its relationship to the mucosa.
    3. Articulate this model to the opposing dentition. This method facilitates proper abutment selection and fabrication.

138. **What is an angulated abutment?**
An angulated abutment is positioned in an angulated direction from the axial position of the fixture. This angulation may vary by up to 30 degrees. Angulated abutments are used when the fixtures have been installed with an unfavorable inclination in relation to the desired position of the prosthesis.

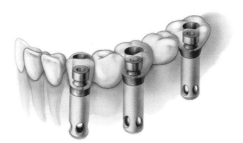

Fig. 9-13. Fixed implant–supported prosthesis. (From Ebersole P, Touhy TA, Hess P, et al.: Toward Health Aging: Human Needs and Nursing Response, ed 7, St. Louis, Mosby, 2008.)

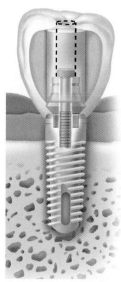

Fig. 9-14. UCLA-type abutment. (From Rosenstiel SF, Land MF, Fujimoto J: Contemporary fixed prosthodontics, ed 4, St. Louis, Mosby, 2006.)

139. **What is the UCLA-type abutment?**

The UCLA abutment is custom-fabricated on the fixture replica. Normally, the fabrication is done so that the final abutment appears like a full-crown preparation on which the prosthesis is cemented. It also may be screw-retained. This customized fabrication technique allows control of angulation, transmucosal shape and height, aesthetic considerations, and interocclusal space (Fig. 9-14).

140. **What is a CAD-CAM abutment?**

CAD-CAM abutments are digitally designed and milled patient-specific custom abutments that are manufactured for most implant brands.

The benefits of CAD-CAM abutments include:
- Customized emergence profile for enhanced soft-tissue management
- Placement of material junction of abutment and crown considering biological principles
- Optimized positioning of the screw access channel for improved esthetics, function, and installation procedure
  Dentsply Sirona Atlantis Abutments and Straumann Cares Abutments are two examples of CAD-CAM abutment brands.

141. **What is platform switching?**

It is fitting and abutment of a smaller circumference compared to the implant in an effort to preserve alveolar crestal bone. This method gained importance when researchers discovered reduced crestal bone loss around implants that had switched platforms. The likely mechanism is that a connective tissue layer develops in the horizontal direction as opposed to the vertical direction with platforms that are matched. Most studies support the use of switched platforms for reducing bone loss.

142. **Can an implant be used for single-tooth replacement?**

Yes. However, careful patient selection and presurgical analysis are critical so that function and aesthetics approximate those of the natural tooth.

143. **Can implants and natural teeth be used together to support a final prosthesis?**

Natural teeth are suspended in bone by the periodontal membrane. This situation allows tooth movement in relationship to bone. An osseointegrated implant, which is fixed rigidly to the bone, allows no movement at its interface. Joining a movable natural tooth and rigid implant with a fixed prosthesis may cause support problems that lead to failure. It is better to separate the prosthesis, if possible (e.g., implant with implant, natural tooth with natural tooth). This strategy may not always be possible. In these cases, there is limited evidence that rigid connection between teeth and implants presents better results when compared with the nonrigid one. The major drawback of nonrigidly connected FDPs is tooth intrusion.

Acknowledgment
The authors gratefully acknowledge the contributions of the previous chapter's author.

BIBLIOGRAPHY

Balshi I, Ekfeldt A, Stember T, Vrielinck L. Three-year evaluation of Branemark implants connected to angulated abutments. *Int J Oral Maxillofac Implants*. 1997;12:52–58.

Bidra AS, Almas K. Mini implants for definitive prosthodontic treatment: a systematic review. *J Prosthet Dent*. 2013;109:156–164.

Bidra AS, Taylor TD, Agar JR. Computer-aided technology for fabricating complete dentures: systematic review of historical background, current status, and future perspectives. *J Prosthet Dent*. 2013;109:361–366.

Chiche GJ, Pinault A. *Esthetics of Anterior Fixed Prosthodontics*. Chicago: Quintessence; 1993.

Gomez-Polo M, Llido B, Rivero A, et al. A 10-year retrospective study of the survival rate of teeth restored with metal prefabricated posts versus cast metal posts and cores. *J Dent*. 2010;38(11):916–920.

Heydecke G, Peters M. The restoration of enodontically treated teeth, single-rooted teeth with cast or direct posts and cores: a systematic review. *J Prosth Dent*. 2002;87(4):380–386.

Lucia VO. *Treatment of the Edentulous Patient*. Chicago: Quintessence; 1986.

Magnussen S, Nilson H, Lindh T. *Branemark Systems: Restorative Dentist's Manual*. Gothenburg, Sweden: Nobel Biocare AB; 1992.

McLaren EA, Schoenbaum T. Combine conventional and digital methods to maximize shade matching. *Compend Contin Educ Dent*. 2011;32(spec no 4):32–33. 30.

McLean JW. *The Science and Art of Dental Ceramics*. vol I. Chicago: Quintessence; 1979.

McLean JW. *The Science and Art of Dental Ceramics*. vol II. Chicago: Quintessence; 1980.

Morrow RM, Rudd KD, Rhoads JE. Dental Laboratory Procedures: Complete Dentures. 2nd ed. vol I. St. Louis: Mosby; 1986.

Phillips R. *Skinner's Science of Dental Materials*. 9th ed. Philadelphia: WB Saunders; 1991.

Rudd KD, Morrow RM, Rhoads JE. *Dental Laboratory Procedures: Removable Partial Dentures*. vol 3. St. Louis: Mosby; 1986.

Shillingburg Jr HT, et al. *Fundamentals of Fixed Prosthodontics*. 2nd ed. Chicago: Quintessence; 1981.

Singh R, Singh SV, Arora V. Platform switching: a narrative review. *Implant Dent*. 2013;22:453–459.

Smith R, Kournjian J. *Understanding Dental Implants*. San Bruno, CA: Kramer Communications; 1989.

Tsaousoglou P, Michalakis K, Kang K, et al. The effect of rigid and non-rigid connections between implants and teeth on biological and technical complications: a systematic review and a meta-analysis. *Clin Oral Implants Res*. 2017;28(7):849–863.

Yamamoto M. *Metal Ceramics: Principles and Methods of Makoto Yamamoto*. Tokyo: Quintessence; 1990.

Yu H, Chen Y, Cheng H, et al. Finish-line designs for ceramic crowns: a systematic review and meta-analysis. *J Prosth Dent*. 2019;122(1):22–30.

CHAPTER 10

PEDIATRIC DENTISTRY AND ORTHODONTICS

Isabelle Chase, James MacLaine

PEDIATRIC DENTISTRY

1. **What is the difference between natal and neonatal teeth?**
   Natal teeth are present at birth, whereas neonatal teeth emerge through the gingiva during the first month of life.

2. **How common are natal teeth?**
   There is a large range in the reported prevalence of natal teeth. One study used two methods of determining prevalence: method 1 prevalence was 1 in 3667 births and method 2 prevalence was 1 in 716 births. In previous studies, the prevalence ranged from 1 in 1000 to 30,000 births.

3. **Summarize the characteristics of natal teeth..**
   - 95% are the actual primary teeth; 5% are supernumerary teeth.
   - All natal teeth observed in one study were mandibular central incisors.
   - A family history of natal teeth has been established in previous studies; the incidence of a positive family history ranges from 8% to 46%.
   - When natal teeth erupt, the enamel is at the normal histologic age for the child. Because the teeth erupt prematurely, the enamel matrix is not fully calcified and wears off quickly. Once the gingival covering is lost, the enamel cannot continue to mature.

4. **How are natal teeth managed?**
   In general, natal teeth are left alone unless they cause difficulty for the infant or mother. Clinical complications include ulceration of the dorsal tongue surface (Riga-Fede disease), lingual frenum, or mother's nipple during breast-feeding. Because natal teeth are usually mobile, some people worry about aspiration. Although no cases of aspiration have been reported, it is generally recommended that highly mobile natal teeth be extracted. On non-mobile natal teeth, treatment may also include smoothing of the incisal edge. If the teeth survive past 4 months of age, the prognosis for continued survival is good; most natal teeth, however, are not aesthetically pleasing because of enamel hypoplasia.

5. **Are any syndromes associated with natal teeth?**
   Four syndromes have been associated with natal teeth: (1) chondroectodermal dysplasia, or Ellis-van Creveld syndrome; (2) oculomandibulodyscephaly with hypotrichosis, or Hallermann-Streiff syndrome; (3) pachyonychia congenita, or Jadassohn-Lewandowski syndrome; and (4) Pierre–Robin syndrome.

6. **What is the definition of early childhood caries (ECC)?**
   The disease of ECC is the presence of one or more decayed (noncavitated or cavitated lesions), missing (because of caries), or filled tooth surfaces in any primary tooth in a child 71 months of age or younger. In children younger than 3 years, any sign of smooth surface caries is indicative of severe early childhood caries (S-ECC). From ages 3 through 5 years, one or more cavitated, missing (because of caries), filled smooth surfaces in primary maxillary anterior teeth or a decayed, missing, or filled score of four or more (age 3), five or more (age 4), or six or more (age 5) surfaces constitutes S-ECC.

7. **What should be included in an infant dental health program?**
   1. Prenatal oral health counseling for parents
      - Counsel parents about their own oral health habits and their effect as role models.
      - Discuss pregnancy-related gingivitis.
      - Review **infant dental care:** (1) clean gums daily before eruption of the first primary tooth to help establish healthy oral flora; and (2) do not use dentifrice to avoid fluoride ingestion.
      - Review **oral care for toddlers** (1-3 years of age): (1) introduce soft toothbrush; (2) use a small "smear" of fluoride-containing toothpaste, twice daily, with the eruption of the first tooth, until 2 years of age, and a pea-sized amount of dentifrice beginning at age 3 years; (3) allow child to begin brushing with supervision (parents should remain primary oral caregiver); and (4) discuss timing of eruption of primary teeth and teething.
      - Review of **preschool oral care** (3-6 years of age): (1) parents should continue to supervise and help with oral hygiene; (2) continue with pea-sized amount of dentifrice; and (3) start flossing if teeth are in contact with each other.

2. Discussion of early childhood caries (baby bottle tooth decay) and how it can be prevented
   - Avoid putting child to sleep with a bottle.
   - Avoid on-demand nocturnal breast-feeding after the first primary tooth begins to erupt.
   - Avoid giving sugar-sweetened beverages by bottle or sippy-cup.
   - Limit sweetened beverages to 4 ounces daily and ideally only with meals.
   - Encourage drinking from a cup around the first birthday.
   - Avoid grazing on processed carbohydrates
3. Discussion of timing of first dental visit (see question 9)

8. **What is meant by anticipatory guidance?**
   Anticipatory guidance is the deliberate and systematic distribution of information to parents as a tool to help them know what to expect, how to prevent unwanted conditions or events, and what to do when an anticipated or unexpected event occurs. Information should include dental and oral development, fluoride status, non-nutritional oral habits (see questions 10 to 12), injury prevention, oral hygiene, and the effects of diet on the dentition.

9. **When should children have their first visit to the dentist?**
   Currently, the American Academy of Pediatric Dentistry (AAPD) and American Dental Association (ADA) recommend an initial oral evaluation within 6 months of the eruption of the first primary tooth and no later than the child's first birthday. At this visit, the dentist should complete thorough medical and dental histories (covering prenatal, perinatal, and postnatal periods) as well as an oral examination. After completing these tasks, the dentist can best formulate a tailored prevention care plan based on the patient's risk of developing oral and dental disease. In addition, the dentist can use this appointment to provide anticipatory guidance (see question 8).

10. **What are non-nutritional sucking habits?**
    Non-nutritional sucking habits are learned patterns of muscular contraction. The most common types are as follows:
    - Finger habit
    - Lip wetting or sucking
    - Abnormal swallowing or tongue thrusting
    - Abnormal muscular habits

    Sucking is the best-developed avenue of sensation for an infant. Deprivation may cause an infant to suck on the thumb or finger for additional gratification.

11. **Are non-nutritional sucking habits harmful to the dentoalveolar structures?**
    If a child stops non-nutritional sucking habits within their first 3 years of life, the risks are low. If there are changes to the dentoalveolar structures, it is usually limited to the maxillary anterior segment and presents as an open bite. If the habit continues past 3 years, the changes may be long-lasting and detrimental to the developing dentoalveolar structures. After 4 years of age, a finger habit can become well established and is much harder to stop. Oral structures can become further deformed by palatal constriction and posterior crossbite.

    Tongue and lip habits are often associated with a finger habit and produce added compensatory forces that can lead to full-blown malocclusion. Thumb and finger habits can cause an anterior open bite, proclination of the upper incisors, lingual movement of the lower incisors, and constriction of the maxillary arch. Lip sucking and lip biting can procline the maxillary incisors, retrocline the mandibular incisors, and increase the amount of overjet.

    Tongue thrusting and mouth breathing may also play a part in the creation of a malocclusion. An anterior open bite is the most common dental problem associated with the anomalies.

12. **Describe intervention therapy for non-nutritional sucking habits..**
    1. Ideally, the patient should understand the problem and want to correct it.
    2. The timing of intervention is controversial. Some authors suggest that therapy should begin around age 4 years to prevent irreversible changes, whereas others suggest waiting until the patient is about 6 to 7 years old to ensure that he or she can understand the intent of therapy.
    3. Patients who decide to accept appliance therapy should have support and encouragement from their parents to help them during treatment.
    4. The dentist should know the patient well to provide intervention and advice at the correct time.
    5. The dentist should be able to evaluate the deformity and extent of its effects so that it can be treated in the best possible manner.

13. **What is the current schedule of systemic fluoride supplementation?**
    See Table 10-1.

14. **Summarize the scientific basis for the use of fluoride varnishes in caries management..**
    1. When used appropriately, varnishes offer a 40% to 56% reduction in the incidence of caries, with a 36% reduction in fissured caries and a 66% reduction in nonfissured (smooth) surfaces.
    2. Varnish results in a 51% reversal of decalcified tooth structure and a reduction in enamel demineralization of 21% to 35%.

Table 10-1. Fluoride Supplementation

AGE	FLUORIDE CONCENTRATION IN LOCAL WATER SUPPLY (ppm)		
	<0.3	0.3-0.6	>0.6
6 mo-3 yr	0.25 mg/day	0	0
3-6 yr	0.50 mg/day	0.25 mg/day	0
6-16 yr	1.00 mg/day	0.50 mg/day	0

3. Varnish application is effective in arresting and reversing active enamel lesions, reducing the need for restorative treatment.
4. Varnishes are as effective as acidulated phosphate fluoride gels in controlling approximal caries.
5. In primary teeth of preschool children, varnishes result in a 44% reduction in caries.

15. **Is prenatal fluoride supplementation effective in decreasing caries rates in the primary dentition?**
No. No studies to date support the administration of prenatal fluorides to protect the primary dentition against caries.

16. **Do home water filtration units have any effect on fluoride content?**
Absolutely. For example, reverse osmosis home filtration systems remove 84%, distillation units remove 99%, and carbon filtration systems remove 81% of the fluoride from water.

17. **Why has the prevalence of fluorosis increased in the United States?**
The increased prevalence is likely because of three factors: (1) inappropriate fluoride supplementation; (2) ingestion of fluoridated toothpaste (most children <5 years ingest all the toothpaste placed on the toothbrush); and (3) high fluoride content of bottled juices. For example, white grape juice may have a fluoride concentration greater than 2 ppm.

18. **What are the common signs of acute fluoride toxicity?**
Acute fluoride toxicity may result in nausea, vomiting, hypersalivation, abdominal pain, and diarrhea.

19. **What is the first step in treating a child who has ingested an amount of fluoride greater than the safely tolerated dose?**
In acute toxicity, set at 5 mg/kg of body weight, the goal is to minimize the amount of fluoride absorbed. Calcium-binding products, such as milk or milk of magnesia, decrease the acidity of the stomach, forming insoluble complexes with the fluoride and thereby decreasing its absorption. For ingestion greater than 5 mg/kg of body weight, syrup of ipecac may be recommended to empty the stomach or gastric lavage.

20. **Are children born with *Streptococcus mutans*?**
Children are not born with *Streptococcus mutans*. Instead, they acquire this caries-causing organism between the ages of about 1 and 3 years. Mothers tend to be the major source of infection. The well-delineated age range of acquisition is referred to as the window of infectivity.
    Transmission of *S. mutans* may be vertical (e.g., from caregiver to child) or horizontal (e.g., between siblings). Transmission may be decreased by reducing habits such as sharing utensils or foods. Additionally, several studies have demonstrated decreasing maternal levels of *S. mutans* decreases the transmission rate to the child.

21. **What variable is the best predictor of caries risk in children?**
Past caries rates are the single best predictor in assessing a child's future risk.

22. **Is milk a contributing factor to early childhood caries?**
Several animal and in vitro studies have suggested that milk and milk components are not cariogenic. Similarly, human breast milk by itself does not cause demineralization. However, when mixed with a sucrose-containing substance, cow's milk and human breast milk promote caries.

23. **What food components reduce the caries-inducing effects of carbohydrates?**
Phosphates, fats, and cheese decrease caries susceptibility. Phosphates apparently have a topical effect that aids in remineralization and improves the structural integrity of the enamel surface. Although the mechanism is not entirely clear, fats may form a protective barrier on the teeth or coat the carbohydrate. Cheese may contribute through a number of mechanisms, including its fat, phosphorus, calcium content, and increased saliva production from chewing.

24. **Is there any dental health benefit to chewing gum?**
One study found that children of mothers who chewed sugar-free gum sweetened with xylitol (in addition to normal oral hygiene measures) had 70% less dental decay than children of mothers who did not chew the gum.

25. Summarize the mechanisms of xylitol's effect..
    - Xylitol has a five-carbon chemical structure not recognized by oral bacteria.
    - Because it is not fermented, no acid production results, and pH levels in the mouth do not decrease (see question 27).
    - Chewing xylitol-sweetened gum promotes stimulation of salivary flow, which in turn helps rinse away excessive sucrose residues and neutralize acids from other foods. In addition, saliva contains calcium and phosphate, which promote remineralization of early caries.
    - Xylitol is a polyol that inhibits the growth of *S. mutans,* thereby reducing caries susceptibility. Continued use helps reduce the number of virulent bacteria in the plaque, although xylitol is not bactericidal.
    - Xylitol reduces plaque in the oral cavity and enhances the proportion of soluble to insoluble polysaccharides.
    - Xylitol complements fluoride in the oral cavity.

26. Who throws a meaner curve, Ryan or Stephan?
    Undoubtedly Stephan! The Stephan curve describes the decrease in pH that occurs following a cariogenic challenge. Hall of Fame pitcher Nolan Ryan, on the other hand, is best remembered for his fastball, although did have a pretty good curve.

27. What is meant by critical pH?
    Critical pH is the pH (~5.5) at which enamel is demineralized.

28. What is the Vipeholm Study? What did it demonstrate?
    In the Vipeholm Study (1954), adult institutionalized patients were followed for several years on a variety of controlled diets. The following results were reported:
    - Caries increased significantly when sucrose-containing foods were ingested between meals.
    - Sucrose in a retentive form produced more caries than forms that were rapidly cleared from the mouth.
    - Sucrose consumed with meals was the least detrimental form.
    - Caries activity differs among people with the same diet.

29. Why does this CAT not have your tongue?
    CAT stands for the *C*aries Risk *A*ssessment *T*ool developed by the AAPD to aid in assessing a child's risk of caries (Table 10-2). Recommendations based on their guidelines are as follows:
    1. Dental caries risk assessment, based on a child's age, biologic and protective factors, and clinical findings, should be a routine component of new and periodic examinations by oral health and medical providers.
    2. There is not enough information at present to carry out quantitative caries risk assessment analyses. However, estimating children at low, moderate, and high caries risk via a preponderance of risk and protective factors will enable a more evidence-based approach to medical provider referrals, as well as establish periodicity and intensity of diagnostic, preventive, and restorative services.
    3. Clinical management protocols, based on a child's age, caries risk, and level of patient and parent cooperation, provide health providers with criteria and protocols for determining the types and frequency of diagnostic, preventive, and restorative care for patient-specific management of dental caries.

30. Why might children with asthma be at higher risk of developing dental caries?
    The two major classes of medications used to treat asthma are anti-inflammatory agents (e.g., corticosteroids, cromolyn sodium) and bronchodilators (beta-adrenergic agonists, such as Ventolin and albuterol). Over the years, numerous studies have shown that all these medications can impair salivary function, causing xerostomia (dry mouth) and thus potentially increasing susceptibility to caries. Evidence suggests that children with asthma may have double the risk of caries in their primary and permanent dentition. Therefore, it is important to implement appropriate preventive measures in asthmatic patients, such as routine fluoride application, extra attention to oral hygiene, and rinsing mouth with water after medication use.

31. What is the earliest macroscopic evidence of dental caries on a smooth enamel surface?
    A white spot lesion results from acid dissolution of the enamel surface, giving it a chalky white appearance. Optimal exposure to topical fluorides may result in the remineralization of such lesions.

32. Which teeth are often spared in early childhood dental caries (nursing caries)?
    The mandibular incisors often remain caries-free as a result of protection by the tongue.

33. Does an explorer stick necessarily indicate the presence of caries?
    Several studies have demonstrated that an explorer stick may often be caused by the anatomy of the pit and fissure and not the presence of caries (poor sensitivity). However, the lack of a stick is a good indication of lack of caries (good specificity). It has been suggested that sharp eyes are more important than sharp explorers in detecting pit and fissure caries.

34. What are the indications for an indirect pulp cap in the primary dentition?
    An indirect pulp cap is indicated in a deep carious lesion approximating the pulp but without signs or symptoms of pulp degeneration. Long-term studies have indicated a higher success rate for indirect pulp caps compared to pulpotomies.

Table 10-2. Caries Risk Assessment Tool (CAT)

CARIES RISK INDICATORS	LOW RISK*	MODERATE RISK†	HIGH RISK‡
Clinical factors	No carious teeth in past 24 mo No enamel demineralization No visible plaque; no gingivitis	Carious teeth in past 24 mo Gingivitis	Carious teeth in past 12 mo Active enamel Demineralization (enamel defect or white spot lesion) or interproximal lesion Visible plaque on anterior (front) teeth Radiographic enamel caries High titers of *Streptococcus mutans* Wearing dental or orthodontic appliances Enamel hypoplasia Defective restorations
Environmental/social characteristics	Optimal systemic and topical fluoride exposure Consumption of simple sugars or foods strongly associated with caries initiation, primarily at mealtimes High socioeconomic status of caregiver Regular use of dental care in an established dental home	Suboptimal systemic fluoride exposure with optimal topical exposure Occasional (one or two) between-meal exposures to simple sugars or foods strongly associated with caries Midlevel socioeconomic status of caregiver (i.e., eligible for school lunch program, CHIP) Irregular use of dental services	Suboptimal topical fluoride exposure Frequent (i.e., 3 or more) between-meal exposures to simple sugars or foods strongly associated with caries Life-time of poverty, low health literacy (i.e., eligible for Medicaid) No dental home Active caries present in the mother Recent immigrant
General health conditions			Children with special health care needs Conditions impairing saliva composition/flow

CHIP, Children's Health Insurance Program.
*Low risk: The child does not have moderate-risk or high-risk indicators.
†Moderate risk: The presence of at least one moderate-risk indicator and no high-risk indicators present results in a moderate-risk classification.
‡High risk: The presence of a single risk indicator in any area of the high-risk category is sufficient to classify a child as being at high risk.
Adapted from American Academy of Pediatric Dentistry: American Academy of Pediatric Dentistry Caries Risk Assessment Tool (CAT). https://www.aapd.org/media/Policies_Guidelines/BP_CariesRiskAssessment.pdf. *Accessed June 7, 2022.*

Calcium hydroxide is a commonly used medication that is applied to the dentin, followed by a restorative material that provides a complete seal.

35. **What are the indications for a direct pulp cap?**
A direct pulp cap may be indicated when there is a small mechanical or traumatic exposure of the pulp. Materials commonly used include calcium hydroxide, glass ionomer and, more recently, mineral trioxide aggregate (MTA). According to one study, successful outcomes are inversely related to the amount of bleeding.

36. **What medication shows the greatest promise for primary tooth pulpotomies?**
Recent studies have suggested that MTA has great potential as a primary tooth pulpotomy medication. It results in less internal root resorption and equal to or improved clinical and radiographic outcomes compared with formocresol or ferric sulfate. (It also smells a lot better than formocresol.)

37. **What are the disadvantages of MTA as a primary tooth pulpotomy medication?**
They are mainly cost considerations. It is at least 20 times more expensive than formocresol.

38. **Which branchial arch gives rise to the maxilla and mandible?**
The first branchial or mandibular arch gives rise to the maxilla, mandible, Meckel's cartilage, incus, malleus, muscles of mastication, and anterior belly of the digastric muscle.

39. How does the palate form?

The paired palatal shelves arise from the intraoral maxillary processes. These shelves, originally in a vertical position, reorient to a horizontal position as the tongue assumes a more inferior position. The shelves then fuse anteriorly with the primary palate, which arises from the median nasal process, and posteriorly and with one another. Failure of fusion results in a cleft palate.

40. When do the primary teeth develop?

At approximately 28 days in utero, a continuous plate of epithelium arises in the maxilla and mandible. By 37 days in utero, a well-defined, thickened layer of epithelium overlying the cell-derived mesenchyme of the neural crest delineates the dental lamina. Ten areas in each jaw become identifiable at the location of each of the primary teeth.

41. After the eruption of a tooth, when is root development completed?

In the primary dentition, root development is complete approximately 18 months after eruption; in the permanent dentition, the period of development is approximately 3 years.

42. Define *ankylosis.* How is it diagnosed?

Ankylosis is the fusion of cementum with alveolar bone and may occur at any time during the course of eruption. Because affected teeth have retarded vertical growth, they appear to be submerged below the occlusal plane. Diagnosis involves visual determination that a tooth may be 1 mm or more below the height of the occlusal plane, radiographic evidence of lack of a periodontal ligament, and/or lack of physiologic mobility. The ankylosed tooth emits an atypical sharp sound on percussion. In addition, children with affected siblings are twice as likely to have submerged teeth compared with the general population. Ankylosis often occurs bilaterally; 67% of affected people have two or more submerged teeth.

43. What causes ankylosis? Which teeth are usually affected?

The definitive cause of ankylosis is unknown. Contributing factors cited in the literature include local mechanical trauma, disturbed local metabolism, localized infection, chemical or thermal irritation, and gaps in the periodontal membrane.

Mandibular first primary molars are usually affected, followed by second mandibular molars, first maxillary molars, and second maxillary molars. The prevalence of infraclusion peaks between 8 and 9 years of age, with a suspected range of 1.3% to 8.9%.

44. How is ankylosis treated?

The severity of submergence dictates the treatment protocol. Therefore, constant vigilance at recall appointments is crucial. The age at which ankylosis begins determines the rate of submergence. The younger the child at onset of ankylosis, the more quickly the tooth submerges because of the increased rate of growth of alveolar bone height. In minor cases, in which the occlusal surface is within 1 mm of the occlusal plane, the tooth needs only monitoring for exfoliation. In rare cases, the ankylosis is severe enough that the occlusal surface meets the interproximal gingival tissue. In such cases, the affected tooth must be extracted, with subsequent space maintenance. For moderate cases, stainless steel crowns or buildup restorations can be used to prevent space loss, due to tipping of adjacent teeth, or supraeruption. With mismanagement or misdiagnosis, the sequelae of infraclusion include space loss, molar tipping, supraeruption of antagonist teeth, and periodontal defects with decreased height of bone.

45. How should dosages of local anesthetic be calculated for a pediatric patient?

Because children's weights vary dramatically for their chronologic age, dosages of local anesthetic should be calculated according to a child's weight. A dosage of 4.4 mg/kg of lidocaine should not be exceeded in pediatric patients.

46. Should the parent be allowed in the operatory with the pediatric patient?

The debate continues. However, some studies have indicated that many pediatric dentists allow the parent to be present in the operatory.

47. What is the treatment for a traumatically intruded primary incisor?

In general, the treatment of choice is to allow the primary tooth to re-erupt. Re-eruption usually occurs within 6 months, but may take up to 1 year. If the primary tooth is displaced into the follicle of the developing permanent incisor, the primary tooth should be extracted.

48. What are the potential sequelae of trauma to a primary tooth?

Potential sequelae include color changes, necrosis, infection, and tooth loss. Color changes include yellow (pulp canal obliteration or metamorphosis), pink (internal resorption), or gray-black (hemosiderin or pulpal necrosis) color changes. Hemosiderin is not uncommon within the first 30 days after the trauma. After 30 days, a gray or gray-black color change in the crown typically indicates pulp necrosis. Necrosis may occur at any time after the injury (weeks, months, years). No treatment is indicated unless other pathologic changes occur (e.g., periapical radiolucency, fistulation, swelling, pain).

Damage to the succedaneous permanent tooth, including hypoplastic defects (Turner's Tooth), dilaceration of the root, or arrest of tooth development, has also been reported.

49. What are the indications for a lingual frenectomy?

Tongue-tie, or ankyloglossia, is relatively rare and usually requires no treatment. Occasionally, however, a short lingual frenum may result in lingual stripping of the periodontium from the lower incisors, which is an indication for frenectomy. A second indication is speech problems secondary to tongue position as diagnosed by a speech pathologist. Inability to latch on or breast-feed has been reported in some infants with a high lingual frenum. Breast-feeding in these patients has been reported to improve following frenectomy.

50. If a child reports a numb lip, can you be certain that the child has a profoundly anesthetized mandibular nerve?

Children, especially young ones, often do not understand what it means to be numb. The mandibular nerve is the only source of sensory innervation to the labial-attached gingiva between the lateral incisor and canine. If probing of this tissue with an explorer evokes no reaction from the patient, a profound mandibular block is present. No other sign can be used to diagnose profound anesthesia of the mandibular nerve.

51. Does slight contact with a healthy approximal surface during preparation of a class II cavity have any significant consequences?

Even slight nicking of the mesial or distal surface of a tooth greatly increases the possibility for future caries. Damaged noncarious primary tooth surfaces are 3.5 times more likely to develop a carious lesion and to require future restoration than undamaged surfaces. Damaged noncarious permanent tooth surfaces are 2.5 times more likely to develop a carious lesion and to require future restoration than undamaged surfaces. Placement of an interproximal wedge before preparation significantly decreases the likelihood of tooth damage and future pathology.

52. Why bother with restoring posterior primary teeth?

Caries is an infectious disease. As at any location in the body, treatment consists of controlling and eliminating the infection. With teeth, caries infection can be eliminated by removing the caries and restoring or extracting the tooth. However, extraction of primary molars in children may result in loss of space needed for permanent teeth. To ensure arch integrity and reduce the risk of pain, infection, and loss of function, decayed primary teeth should be treated with well-placed restorations.

53. What is the most durable restoration for a primary molar with multisurface caries?

Stainless steel crowns have the greatest longevity and durability. Their 4.5-year survival rate is more than twice that of amalgam (90% vs. 40%).

54. How should a primary tooth be extracted if it is next to a newly placed class II amalgam?

Three steps can be taken to eliminate the possibility of fracturing the newly placed amalgam:

1. The primary tooth to be extracted can be disked to remove bulk from the proximal surface. Care still must be taken to avoid contacting the new restoration.
2. Placing a matrix band (T-band) around the newly restored tooth offers additional protection.
3. When luxating the primary tooth, ensure that the elevator is placed subgingivally so that the forces are against alveolar bone rather than the adjacent amalgam.

55. Can composites be used to restore primary teeth?

Yes, if good technique is followed, composite material may be used. There are several factors that may affect longevity, including operator experience, size of restoration, and tooth position. Interproximally, it may be difficult to get the type of isolation required for optimal bonding, thus in cases where isolation or patient cooperation is in question, resin-based composite may not be an ideal restoration choice.

56. What are the indications and contraindications for pulpectomy in a primary tooth?

Indications
- Teeth with irreversible inflammation or necrosis of the radicular pulp due to caries or trauma
- Often attempted on the primary second molar before eruption of the first permanent molar

Contraindications
- Teeth with advanced resorption (internal or external), loss of root structure, or evidence of periapical infection involving the crypt of the succedaneous tooth
- Primary root canals that are difficult to prepare because of variable and complex morphology
- Proximity of succedaneous tooth bud (unwanted damage may result from instrumentation, medication, or filling materials)

57. How successful is pulpectomy in a primary tooth?

A recent systematic review and meta-analysis indicated an 18-month success rate in primary teeth treated with zinc oxide–eugenol (ZOE) or ZOE plus iodoform pulpectomies, of 90% compared to 71% or less for iodoform paste. The most important preoperative predictor of success is amount of tooth root absorption (>23% resorption reduces the success rate to only 23%). If correctly done, pulpectomy does not cause adverse effects on succedaneous tooth formation, but it does involve a 20% chance of altering the eruption path of the permanent tooth.

58. **What filling materials may be used for pulpectomy in a primary tooth?**
The ideal properties of the filling material for pulpectomy in a primary tooth include a resorption rate similar to that of primary root, no damage or irritation of periapical tissues or the permanent tooth bud, antiseptic nature, and no discoloring of teeth. The two most commonly used materials are as follows:
- ZOE paste—different rate of resorption, potential underfilling, mild foreign body reaction with overfilling
- Calcium hydroxide and iodoform paste—rapid resorption, no deleterious effects on succedaneous tooth

59. **Which syndromes or conditions are associated with supernumerary teeth?**

Apert syndrome	Gardner syndrome
Cleft lip and palate	Hallermann-Streiff syndrome
Cleidocranial dysplasia	Oral-facial-digital syndrome type 1
Crouzon syndrome	Sturge-Weber syndrome

60. **Which syndromes or conditions are associated with congenitally missing teeth?**

Achondroplasia	Incontinentia pigmenti
Ectodermal dysplasia	Chondroectodermal dysplasia
Cleft lip and palate	Oral-facial-digital syndrome type 1
Hallermann-Streiff syndrome	Down syndrome
Crouzon syndrome	Rieger syndrome

61. **In the case of a congenitally missing second premolar, how long can the second primary molar be retained?**
Most second primary molars lacking succedaneous teeth can be retained indefinitely, provided there is adequate root support in the plane of occlusion.

62. **What are the differences among fusion, gemination, and concrescence?**
Fusion is the union of two teeth, resulting in a double tooth, usually with two separate pulp chambers. Fusion is usually observed in the primary dentition.
Gemination is the attempt of a single tooth bud to give rise to two teeth. The condition usually presents as a bifid crown with a single pulp chamber in the primary dentition.
Concrescence is the cemental union of two teeth, usually the result of trauma.

63. **What is the incidence of inclusion cysts in the infant?**
It is approximately 75%.

64. **What are the three most common types of inclusion cysts and their cause?**
1. **Epstein's pearls** are caused by entrapped epithelium along the palatal rapine.
2. **Bohn's nodules** are ectopic mucous glands on the labial and lingual surfaces of the alveolus.
3. **Dental lamina cysts** are remnants of the dental lamina along the crest of the alveolus.

65. **What are the most common systemic causes of delayed exfoliation of the primary teeth and delayed eruption of the permanent dentition?**

Achondroplasia	Gardner syndrome
Apert syndrome	Hypopituitarism
Chondroectodermal dysplasia	Hypothyroidism
Cleidocranial dysplasia	Ichthyosis
De Lange syndrome	Osteogenesis imperfecta
Down syndrome	Vitamin D–resistant rickets

66. **What are the most common systemic causes of premature exfoliation of the primary dentition?**

Fibrous dysplasia	Hypophosphatasia
Cyclic neutropenia	Juvenile diabetes
Acatalasia	Odontodysplasia
Chediak-Higashi disease	Papillon-Lefèvre syndrome
Dentin dysplasia	Prepubertal periodontitis
Gaucher disease	Scurvy
Histiocytosis	Vitamin D–resistant rickets

67. Give the appropriate splinting times for the following traumatic dental injuries: luxation, avulsion, root fracture, and alveolar fracture..

    Luxation: 4 weeks

    Avulsion: Recent guidelines have standardized splinting times for all permanent teeth regardless of root development. A flexible splint for 2 weeks is recommended for reimplanted teeth, unless there is an associated jaw or alveolar fracture, then splinting for 4 weeks is recommended.

    Root fracture and alveolar fracture: 4 weeks for alveolar fractures and root fractures limited to the apical third and midroot. For cervical third root fractures, a longer splinting time (up to 4 months) may be beneficial.

    In all cases, a flexible splint should be used to allow physiologic movement of the teeth. In addition, sound clinical judgment should be exercised to help decide whether longer splinting times are necessary. For example, an avulsed tooth that is still +3 mobile after 2 weeks may need to be splinted for additional time.

68. What can be done to prevent impaction of permanent maxillary canines?

    Within 1 year after the total eruption of the maxillary lateral incisors, the maxillary canines should be palpable. Additionally, a panoramic radiograph or intraoral radiographs should be taken to determine the axial inclination of the developing permanent canine. If mesial angulation is noted with overlap of the maxillary lateral incisor root, extraction of the maxillary primary canine and maxillary first primary molars may often eliminate the impaction of the maxillary canine.

69. What is the most important technique of behavioral guidance in pediatric dentistry?

    It is "tell-show-do." Tell the child what is going to happen, show the child what is going to happen, and then perform the actual procedure intraorally. The major fear in pediatric dental patients is the unknown. The tell, show, and do technique eliminates fear and enhances the patient's behavioral capabilities.

70. What pharmacologic agents are indicated for behavioral control of the pediatric dental patient in an office setting?

    With the exception of general anesthesia, there are no absolutely predictable pharmacologic agents for controlling the behavior of pediatric dental patients. Unless the operator has received specific training in sedation techniques for children, patients with anxiety or behavioral problems are best referred to a specialist in pediatric dentistry.

71. Do hypertrophic adenoids and tonsils affect dental occlusion?

    The incidence of posterior crossbite is increased in children with significant tonsillar and adenoid obstruction. Of children with a grade 3 obstruction, 80% have a posterior crossbite.

72. What technique may be used if a pediatric patient cannot tolerate a conventional bitewing radiograph?

    To help reduce gagging and pushing the film out of the mouth with the tongue, try placing the film while the patient watches in a small hand mirror. This distracts the child and allows them to see that the film is not going into the throat. A Snap-a-Ray film holder may also help the child better tolerate the film position because it reduces the vertical height and minimizes discomfort in the floor of the mouth. Digital sensors make it even more challenging due to their increased bulk.

    If these techniques don't work, a buccal bitewing is taken. The tab of the film is placed on the occlusal surfaces of the molar teeth, and the film itself is positioned between the buccal surfaces of the teeth and cheek. The cone is directed from 1 inch behind and below the mandible upward to the area of the second primary molar on the contralateral side. The setting is three times that which is normally used for a conventional bitewing exposure.

73. What are the morphologic differences between primary and secondary teeth? How does each difference affect amalgam preparation?

    1. The occlusal anatomy of primary teeth is generally not as defined as that of secondary teeth, and supplemental grooves are less common. The amalgam preparation therefore can be more conservative.
    2. The enamel in primary teeth is thinner than in secondary teeth (usually 1 mm thick); therefore, the amalgam preparation is shallower in primary teeth. A depth of 1.5 mm from the occlusal surface will place the preparation 0.5 mm into dentin, which allows for sufficient bulk of the amalgam. This depth is easy to approximate using a 330 bur because the head length of this bur is 1.6 mm.
    3. Pulp horns in primary teeth extend higher into the crown of the tooth than pulp horns in secondary teeth; therefore, the amalgam preparation must be conservative to avoid a pulp exposure. The most common pulp exposure is the mesial buccal pulp horn of the mandibular first molar.
    4. Primary molar teeth have an exaggerated cervical bulge that makes matrix adaptation more difficult.
    5. The generally broad interproximal contacts in primary molar teeth require wider proximal amalgam preparation than those in secondary teeth.
    6. Enamel rods in the gingival third of the primary teeth extend occlusally from the dentinoenamel junction, eliminating the need in class II preparations for the gingival bevel that is required in secondary teeth.

74. **What is the purpose of the pulpotomy procedure in primary teeth?**
The pulpotomy procedure preserves the radicular vital pulp tissue when the entire coronal pulp is amputated. The remaining radicular pulp tissue is treated with an agent such as formocresol or MTA.

75. **What is the advantage of the pulpotomy procedure on primary teeth?**
The pulpotomy procedure allows resorption and exfoliation of the primary tooth but preserves its role as a natural space maintainer.

76. **What are the indications for the pulpotomy procedure in primary teeth?**
   1. Primary tooth that is restorable with carious or iatrogenic pulp exposure
   2. Deep carious lesions without spontaneous pulpal pain
   3. Absence of pathologic internal or external resorption but intact lamina aura
   4. No radiographic evidence of furcal or periapical pathology
   5. Clinical signs of a normal pulp during treatment (e.g., controlled hemorrhage after coronal amputation)

77. **What are the contraindications for pulpotomy in primary teeth?**
   1. Interradicular (molar) or periapical (canine and incisor) radiolucency
   2. Internal or external resorption
   3. Advanced root resorption, indicating imminent exfoliation
   4. Uncontrolled hemorrhage after coronal pulp extirpation
   5. Necrotic dry pulp tissue or purulent exudate in pulp canals
   6. Sinus tracks or abscess formation
   7. Medical condition (e.g., immunosuppression, severe cardiac disease)

78. **How does rubber dam isolation of the tooth improve management of pediatric patients?**
   1. The rubber dam seems to calm the child because it acts as a physical and psychological barrier, separating the child from the procedure being performed.
   2. Gagging from the water spray or suction is alleviated.
   3. Access is improved because of tongue, lip, and cheek retraction.
   4. The rubber dam reminds the child to open the mouth.
   5. The rubber dam ensures a dry field that otherwise would be impossible in many children.
   6. It helps prevent inadvertent swallowing and/or aspiration of materials.

79. **When do the primary and permanent teeth begin to develop?**
The primary dentition begins to develop during the sixth week in utero; formation of hard tissue begins during the 14th week in utero. Permanent teeth begin to develop during the 12th week in utero. Formation of hard tissue begins about the time of birth for the permanent first molars and during the first year of life for the permanent incisors.

80. **Summarize the chronology of development and eruption of the primary and permanent teeth..**
See Table 10-3.

81. **What is leeway space?**
Leeway space is the difference in the total of the mesiodistal widths between the primary canine, first molar, and second molar and the permanent canine, first premolar, and second premolar. In the mandible, leeway space averages 1.7 mm (unilaterally); it is usually about 0.9 to 1.1 mm (unilaterally) in the maxilla.

82. **What changes occur in the size of the dental arch during growth?**
From birth until about 2 years of age, the incisor region widens, and growth occurs in the posterior region of both arches. During the period of the full primary dentition, arch length and width remain constant. Arch length does not increase once the second primary molars have erupted; any growth in length occurs distal to the second primary molars and not in the alveolar portion of the maxilla or mandible. There is a slight decrease in arch length with the eruption of the first permanent molars and a slight increase in intercanine width (and some forward extension of the anterior segment of the maxilla) with the eruption of the incisors. A further decrease in arch length may occur with molar adjustments and the loss of leeway space when the second primary molar exfoliates.

83. **What is the pink tooth of Mummery?**
It is the pink appearance of a tooth caused by internal resorption.

84. **What intervention is indicated when permanent maxillary canines are observed radiographically to be erupting palatally?**
It is extraction of the primary maxillary canine. About 75% of ectopic canines show normalization of eruption at 12 months.

85. **Does teething cause systemic manifestations?**
Although teething may be associated with drooling, gum rubbing, or changes in dietary intake, no evidence indicates that it causes systemic illness (e.g., diarrhea, fever, rashes, seizures, bronchitis). Fever associated with teething may be a manifestation of undiagnosed primary herpes gingivostomatitis.

Table 10-3. Chronology of Development and Eruption of Teeth*

TOOTH	TOOTH GERM COMPLETED	CALCIFICATION COMMENCES	CROWN COMPLETED	ERUPTION IN MOUTH	ROOT COMPLETED
Primary					
Incisor	3-4 mo i.u.	2-4 mo	6-8 mo	6 mo-2 yr	
Canines	5 mo i.u.	9 mo	16-20 mo	2½-3 yr	
First molars	12-16 wk i.u.	5 mo i.u.	6 mo	12-15 mo	2-2½ yr
Second molars	6-7 mo i.u.	11-12 mo	20-30 mo	3 yr	
Permanent					
Central incisors	30 wk i.u.	3-4 mo	4-5 yr	Max, 7-9 yr	9-10 yr
				Mand, 6-8 yr	
Lateral incisors	32 wk i.u.	Max, 10-12 mo	4-5 yr	7-9 yr	10-11 yr
		Mand, 3-4 mo			
Canines	30 wk i.u.	4-5 mo	6-7 yr	Max, 11-12 yr	12-15 yr
				Mand, 9-10 yr	
First premolars	30 wk i.u.	1½-2 yr	5-6 yr	10-12 yr	12-14 yr
Second premolars	31 wk i.u.	2-2½ yr	6-7 yr	10-12 yr	12-14 yr
First molars	24 wk i.u.	Birth	3-5 yr	6-7 yr	9-10 yr
Second molars	6 mo	2½-3 yr	7-8 yr	12-13 yr	14-16 yr
Third molars	6 yr	7-10 yr	12-16 yr	17-21 yr	18-25 yr

Mand, Mandibular; *Max,* maxillary.
*All dates postnatal, except where designated intrauterine (i.u.).
Adapted from Bishara SE: Textbook of Orthodontics, Philadelphia, WB Saunders, 2001.

86. **Should dental implants be placed in the growing child?**
Generally, placing implants should be deferred until growth is completed. In a growing child, the implant may become submerged or embedded. In addition, an implant that crosses the midline may limit transverse growth.

87. **Should an avulsed primary tooth be reimplanted?**
No. The prognosis of reimplanted primary teeth is poor and may adversely affect the developing succedaneous tooth.

88. **How should an avulsed primary tooth be managed?**
Rinse the tooth with water, and place it under the child's pillow.

89. **What variable is most important in the prognosis of an avulsed permanent tooth?**
Time out of the mouth is most critical. After a dry time of 30 minutes, most PDL cells are nonviable. With an extra-alveolar time less than 1 hour, partial periodontal ligament (PDL) healing is possible; an extra-alveolar time longer than 1 hour results in total PDL death and progressive root resorption.

90. **What other factors affect prognosis?**
Storage/transportation in a physiologic storage medium (e.g., tissue culture or cell transport media) or osmolality-balanced media (e.g., milk or Hanks Balanced Salt Solution) improves prognosis. In addition, the maturity of the root (open vs. closed apex) will affect prognosis. Immature teeth with open apices have an improved prognosis as spontaneous revascularization may occur.

91. **If an avulsed tooth cannot be reimplanted immediately, which transport medium is best?**
In order of preference, they are Hank's balanced salt solution, milk, saliva or saline. Water is a poor medium but better than keeping the tooth dry.

92. **How do closed versus open apices affect prognosis?**
Closed apices
• Revascularization is not likely.
• Pulp extirpation should occur in 7 to 10 days.
• Pulpal necrosis (radiolucency) is usually noted as early as 3 to 4 weeks (usually, apical third within 1 year).
Open apices
• Revascularization is possible.
• Pulp necrosis is evident after 2 to 4 weeks and presents with periapical pathology, sometimes with signs of internal root resorption (IRR).

93. What are the most common complications after reimplantation of an avulsed tooth?
    - Pulpal necrosis
    - Inflammatory resorption, replacement resorption (ankylosis)
    - Internal calcification with pulpal obliteration (common in non–endodontically treated reimplants)

94. Describe the occurrence of ankylosis after reimplantation of an avulsed tooth..
    - Irreversible and progressive
    - More rapid progression with younger age
    - Mobility and dull percussion noted as early as 5 weeks (on radiographs at 8 weeks)
    - Small areas of ankylosis are reversible with functional mobility
    - The tooth loss is rapid and typically occurs within 1 to 5 years.

95. What is the most reliable diagnostic test for ankylosis?
    It is percussion.

96. Do all discolored primary incisors require treatment?
    The gray discoloration of primary teeth is usually the result of a traumatic episode. This discoloration is caused by hemorrhage into the dentinal tubules or a necrotic pulp. In the case of hemorrhage into the dentinal tubules, the discoloration usually appears within 1 month of the injury. Often, the teeth return to their original color as the blood breakdown products are removed from the site. Discoloration caused by a necrotic pulp may take days, weeks, months, or even years to develop. It does not improve with time and may actually worsen. A tooth that is light gray may progress to dark gray. A yellow opaque discoloration is usually indicative of calcific degeneration of the pulp. Discolored teeth do not require treatment unless there is radiographic and/or clinical evidence of pathology of the periodontium (soft and/or hard tissues).

97. Which two dentists have appeared on the cover of *Time* magazine?
    They are Dr. Harold Kane Addelson, the originator of the tell-show-do technique, and Dr. Barney Clark, the first human recipient of a mechanical heart.

ORTHODONTIC TREATMENT

98. What is the relationship between overjet and dental trauma?
    Because of the high prevalence of dental trauma involving maxillary incisors, it is important to determine whether any interceptive treatment can lower a patient's risk for trauma. Children with class II malocclusions and increased overjet face a greater risk of maxillary incisor trauma. A tendency to a skeletal open bite with a negative overbite and excessive overjet predispose patients to dental trauma. Children with overjets more than 3 mm are twice as likely to injure the anterior teeth as children with overjets less than 3 mm, and a 6-mm overjet results in four times the risk of trauma. The risk of trauma increases with increasing overjet measurements.
    Although definitive guidelines are not available, high-risk children with a large overjet, excessive maxillary incisor proclination, and high facial angle may benefit from an evaluation for early orthodontic intervention. It is the dentist's role to provide anticipatory guidance about injury prevention and the use of a mouth guard.
    NOTE: The American Association of Orthodontists recommends that all children be seen by an orthodontist by age 7 years.

99. What are the advantages of fixed versus removable orthodontic appliances?
    Fixed orthodontic appliances offer controlled tooth movement in all planes of space. Removable appliances are generally restricted to tipping teeth.

100. What is the straight-wire appliance?
    The straight-wire appliance, invented by Dr. Larry Andrews in the 1970s, is the most common type of fixed orthodontic appliance, consisting of a complete set of orthodontic brackets. The brackets have in-built features (known as a prescription) that allow placement of an ideal arch wire without bends (a so-called straight wire). Expression of the bracket prescription will position the individual teeth in correct relation to each other to best facilitate optimal aesthetics and occlusion. These features include the following: (1) variations in bracket thickness to compensate for differences in the labiolingual position and thickness of individual teeth; (2) variations in angulation of the bracket slot relative to the long axis of the tooth to allow mesiodistal differences in the root angulation of individual teeth; and (3) variations in torque of the bracket slot to compensate for buccal-lingual differences in the root angulation of individual teeth. Previous to the straight-wire appliance, the orthodontist had to spend considerable chair-side time bending each individual wire to achieve the desired tooth positions.

101. What is a bracket prescription for the straight-wire appliance?
    The variations of a particular set of brackets are known as a prescription. Until recently, sets of brackets were limited to off-the-shelf prescriptions, designed with average population values. The orthodontist would still need to place bends in the arch wire during the finishing stage of treatment to account for individual characteristics of that occlusion. However, it is now possible to obtain brackets with custom prescriptions for the individual patient. The purported benefit is a shorter overall treatment time and even less wire bending from the orthodontist!

102. **What are so-called functional appliances? Do they work?**

Functional appliances are a group of fixed and removable appliances that were originally purported to promote or inhibit jaw growth, usually for class 2 malocclusions. These appliances have been shown to be effective in correcting class II malocclusions. Controversy surrounds the question of whether or not there is long-term extra growth of the mandible: most studies indicate that their effects are mainly dentoalveolar, with little effect on the growth of the mandible. However, with treatment, facial convexity is generally reduced and the occlusion corrected, so many clinicians utilize functional appliances irrespective of whether they believe in the added growth benefits.

103. **When should orthodontic therapy be initiated?**

There is no one optimal time to initiate treatment for every orthodontic problem. For example, a patient in primary dentition with a bilateral posterior crossbite may benefit from palatal expansion at age 4 years. Conversely, the same-aged patient with a class III malocclusion caused by mandibular prognathism is best treated by waiting until all craniofacial growth is completed.

104. **What is the difference between a skeletal and dental malocclusion?**

Skeletal malocclusion refers to a disharmony between the jaws in a transverse, sagittal, or vertical dimension or any combination thereof. Examples of skeletal malocclusions include retrognathism, prognathism, open bites, and bilateral posterior crossbites. Dental malocclusion refers to malpositioned teeth, generally the result of a discrepancy between tooth size and arch length. This discrepancy often results in crowding, rotations, or spacing of the teeth. Most malocclusions are neither purely skeletal nor purely dental but rather a combination of the two.

105. **If a primary first molar is lost, is a space maintainer necessary?**

Before eruption of the 6-year molar and its establishment of intercuspation, mesial migration of the second primary molar will occur, and a space maintainer is indicated to prevent space loss.

106. **When should a crossbite be corrected?**

Whenever a crossbite with an associated functional shift of the mandible upon closing is noted, and the patient is amenable to intraoral therapy, correction is indicated. Correction of a crossbite without an associated functional shift may be treated as soon as noted, or deferred until the early permanent dentition so that the intercuspation of the buccal segments maintains the result.

107. **When is the proper time to consider diastema treatment?**

A thick maxillary frenum with a high attachment (sometimes extending to the palate) is common in the primary dentition and does not require treatment. However, a large midline diastema in the primary dentition may indicate the presence of an unerupted midline supernumerary tooth (mesiodens) and often warrants an appropriate radiograph.

The permanent maxillary central incisors erupt labial to the primary incisors and often exhibit a slight distal inclination that results in a midline diastema. This midline space is normal and decreases with the eruption of the lateral incisors. Complete closure of the midline diastema, however, does not occur until the permanent canines erupt. Treatment of residual midline space is addressed orthodontically at this time.

108. **What is ectopic eruption? How is it treated?**

Ectopic eruption occurs when the erupting first permanent molar begins to resorb the distal root of the second primary molar. Its occurrence is much more common in the maxilla, and it is often associated with a developing skeletal class II pattern. It is seen in about 2% to 6% of the general population and 25% in patients with cleft lip and palate; it spontaneously corrects itself in about 60% of cases. If the path of eruption of the first permanent molar does not self-correct, a brass wire or orthodontic separating elastic can be placed between the first permanent molar and second primary molar, if possible. In severe cases, one may use a Halterman appliance to upright the ectopic tooth or the second primary molar may exfoliate early because of severe resorption or require extraction, necessitating the need for space maintenance or space regaining.

109. **What is the effect of early extraction of a primary tooth on the eruption of the succedaneous tooth?**

If a primary tooth must be extracted prematurely, and 50% of the root of the permanent successor has developed, eruption of the permanent tooth is usually delayed. If more than 50% of the root of the permanent tooth has formed at the time of extraction of the primary tooth, eruption is accelerated.

110. **Where are the primate spaces located?**

In the maxilla, primate spaces are located distal to the primary lateral incisors. In the mandible, primate spacing is found distal to the primary canines.

111. **What is the normal molar relationship in the primary dentition?**

Historically, both the flush terminal plane and mesial step have been considered normal. More recent studies have demonstrated that this may not be the case, because about 45% of children with a flush terminal plane go on to develop a class II molar relationship in the permanent dentition.

112. What is meant by the term *pseudo–class III*?

    This term refers to the condition in which the maxillary incisors are in crossbite with the mandibular incisors. Although the patient appears to have a prognathic mandible, it is caused not by a skeletal disharmony but rather by the anterior positioning of the jaw as a result of occlusal interference. The ability of the patient to retrude the mandible to the edge-to-edge incisal relationship is often considered diagnostic.

113. What is the space maintainer of choice for a 7-year-old child who has lost a lower primary second molar to caries?

    The lower lingual arch (LLA) is the maintainer of choice. The 6-year-old molars are banded. The connecting wire lies lingual to the permanent lower incisors in the gingival third and prevents mesial migration of the banded molars. Unlike the band and loop space maintainer, the LLA is independent of eruption sequence. (The band and loop serve no purpose after the primary first molar exfoliates.) However, the LLA should not be used if the permanent mandibular incisors are absent because the lingual arch may prevent the eruption of these teeth.

114. What is the space maintainer of choice for a 5-year-old child who has lost an upper primary second molar to caries prior to the eruption of the first permanent molar?

    The distal shoe is the appliance of choice. This appliance extends backward from a crown on the primary first molar and subgingivally to the mesial line of the unerupted first permanent molar, thus preventing mesial migration.

115. A 4-year-old child with generalized spacing loses three primary upper incisors to trauma. What space maintainer is needed?

    No space maintainer is necessary.

116. What is the best space maintainer for any pulpally involved primary tooth?

    Restoring the tooth with pulpal therapy is the best way to preserve arch length and integrity.

117. If a primary tooth is lost to caries but has no successor, is it necessary to maintain space?

    Sometimes it is necessary to maintain the space, but not always. The decision is based on the patient's skeletal and dental development. Either way, orthodontic evaluation is of the utmost importance to formulate the future plan for this space.

118. When do you remove a space maintainer once it is inserted?

    The space maintainer can be removed as soon as the succedaneous tooth begins to erupt through the gingiva. Space maintainers left in place too long make it more difficult for patients to clean their teeth. Furthermore, it may be necessary to replace a distal shoe with another form of space maintainer once the 6-year molar has erupted to prevent rotation of the molar around the bar arm.

119. What are the various types of headgear and their indications?

    There are four basic types of headgear. Each type of headgear has two major components, intraoral and extraoral. The extraoral component is what generally categorizes the type of headgear.

    1. **Cervical-pull headgear.** The intraoral component of cervical-pull headgear is composed of a heavy bow that engages the maxillary molars through some variation on a male-female connector. The anterior part of the bow is welded to an extraoral portion connected to an elasticized neck strap, which provides the force system for the appliance. The force application is in a down and backward direction. This headgear is generally used in a class II, division 1 malocclusion, in which distalization of the maxillary molars and/or restriction of maxillary growth, as well as anterior bite opening, is desired.
    2. **Straight-pull headgear.** The intraoral component is similar to the cervical-pull headgear. However, the force application is in a straight backward direction from the maxillary molar, parallel to the occlusal plane. Like cervical-pull headgear, this appliance is also used for a class II, division 1 malocclusion. Because of the direction of force application, this appliance may be chosen when excessive bite opening is undesirable.
    3. **High-pull headgear.** The intraoral components of high-pull headgear are similar to those described. However, the force application is in a back and upward direction. Consequently, it is usually chosen for a class II, division 1 malocclusion in which a bite opening is contraindicated (class II malocclusion with an open bite).
    4. **Reverse-pull headgear.** Unlike the other headgears, the extraoral component of reverse-pull headgear is supported by the chin, cheeks, forehead, or a combination of these structures. The intraoral component usually attaches to a fixed appliance in the maxillary appliance via elastics. Reverse-pull headgear is generally used for a class III malocclusion, in which protraction of the maxilla is desirable.

120. Does anyone use headgear anymore?

    Headgear is a useful part of an orthodontist's armamentarium, however, its use has declined in modern practice due to various reasons: (a) most orthodontists now routinely use bonded tubes on the molar teeth, rather than traditional bands, which are not able to withstand headgear forces; (b) orthodontists use alternate Class 2 correctors; (c) orthodontists fear losing patients to another provider who does not use headgear; (d) the rise of Aligner therapy.

121. **What is the traditional sequence of orthodontic treatment in straight-wire technique?**
    1. **Level and align.** This phase establishes preliminary bracket alignment, generally with a light nickel-titanium arch wire.
    2. **Working arch wires.** This phase corrects vertical discrepancies (e.g., bite opening) and sagittal position of the teeth. A heavy round or rectangular arch wire is generally used.
    3. **Finishing arch wires.** This phase idealizes the position of the teeth. Generally, light, formable, round, or rectangular arch wires are used.
    4. **Retention.** Retention of teeth in their final position may be accomplished with a fixed or removable retainer.

122. **What are the dental health benefits of orthodontic treatment?**
    Ironically, few studies have shown any dental health benefit to orthodontic treatment. Positive effects on caries susceptibility, periodontal disease, and temporomandibular disorders (TMDs) are largely unsupported by the literature. The exception would be susceptibility to trauma, for which studies have suggested a direct relationship between overjet and trauma to the maxillary incisors.

123. **What is Aligner therapy?**
    Aligner therapy is a more cosmetic alternative to the traditional wires-and-brackets techniques. First an intra-oral scan provides a computer-rendered version of the patient's teeth. Proprietary software is then used to segment and incrementally move the individual teeth into ideal occlusion, according to the orthodontist's instructions. Each incremental movement of the set of teeth is captured as a newly rendered 3D model which can be 3D printed. And so, a series of 3D-printed dental models are created. A plastic sheet is thermoformed over each model, then trimmed around the gingival level. This creates a series of "Aligners," which, when worn sequentially by the patient, move the teeth into alignment.

124. **That sounds easy! Why do people still use the metal wires and brackets?**
    Aligner therapy has come a long way over the last 20 years, however, mechanically, it is still not as capable as traditional wires and brackets, especially in younger patients who will have shorter crown heights. Additionally, a high level of patient compliance is essential for treatment success, which is not always achievable.

125. **What is DTC orthodontics?**
    DTC stands for direct-to-consumer. It is a business model adopted by several companies that market Aligner therapy directly to patients. In some instances, direct-to-consumer orthodontic companies do not involve the in-person evaluation and/or in-person supervision of orthodontic treatment by an orthodontist.
    The American Association of Orthodontists warns patients to carefully consider what may be missing with direct-to-consumer orthodontic treatment. They ask patients to consider potentially irreversible and expensive damage such as tooth and gum loss, changed bites, and other issues if treatment is not performed correctly.
    What other transforming medical treatment, they ask, would you undergo without an in-person, pretreatment evaluation, or ongoing in-person supervision from a medical professional?

126. **How stable is the orthodontic correction of crowding?**
    Approximately two-thirds of all patients treated for crowding experience significant relapse without some form of permanent retention. This relapse rate is about the same whether the patient is treated with a nonextraction or extraction approach; whether third molars are present, congenitally missing, or extracted; and whether treatment is started in the mixed dentition or permanent dentition. Unfortunately, no variables that correlate with relapse potential have been identified. Also, relapse potential continues throughout life.

127. **What is the best way to prevent relapse?**
    It is lifelong retention. The type of retainer appears less important than the length of retention.

128. **Does eruption of third molars cause crowding of the incisors?**
    No. The eruption of third molars with a real or perceived increase in crowding of the incisors is coincidental. Studies have revealed that patients who are congenitally missing third molars experience the same crowding phenomenon.

129. **What is the ideal molar relationship in the primary dentition?**
    It is the mesial step. Although many pediatric dentistry and orthodontic texts suggest that the mesial step relationship and the flush terminal plane are considered normal, a longitudinal study has revealed that almost 50% of flush terminal plane relationships in the primary dentition later develop into class II malocclusions.

130. **Define *early mesial shift* and *late mesial shift*.**
    These terms date back to the work of Baume in the late 1950s. The *early mesial shift* refers to the closure of the generalized spacing frequently observed in the primary dentition that closes with the eruption of the permanent first molars, causing a shift of the primary molars mesially. The *late mesial shift* occurs with the exfoliation of the second primary molars and the mesial drift of the first permanent molars into the leeway space.

ACKNOWLEDGMENT

The authors gratefully acknowledge the contribution of the previous chapter author.

BIBLIOGRAPHY

Aeinehchi M, Dadvand S, Fayazi S, Bayat-Movahed S. Randomized controlled trial of mineral trioxide aggregate and formocresol for pulpotomy in primary molar teeth. *Int Endod J.* 2007;40:261–267.

Alavaikko S, Jaakkola MS, Tjaderhane L, Jaakkola JJ. Asthma and caries: a systematic review and meta analysis. *Am J Epidemiol.* 2011;174:631–641.

Al-Zayer MA, Straffon LH, Feigal RJ, Welch KB. Indirect pulp treatment of primary posterior teeth: a retrospective study. *Pediatr Dent.* 2003;25:29–36.

American Academy of Pediatric Dentistry. *Guideline on infant oral health care*; 2012. http://www.aapd.org/media/Policies_Guidelines/G_InfantOralHealthCare.pdf. Accessed June 7, 2022.

American Academy of Pediatric Dentistry. Pediatric restorative dentistry. In: *The Reference Manual of Pediatric Dentistry.* Chicago: American Academy of Pediatric Dentistry; 2021:386–398.

American Academy of Pediatric Dentistry. Pulp therapy for primary and immature permanent teeth. In: *The Reference Manual of Pediatric Dentistry.* Chicago, 2021: American Academy of Pediatric Dentistry; 2021:399–407.

American Academy of Pediatric Dentistry. Pulp therapy for primary and immature permanent teeth. In: *The Reference Manual of Pediatric Dentistry.* Chicago, IL: American Academy of Pediatric Dentistry; 2022:415–423.

American Dental Association. Baby's first dental visit. *ADA News*; 2001.

Baccetti T, Antonini A. Dentofacial characteristics associated with trauma to maxillary incisors in the mixed dentition. *J Clin Pediatr Dent.* 1998;22:281–284.

Bishara SE. *Textbook of Orthodontics.* Philadelphia: WB Saunders; 2001.

Bishara SE, Hoppens BJ, Jakobsen JR, Kohout FJ. Changes in the molar relationship between the deciduous and permanent dentitions: a longitudinal study. *Am J Orthod Dentofac Orthop.* 1988;93:19–28.

Bourguignon C, Cohenca N, Lauridsen E, et al. International Association of Dental Traumatology guidelines for the management of traumatic dental injuries: 1. Fractures and luxations. *Dent Traumatol.* 2020;36(4):314–330.

Brown MD, Aaron G. The effect of point-of-use water conditioning systems on community fluoridated water. *Pediatr Dent.* 1991;13:35–38.

Casamassimo PS, Fields HW, McTigue DJ, et al. *Pediatric Dentistry: Infancy Through Adolescence.* 5th ed. St. Louis: Saunders; 2013.

Caulfield PW, Cutter GR, et al. Initial acquisitions of mutans streptococci by infants: evidence for a discrete window of infectivity. *J Dent Res.* 1993;72:37–45.

Coll JA, Sadrian R. Predicting pulpectomy success and its relationship to exfoliation and succedaneous dentition. *Pediatr Dent.* 1996;18:57–63.

Day PF, Flores MT, O'Connell AC, et al. International Association of Dental Traumatology guidelines for the management of traumatic dental injuries: 3. Injuries in the primary dentition. *Dent Traumatol.* 2020;36(4):343–359.

Disney JA, Graves RC, Stamm JW, et al. The University of North Carolina Caries Risk Assessment study: further developments in caries risk prediction. *Community Dent Oral Epidemiol.* 1992;20:64–75.

Douglas J, Tinanoff N. The etiology, prevalence and sequelae of infraclusion of primary molars. *ASDC J Dent Child.* 1991;58:381–483.

Edelstein B. Evidence-based dental care for children and the age 1 dental visit. *Pediatr Ann.* 1998;27:569–574.

Einwag J, Dunninger F. Stainless steel crowns versus multisurface amalgam restorations: an 8-year longitudinal clinical study. *Quintessence Int.* 1996;27:321–323.

Enlow DH. *Facial Growth.* 3rd ed. Philadelphia: WB Saunders; 1990.

Ericson S, Kurol J. Early treatment of palatally erupting maxillary canines by extraction of the primary canines. *Eur J Orthod.* 1988;10:282–295.

Flores MT, Andreasen JO, Bakland LK, et al. Guidelines for the evaluation and management of traumatic dental injuries. *Dent Traumatol.* 2001;17:193–198.

Fouad AF, Abbott PV, Tsilingaridis G, et al. International Association of Dental Traumatology guidelines for the management of traumatic dental injuries: 2. Avulsion of permanent teeth. *Dent Traumatol.* 2020;36(4):331–342.

Fuks AB. Pulp therapy for the primary and young permanent dentitions. *Dent Clin North Am.* 2000;44:571–596.

Gorlin RJ, Cohen Jr MM, Levin LS. *Syndromes of the Head and Neck.* New York: Oxford University Press; 1990.

Gustafson BE, Quensel CE, Lanke LS, et al. The Vipeholm Dental Caries Study: The effect of different levels of carbohydrate intake on caries activity in 436 individuals observed for five years. *Acta Odontol Scand.* 1954;11:232–364.

Hupp J, Ellis E, Tucker MR. *Contemporary and Maxillofacial Surgery.* 6th ed. St. Louis: Mosby; 2014.

Isokangas P, et al. Occurrence of dental decay in children after maternal consumption of xylitol chewing gum, a follow-up from 0 to 5 years of age. *J Dent Res.* 2000;79:1885–1889.

Kaban LB. *Pediatric Oral and Maxillofacial Surgery.* Philadelphia: WB Saunders; 1990.

Kates GA, Needleman HL, Holmes LB. Natal and neonatal teeth: a clinical study. *J Am Dent Assoc.* 1984;109:441–443.

King DL, Steinhauer W, Garcia-Godoy F, Elkins CJ. Herpetic gingivostomatitis and teething difficulty in infants. *Pediatr Dent.* 1992;14:82–85.

King NM, Lee AMP. Natal teeth and steatocystoma multiplex: a newly recognized syndrome. *J Craniofac Genet Dev Biol.* 1987;7:311–317.

Marcum BK, Turner C, et al. Pediatric dentists' attitudes regarding parental presence during dental procedures. *Pediatr Dent.* 1995;17:432–436.

Matsuo T, Nakanishi T, Shimizu H, Ebisu S. A clinical study of direct pulp capping applied to carious-exposed pulps. *J Endod.* 1996;22:551–556.

McDonald RE, Avery DR. *Dentistry for the Child and Adolescent.* St. Louis: Mosby; 1994.

Messer LB, Cline JT. Ankylosed primary molars: results and treatment recommendations from an eight-year longitudinal study. *Pediatr Dent.* 1990;2:34–47.

Mortazavi M, Mesbahi M. Comparison of zinc oxide and eugenol, and Vitapex for root canal treatment of necrotic primary teeth. *Int J Paediatr Dent.* 2004;14:417–424.

Moyers R. *Handbook of Orthodontics.* Chicago: YearBook; 1986.

Nguyen QV, Bezemer PD, Habets L, Prahl-Anderson B. A systematic review of the relationship between overjet size and traumatic dental injuries. *Eur J Orthodont.* 1999;21:502–515.

Noorollahian H. Comparison of mineral trioxide aggregate and formocresol as pulp medicaments for pulpotomies in primary molars. *Br Dent J.* 2008;204:E20.

Oulis CJ, Vadiakas GP, et al. The effect of hypertrophic adenoids and tonsils on the development of posterior crossbites and oral habits. *J Clin Pediatr Dent.* 1994;18:197–201.

Peng L, Ye L, Guo X, et al. Evaluation of formocresol versus ferric sulphate primary molar pulpotomy: a systematic review and meta-analysis. *Int Endod J.* 2007;40:751–757.

Proffit WR, Fields HW, Sarver DM. *Contemporary Orthodontics.* 5th ed. St. Louis: Mosby; 2013.

Ryburg M, Moller C, Ericson T. Saliva composition and caries development in asthmatic patients treated with beta 2-adrenergic agonists: a 4-year follow-up study. *Scand J Dent Res.* 1991;99:212–219.

Sanchez DM, Childers NK. *Anticipatory Guidance in Oral Health: Rationale and Recommendations.* American Academy of Family Physicians; 2001.

Schatz J-P, Hakeberg M, et al. Prevalence of traumatic injuries to permanent dentition and its association with overjet in a Swiss child population. *Dent Traumatol.* 2013;29:110–114.

Scully C, Welbury R. *Color Atlas of Oral Diseases in Children and Adolescents.* London: Mosby-Year Book Europe; 1994.

Stephan RM. Changes in the hydrogen ion concentration on tooth surfaces in carious lesions. *J Am Dent Assoc.* 1940;27:718.

Tuna D, Olmez A. Clinical long-term evaluation of MTA as a direct pulp capping material in primary teeth. *Int Endod J.* 2008;41:273–278.

Vaikuntam J. Fluoride varnishes: should we be using them? *Pediatr Dent.* 2000;22:513–516.

Vij R, Coll JA, Shelton P, Farooq NS. Caries control and other variables associated with success of primary molar vital pulp therapy. *Pediatr Dent.* 2004;26:214–220.

CHAPTER 11

ORAL AND MAXILLOFACIAL SURGERY

Bonnie L. Padwa, Mark A. Green

GENERAL CONSIDERATIONS

1. **What conditions do the American Heart Association (AHA) currently recommend antibiotic prophylaxis for prior to dental procedures?**
   - Congenital heart disease
     - Unrepaired cyanotic heart defect
     - Repaired congenital heart defect with prosthetic material or device during the first 6 months from repair
     - Repaired congenital heart defect with residual defects adjacent to area of prosthetic material
   - Recipient of a cardiac transplant with associated cardiac valvulopathy
   - Prosthetic cardiac valves/material
   - Previous, relapse or recurrent infective endocarditis

2. **When should antibiotic prophylaxis be given for a dental procedure?**
   A single dose should be given 30 to 60 minutes prior to all dental procedures when the above-mentioned criteria have been met.

3. **What are the standard antibiotic prophylactic doses recommended by the AHA prior to dental procedures when indicated?**
   - Amoxicillin 2 g (adults) or 50 mg/kg (pediatrics)
   - Ampicillin 2 g (adults) or 50 mg/kg (pediatrics)
   - Cefazolin or ceftriaxone 1 g (adults) or 50 mg/kg (pediatrics)
   - Azithromycin or clarithromycin 500 mg (adults) or 15 mg/kg (pediatrics)
   - Doxycycline 100 mg (adults or >45 kg) or 2.2 mg/kg (<45 kg)
   *Note that clindamycin is no longer a recommended antibiotic prophylaxis for dental procedures

4. **List common findings in a patient with obstructive sleep apnea (OSA)..**
   - Snoring
   - Excessive daytime sleepiness
   - Impaired cognition and memory loss
   - Hypertension
   - Heart failure (cor pulmonale)
   - Cardiac arrythmias
   - Sexual dysfunction

5. **How is STOP-BANG calculated for patients with OSA?**
   STOP-BANG is a score that is calculated by answering 8 yes or no questions to assess the likelihood of having sleep apnea. Yes answers to 5 or more of the following questions places a patient at high risk for OSA: **S**noring, **T**ired, **O**bserved apnea, **P**ressure (high), **B**MI > 35 kg/m², **A**ge > 50 years, **N**eck > 40 cm in circumference, **G**ender (male).

6. **When undergoing outpatient sedation or general anesthesia, what are some risk factors for aspiration?**
   In general, conditions associated with delayed gastric emptying place patients at higher risk. These include diabetes (gastroparesis), gastroesophageal reflux, gastrointestinal obstructions, pregnancy, obesity, and liver failure (ascites). Procedures involving the posterior nasopharynx or oropharynx may pose a risk to bleeding into the airway.

7. **What factors influence the risk of osteonecrosis following a dental extraction in a patient treated with radiation for management of head and neck malignancy?**
   - Location of radiation field
   - Amount of radiation
   - Type of tumor
   - Systemic comorbidities
   - Time since radiation therapy
   - History of hyperbaric oxygen therapy

8. **What is osteoradionecrosis of the jaw?**
   Osteoradionecrosis of the jaw occurs when bone dies due to compromised vascularity and bone metabolism following exposure to radiation. It is typically preceded by an infection, trauma, or procedure to the area (such as

a dental extraction). The risk of osteoradionecrosis is dose dependent with radiation doses greater than 50 gray (Gy) posing the most risk.

9. **How is medication-related osteonecrosis of the Jaw (MRONJ) diagnosed?**
A patient must have a current or previous treatment with an anti-resorptive or anti-angiogenic agent, have an area of exposed bone or fistula tract to bone for 8 or more weeks, and have no prior history of radiation therapy or malignancy in the jaws.

10. **Name common medications that have been linked to MRONJ..**
    - Bisphosphonates (e.g., pamidronate, alendronate, zoledronate)
    - Denosumab
    - Sunitinib
    - Bevacizumab

11. **What is the most common adverse reaction observed at the dental office?**
Syncope, or fainting, is one of the most common adverse reactions in the dental setting, accounting for nearly half of all medical emergencies in the dental practice. This is usually a result of a vasovagal reaction by the body. Early recognition is important and supportive treatment should be initiated. Patients may confess they feel lightheaded, uneasy, nauseous, or seeing spots. Provide reassurance and position into the Trendelenburg position (lying back with feet above their head). If pregnant, the patient should be positioned in left lateral decubitus position to avoid aortocaval compression from the gravid uterus. Oxygen should be administered, cold compresses applied to the forehead/back of neck and tight clothing loosened when possible. Vitals should be monitored until symptoms pass.

LOCAL ANESTHESIA

12. **What is the difference between anesthesia and analgesia?**
Anesthesia denotes a lack of perception to stimuli or touch, whether it be a painful stimulus or not. Analgesia is the absence of pain in the setting of a painful stimulus.

13. **What is the difference between an amide and an ester local anesthesia?**
Amide local anesthetics (e.g., xylocaine, mepivacaine) are the most commonly used local anesthetics. Local anesthetic properties are derived from their lipophilic aromatic ring, terminal amine, and intermediate ester or amide chain. Ester local anesthetics (e.g., procaine) are hydrolyzed by plasma esterases while amide local anesthetics are biotransformed in the liver.

14. **Why do the effects of some local anesthetics last longer than others?**
Local anesthetic effects are based on the ability of drugs to penetrate into nerve cells (lipid solubility) and then remain bound to those cells (protein binding ability). Bupivacaine-epinephrine is a long-acting local anesthetic used for prolonged surgical-grade anesthesia.

15. **What is the purpose of epinephrine in local anesthesia?**
Epinephrine is a vasoconstrictor and prevents the dissipation of the local anesthetic outside of the intended site. It also aids in the constriction of blood vessels, improving hemostatic control.

16. **What is methemoglobinemia and how is it treated?**
Methemoglobinemia can occur when larger doses of local anesthetic are given and hemoglobin becomes oxidized from its ferric state to its ferrous state, disrupting hemoglobin's ability to transport and release oxygen at tissues. Cyanosis, lethargy, and respiratory depression are all signs of methemoglobinemia. Treatment includes intravenous methylene blue to convert hemoglobin back to its ferric state.

17. **What are the max doses of commonly used local anesthetics in a healthy patient?**
    - Lidocaine without epinephrine 4.5 mg/kg or 300 mg in adults
    - Lidocaine with epinephrine 7.0 mg/kg or 500 mg in adults
    - Mepivacaine without epinephrine 6.6 mg/kg or 400 mg in adults
    - Articaine with epinephrine 7 mg/kg or 500 mg in adults
    - Bupivacaine with epinephrine 3 mg/kg or 225 mg in adults

18. **How many carpules of 2% lidocaine with 1:100,000 epinephrine can be used in a healthy 70 kg healthy adult?**
A standard carpule of local anesthetic contains 1.8 mL of solution. 2% lidocaine means there is 36 mg of lidocaine in each carpule. If the max dose is 7 mg/kg (for lidocaine with epinephrine) × 70 kg, then the patient can receive 490 mg of lidocaine or 13 carpules.

19. **What populations are at greatest risk of local anesthetic overdose or toxicity?**
Pediatric and geriatric populations. Geriatric patients undergo slower metabolism of local anesthetics. They may also be on multiple medications that can alter the metabolic breakdown of local anesthetics. Larger volumes

of local anesthetics used for routine operations in adults may exceed the acceptable dosage allowed in smaller pediatric patients.

20. **Where should local anesthetic be injected to extract the maxillary central incisor, maxillary second molar, mandibular canine, or mandibular third molar?**
    - Maxillary central incisor: 1. Local infiltration along the facial of the tooth near apex, 2. Nasopalatine block
    - Maxillary second molar: 1. Local infiltration along the facial of the tooth near apex, 2. Posterior superior alveolar nerve block, 3. Greater palatine nerve block
    - Mandibular canine: 1. Inferior alveolar nerve block, 2. Lingual nerve block
    - Mandibular third molar: 1. Inferior alveolar nerve block, 2. Lingual nerve block, 3. Long buccal nerve block

21. **What are some complications that may result from an inferior alveolar nerve block being injected improperly?**
    If injected too posteriorly, behind the ramus of the mandible, the facial nerve may become anesthetized which results in hemifacial paralysis. Symptoms resolve once the effects of the anesthesia wear off. Provide the patient with reassurance and protect the eye if unable to blink (e.g., taping, ophthalmic ointment). Injection into the inferior alveolar blood vessels may result in cardiac arrythmias or heart palpitations felt by the patient. Damage to the inferior alveolar blood vessels may result in a hematoma and care must be taken when patients have a coagulopathy or are anti-coagulated. The use of articaine for inferior alveolar nerve blocks has been associated with a greater incidence of post-injection nerve injury.

DENTOALVEOLAR SURGERY

22. **What are some common indications for dental extractions?**
    - Pain
    - Nonrestorable teeth (e.g., fractures, dental caries)
    - Periodontal disease or mobility
    - Trauma
    - Crowding
    - Hygiene
    - Pathology
    - Supernumerary teeth (when indicated, not all supernumerary teeth necessitate extraction)
    - Impacted teeth (when indicated, not all impacted teeth necessitate extraction)
    - Prosthetic driven
    - Health reasons (e.g., endocarditis, radiation)

23. **What factors are essential for exodontia?**
    When removing a tooth, the operator must ensure they have sufficient access to the tooth and the tooth has an unimpeded path for delivery. Extractions should always be performed with controlled force.

24. **What is the benefit of using a bite block or mouth prop when extracting a mandibular tooth?**
    The bite block will prevent overutilization of the lateral pterygoid muscles to maintain mouth opening. It also prevents stress on the contralateral temporomandibular joint.

25. **What are some contraindications to dental extractions?**
    Most contraindications are relative and the risk of NOT performing a tooth extraction should be weighed against the risks of extraction. Some contraindications to routine dental extraction include poorly controlled diabetes, coagulopathy, immune compromise (ANC < 500), hematologic malignancy such as leukemia, unstable cardiac disease (myocardial infarction within the last 6 months), radiation, or drug therapies (e.g., certain chemotherapies).

26. **What are some of the benefits of removing third molars in younger patients rather than waiting until they are older?**
    In younger patients, third molars are typically still developing. They contain a large follicle around the crown of the tooth and the roots are not completely formed resulting in less bony attachment. Overall, this reduces the complexity of the extraction procedure. Recovery following the procedure is shorter for younger patients and the risk of complications increases with age.

27. **What are some factors that may influence difficulty when extracting a tooth?**
    - Mobility of the tooth (ankylosis, or fusion of the tooth to the adjacent alveolar bone, increases the difficulty)
    - Extent of decay or fractured crowns
    - External or internal root resorption
    - The number, shape, and length of roots
    - Prior endodontic therapy
    - Proximity to vital structures (inferior alveolar nerve and maxillary sinus may be at risk during extraction of posterior teeth, particularly third molars)
    - Patient health, anxiety, and cooperation level

28. **What class of lever is most common for exodontia?**
A class I lever involves the utilization of a fulcrum with the force (operator's hand) applied to one side and the resistance (tooth) on the other side of the fulcrum (alveolar bone). An elevator can also be used as a wedge, where force is applied apically, to result in widening of the periodontal ligament (PDL) space around the root and driving the root in the opposite direction as the force applied. Other elevators can utilize the wheel and axle principle, rotating the elevator and generating force around an arc of rotation.

29. **How should extractions sockets be managed after a tooth is removed?**
The socket should be irrigated out with normal saline. The site should be inspected to confirm there are no residual tooth fragments or bone spicules remaining. A curette can be used to remove granulation tissue if present but aggressive curettage of the socket is not advised. Compress alveolar bone when widening occurs during the extraction process. A suture may be necessary to reapproximate the papillae surrounding the sockets but primary closure is not necessary.

30. **What are the indications for third molar extractions?**
    - Pericoronitis
    - Dental caries
    - Periodontal disease
    - Position prevents appropriate hygiene in the area
    - Pathology (e.g., tumor or cyst)
    - Pain
    - Resorption of adjacent tooth or roots

31. **How should third molars be managed when they don't meet criteria for removal?**
Third molars that are erupted and in function should be monitored per the patient's routine dental maintenance plan. In some cases, these teeth may require a more frequent maintenance plan to address hygiene or caries risk. For unerupted and impacted third molars that are free of symptoms and signs of disease, they should be monitored with active surveillance. This requires clinical and periodic radiologic exams to ensure pathology does not develop. The interval for radiographic re-evaluation can vary depending on patient factors.

32. **When would a coronectomy be considered contraindicated for a deeply impacted mandibular third molar?**
A coronectomy requires 3 mm of coronal bone above the retained roots to allow for appropriate healing. Coronectomy should not be performed when there is an active infection at the site or when the roots of the tooth are mobile. One should also consider the location of the inferior alveolar nerve and lingual nerve in relation to the cementoenamel junction of the impacted third molar in order to avoid injury during de-coronation.

33. **How should impacted mandibular second molars be managed?**
Lower second molars are most often impacted due to inadequate space in the arch. The mandibular third molar may develop in a position that impedes the eruption of the mandibular second molar. In these cases, early identification is important and the mandibular third molar may be removed early to allow eruption of the second molar. Surgical repositioning or uprighting of the mandibular second molars is indicated when angulation of the teeth prevents a normal eruption. This should be done before the roots fully develop to optimize the success of the operation. Teeth should be repositioned above the height of contour of the adjacent first molar but not be in traumatic occlusion with the opposing maxillary molar.

34. **What are some signs of impacted maxillary canines?**
    - Delayed eruption
    - Over-retained deciduous canines past 14 to 15 years of age
    - Tipping of the lateral incisor
    - Absence of normal labial canine bulge
    - Canine crown palpable on the palatal aspect of the alveolus

35. **Where are impacted maxillary canines most often positioned?**
Palatal to the dental arch.

36. **What is the difference between an open versus a closed surgical exposure technique for a palatally impacted maxillary canine?**
The main difference between these two techniques is the use of active orthodontic traction. In an open technique, bone and tissue are removed around the crown of the impacted canine and a window is left for spontaneous and passive eruption of the tooth. With a closed technique, a chain is bonded to the crown of the palatally displaced canine and the tooth is moved orthodontically under the mucosa until it erupts.

37. **What are the most common areas for supernumerary teeth? Do they need to be removed?**
The most common supernumerary teeth are maxillary incisors (mesiodens), fourth molars, and mandibular premolars. Not all supernumerary teeth need to be removed and their indications mirror that of other impacted teeth. Signs of periodontal bone loss on adjacent teeth, root resorption, displacement of teeth, pathology

associated with supernumerary tooth, and need for orthodontic therapy with movement of teeth into the area of the supernumerary tooth are indications that warrant extraction of supernumerary teeth.

38. **Where is the most common site for an impacted maxillary mesiodens to be positioned?**
Palatal to the maxillary central incisors.

39. **What are the most common complications during or after dental extractions?**
    - Bleeding
    - Infection
    - Alveolar osteitis (dry socket)
    - Trauma to surrounding soft tissue
    - Communication into the maxillary sinus
    - Injury to the inferior alveolar or lingual nerve
    - Displacement of root or tooth fragments
    - Fractured root, unintentionally retained tooth fragments at the extraction site
    - Fractured alveolar bone or maxillary tuberosity

40. **Which root of a maxillary first molar is most likely to be displaced into the maxillary sinus? How is it managed?**
The palatal root of the maxillary first molar sits in close proximity to the maxillary sinus and is most prone to displacement when luxation is attempted with uncontrolled force in an apical direction. Retrieval may be possible with the help of sitting the patient upright and suctioning at the communication into the sinus. A small hemostat or irrigation may be helpful to deliver the root tip to the communication site. In some cases, a Caldwell Luc procedure may be required to create a separate window into the maxillary sinus to remove the displaced root tip.

41. **How should root tips that are displaced into the inferior alveolar nerve canal be managed?**
When a root tip is suspected to be displaced into the inferior alveolar nerve canal, careful removal is indicated when it can be visualized. This is best performed by removing surrounding bone and grabbing the root with a small hemostat. If the root can't be visualized, radiologic verification should be obtained using cone beam computed tomography (CBCT). Root tips can be displaced into marrow spaces, submandibular space, floor of mouth, or under the buccal mucosa. If confirmed on CBCT, delayed removal may be recommended when infection or neurologic changes are observed. If small and asymptomatic, observation is a viable option.

42. **How should a communication into the maxillary sinus upon removal of a maxillary tooth be managed?**
Tension-free watertight closure of the extraction site is essential. Gel foam or a hemostatic agent may be placed into the socket to help stabilize the blood clot postoperatively. The patient should refrain from using a straw or blowing their nose for 2 weeks after the procedure. Antibiotics are used to prevent an infection in the sinus and decongestants decrease swelling at the nasal ostium and improve maxillary sinus drainage.

43. **How can a root fracture be avoided during a tooth extraction?**
Roots may become brittle with age or if root canal treated. Care should be taken to avoid applying uncontrolled force against the tooth. Surgical exposure and removal of surrounding bone can be helpful in reducing the risk of root fracture.

44. **What is the risk when extracting a free-standing molar in the maxilla?**
These teeth are at risk of causing an alveolar process fracture or fracture of the maxillary tuberosity.

45. **What are the risks of inferior alveolar nerve (IAN) injury and lingual nerve injury following mandibular third molar extractions? How is it treated?**
The risk of IAN or lingual nerve injury varies by patient-specific factors and surgical technique. The risk of permanent injury to the inferior alveolar nerve ranges from 0% to 0.9% and the risk of permanent lingual nerve injury is less common, reported 0% to 0.5%. Most cases resolve on their own and should be followed closely. Steroid therapy may assist in resolving symptoms faster but prolonged hypoesthesia or anesthesia after 3 months warrants surgical intervention consideration.

46. **What causes a dry socket?**
A dry socket, also known as alveolar osteitis, is an inflammatory condition that typically occurs at an extraction site 3 to 5 days after the extraction. It is caused by the disruption of the blood clot that protects the underlying socket. The frequency of a dry socket occurs in less than 5% of patients who have a mandibular third molar removed. Risk factors that increase the risk of developing a dry socket include smoking in the perioperative period, poor oral hygiene, oral contraception use, improper home care, and surgeon inexperience.

47. **What can be done to prevent a dry socket?**
In general, most people agree that good surgical technique is important in preventing the development of a dry socket. Proper oral hygiene and perioperative 0.12% chlorhexidine rinse may be of benefit. Postoperative

antibiotics have been shown to reduce the risk of dry socket but the risks of taking antibiotics may not justify this benefit. Smoking should be avoided leading up to and after a tooth is extracted until the mucosa has healed.

48. **How are dry sockets treated?**
Curettage to reestablish a blood clot was previously performed but this is no longer advocated. Gentle irrigation with warm salt water helps to prevent food impaction and improve overall hygiene in the area. Therapy is mostly supportive and a medicated dressing impregnated with eugenol, benzocaine, and balsam of Peru can be helpful in managing discomfort. Nonsteroidal anti-inflammatories, such as ibuprofen, can provide systemic pain control until symptoms subside.

49. **What are some findings seen on a panoramic radiograph that correlate with an injury risk to the inferior alveolar nerve during extraction of mandibular third molars?**
    - Root darkening
    - Root deflection
    - Interruption of canal outline
    - Narrowing of the canal
    - Diversion of canal
    - Bifid root apex

50. **What is paresthesia?**
Paresthesia is an abnormal sensation that is not necessarily painful or unpleasant which may or may not be triggered by a stimulus.

51. **What is dysesthesia?**
Dysesthesia is an abnormal and unpleasant sensation that is triggered by a normal stimulus.

52. **How often does the lingual nerve sit above the lingual crest of bone in the area of the mandibular third molar?**
Approximately 10%. It is in direct contact with the crest 25% of the time.

53. **When are sinus precautions recommended following a dental extraction and what are they?**
Sinus precautions are recommended when a hole or communication forms between the oral cavity and the maxillary sinus following an extraction or surgical procedure. Risk factors for a communication include pneumatization of the sinus, alveolar bone loss, and solitary maxillary molars. Sinus precautions minimize a pressure gradient between the sinus and the oral cavity. Recommendations include no blowing your nose, sneezing with your mouth open, no using straws, no popping your ears, no spitting, and no activities where air pressure is increased (e.g., airplane, scuba diving).

54. **How soon after a dental extraction is bone healing observed on a radiograph?**
Bone formation takes approximately 6 to 8 weeks to form in an extraction socket. Early bone is not well mineralized and it takes up to 6 months for complete healing to be evident on radiographs.

WOUND CLOSURE AND MANAGEMENT

55. **What factors are important when planning an incision for an oral surgical procedure?**
    - Location of vital structures
    - Access
    - Blood supply to tissue

56. **How are incisional and excisional biopsies different?**
An incisional biopsy obtains a representative sample of the lesion biopsied. It does not remove the entire lesion and minimizes distortion for future definitive treatment. An excisional biopsy completely removes a lesion with a margin of healthy tissue, yielding both a pathologic diagnosis and definitive treatment in one operation.

57. **What is the most common reason for tearing a mucogingival flap?**
    - Incision or flap is too small
    - Too much force or retraction
    - Flap is not reflected in a subperiosteal fashion

58. **When resecting around a lesion in a lenticular fashion, the length of the ellipse should be how many times longer than the width of the resection?**
The length should be three times longer than the width to allow for optimal closure.

59. **What are some reasons for persistent bleeding after an oral surgical procedure?**
    - Coagulopathy
    - Traumatic procedure

- Anticoagulant therapy including nonsteroidal anti-inflammatories (NSAIDs)
- Malnutrition
- Renal disease
- OTC vitamins or homeopathic medications

60. **Name some ways to achieve hemostasis..**
    - Pressure
    - Thermal cautery
    - Electrocautery
    - Suture ligation
    - Bone wax
    - Application of vasoactive agents (e.g., epinephrine)
    - Topical thrombotic agent (e.g., Gelfoam™, Surgicel™, Avitene™)

61. **How is bleeding from a nutrient vessel from bone managed?**
    For smaller vessels, electrocautery can be used to achieve hemostasis. The bone can also be burnished or bone wax applied over the vessel to control the bleeding.

62. **What is a hematoma? How is it treated?**
    A hematoma is when blood accumulates under tissue in an area of "dead space" or area of a wound that can't be brought together. Blood accumulates until the pressure builds and bleeding stops. In some cases, the bleeding may persist resulting in failure of wound closure. If small, the hematoma can be allowed to resolve on its own; however, larger hematomas can be a nidus for infection.

63. **How can a hematoma be avoided?**
    - Use sutures to bring tissue planes together to obliterate dead space
    - Identify sources of bleeding in the wound and cauterize/ligate as necessary
    - Packing can be placed into a wound and later removed after bleeding has stopped
    - Pressure dressing to collapse dead space
    - Drain placement allows passive flow of fluids out of the dead space to reduce fluid accumulation

64. **What is the difference between a hematoma and ecchymosis?**
    A hematoma is a collection of blood under tissues that can result in serious swelling whereas ecchymosis represents an accumulation of blood submucosally or under skin after surgical manipulation and only results in mild swelling. Ecchymosis has a black and blue appearance that resolves over time with the help of moist heat.

65. **What is layered closure of a laceration?**
    Lacerations can transverse multiple tissue planes. Layered wound closure reapproximates the tissue planes with absorbable sutures to enable reapproximation of the skin or mucosa in a tension-free manner.

66. **Name the advantages and disadvantages of a continuous suture..**
    Continuous sutures, also known as running sutures, allow for quick closure with relative ease. The wound can be closed in a watertight fashion with distribution of tension along the entire suture line. The main disadvantage is that if the suture fails or rips in any one area, the integrity of the wound closure is compromised. For this reason, running sutures are best used when additional sutures are placed in deeper tissue layers.

67. **What is the benefit of a monofilament suture over a polyfilament suture?**
    A monofilament suture consists of a single strand of material that prevents the harboring of organisms in the suture material and is less prone to infection. Polyfilament sutures are comprised of multiple fiber strands that are braided or twisted together resulting in more surface area for bacteria adherence. Monofilament sutures also tend to pass through tissue more effortlessly and are less likely to tear tissue.

INFECTIONS

68. **What is the most common source of bacteria in orofacial infections?**
    Indigenous bacteria that normally live on or in the host. Oral flora are the most common bacteria involved in odontogenic infections.

69. **What does empiric antibiotic treatment mean?**
    Many infections are initially treated with broad-spectrum antibiotics that target presumed causative organisms based on the site of the infection (e.g., oral flora). Antibiotic therapy is then narrowed based on available gram stain and culture data to target causative organisms.

70. **How does an odontogenic infection progress?**
    Early infection presents as a cellulitis. This is induced by highly virulent bacteria (often streptococci). The composition of bacteria that make up the cellulitis then shifts from aerobic to more anaerobic. Over time, anaerobic bacteria predominate and form an abscess.

71. **What is an abscess?**
An abscess is a pocket of necrotic tissue, bacteria, and dead white blood cells. The area of the abscess often feels fluctuant on palpation.

72. **How is an odontogenic abscess best treated?**
The most important therapy is to eliminate the source of the infection. In the case of an infected tooth, it can either be treated with root canal therapy or extraction. Incision and drainage of the soft tissue at the site of the abscess will help alleviate swelling and improve effectiveness of antibiotic therapy but will not address the source of the infection. Antibiotics alone have poor success with treating a well-localized abscess.

73. **What are the steps when performing an incision and drainage procedure for an odontogenic abscess?**
Locate the abscess and administer local anesthesia around the site. Do not inject through the infection as this can seed bacteria to other areas. An incision is placed at the most dependent part of the swelling. The incision should be wide enough to allow sufficient drainage. The abscess is then dissected bluntly with a hemostat down to bone and the source of the infection. The wound should be copiously irrigated with normal saline to dilute bacterial pollutants. The wound is then packed with iodoform gauze or a drain is placed to maintain wound patency. Postoperative care involves frequent rinses and antibiotic therapy (when indicated). Patients should return 24 to 48 hours for drain or packing removal. When the abscess cavity is larger, drains may be advanced or the packing changed over several days.

74. **When should antibiotics be administered for orofacial infections?**
    - Systemic involvement with fever, lethargy, malaise, weakness, or change in vitals
    - Spreading to other sites or distal progression
    - Failure of standard surgical intervention for source control (e.g., extraction)
    - Immune compromised
    - History of endocarditis or prosthetic heart valve

75. **What antibiotic should be used as the first-line therapy in an odontogenic infection?**
Penicillin is the preferred drug since greater than 95% of bacteria causing odontogenic infections respond to penicillin.

76. **What characteristics of penicillin make it the ideal first-line therapy for odontogenic infections?**
    - Bactericidal
    - Low toxicity
    - Cost-effective

77. **What are some alternative empiric antibiotics for patients who are allergic to penicillin?**
A combination of multiple agents may be necessary to achieve the same antibiotic profile as penicillin. Erythromycin, azithromycin, clindamycin, vancomycin, and metronidazole are all common antibiotics used in the treatment of odontogenic infections.

78. **What is antibiotic-associated colitis (AAC)?**
AAC can occur in the setting of antibiotic use and is a disruption in the normal enteral flora of the colon leading to overgrowth of *Clostridium difficile*. *C. difficile* produces toxins resulting in pseudomembranous colitis. Signs and symptoms include diarrhea, fever, leukocytosis, and painful, cramping abdominal pain. Treatment includes metronidazole or oral vancomycin to combat the overgrowth of *C. difficile*.

79. **Which antibiotic commonly used in dental practice is associated with increased risk of ACC?**
Clindamycin

80. **Do cultures need to be obtained when performing an incision and drainage of an abscess?**
Cultures are not always necessary but should be strongly considered when a patient is immunocompromised, already failed prior therapy, demonstrates a systemic infection, or is planning an antibiotic change.

81. **When should a patient be hospitalized for an infection?**
    - Fever greater than 38°C
    - Dehydration
    - Mental status changes
    - Pain out of proportion to clinical exam
    - Vital sign changes (hypotension, tachycardia)
    - Trismus
    - Leukocytosis with WBC > 10,000
    - Difficulty with swallowing or elevation of tongue
    - Voice changes

- Difficulty breathing
- Submandibular swelling
- Failed outpatient therapy
- Need for parental antibiotic therapy

82. **What is Ludwig's angina?**
    - Bilateral submandibular and submental space cellulitis. Patients develop marked edema involving the floor of mouth with displacement of the tongue posteriorly resulting in airway compromise.

83. **What bacteria are responsible for acute maxillary sinusitis?**
    Haemophilus influenzae, Streptococcus pneumoniae, and *Streptococcus pyogenes.*

84. **What is the treatment for acute maxillary sinusitis?**
    Nasal decongestants (e.g., pseudoephedrine, phenylephrine, oxymetazoline) help shrink the nasal mucosa and widen the paranasal sinus ostia to improve drainage. Saline irrigation helps clear purulent exudates. If bacterial sinusitis is suspected, an antibiotic such as amoxicillin/clavulanate or moxifloxacin, should be initiated. Surgical intervention may be necessary in severe cases to reestablish adequate drainage.

TRAUMA

85. **Describe the different types of displacement injuries to teeth and appropriate treatment regimens.**
    See Table 11-1.

86. **How is an avulsed primary tooth managed?**
    Supportive care and pain management. A primary tooth should not be reimplanted.

87. **How can an avulsed tooth be preserved until it can be reimplanted and splinted?**
    Hank's balanced salt solution (HBSS) is the ideal isotonic media to transport and preserve an avulsed tooth. When not available, saliva, milk, or another isotonic salt solution should be used. The goal of these solutions is to preserve the viability of periodontal ligament (PDL) cells. Avulsed teeth should not be stored in water, which due to osmosis, causes cell lysis and death of PDL cells.

Table 11-1. Types of Dental Injuries and Management

TYPE OF INJURY	DESCRIPTION	TREATMENT
Concussion	Injury to supporting periodontal ligament but tooth remains in the socket	Soft diet, occlusal adjustment if needed
Subluxation	Mobility of the involved tooth without displacement	Soft diet, occlusal adjustment if needed
Intrusion	Tooth is displaced in an apical position in the bone	When root is not fully formed, the tooth can be monitored for re-eruption. If greater than 3 mm, surgical repositioning may be necessary. When root is fully formed, tooth should be repositioned and splinted for 2-4 weeks depending on degree of displacement
Extrusion	Tooth is partially displaced out of the socket	Tooth should be repositioned into the socket and splinted for 2 weeks (flexible splint)
Lateral luxation	Tooth is displaced horizontally with fracture of surrounding alveolar bone	Tooth should be repositioned into the socket and splinted for 2-4 weeks depending on degree of displacement (flexible splint)
Avulsion	Total displacement of the tooth out of the socket	Immediate reimplantation is ideal with semi-rigid splint for 7-14 days. Root surface should not be manipulated or debrided to preserve vitality of PDL. Patient should be placed on antibiotics. If apex is closed, calcium hydroxide pulpectomy should be initiated within 2 weeks. If tooth is unable to be reimplanted immediately (>60 minutes), it should be soaked in doxycycline and fluoride prior to insertion and extraoral root canal therapy can be initiated prior to reinsertion

88. **What is the difference between root inflammatory external resorption and replacement resorption following trauma?**

Inflammatory external resorption results from pulpal necrosis and infection, usually following a trauma. This leads to resorption of the external root surface (and/or internal surface of the pulp canal/chamber). Treatment with calcium hydroxide pulpectomy can halt progression of the resorption. Replacement resorption occurs after damage to PDL fibers, leading to direct contact between cementum and bone. Tooth cementum resorbs and is then replaced by bone, leading to ankylosis of the tooth.

89. **How soon can inflammatory root resorption or replacement resorption be observed on radiographs?**

Periapical radiolucency in cases of inflammatory root resorption can be observed as early as 3 weeks after an injury. Replacement resorption may not present until 6 weeks after the injury. Interval radiographs after dental trauma are necessary to identify these processes early.

90. **How long should dentoalveolar fractures be splinted?**

Four to six weeks with rigid splinting or arch bars.

91. **What is the most common facial bone fracture?**

The nasal bone.

92. **What is a nasal septal hematoma?**

Trauma (most common), surgery, or medication can lead to the formation of a hematoma or collection of blood under the mucoperichondrium of the nasal septal cartilage. The nasal septal cartilage receives its blood supply from the overlying perichondrium. Prompt intervention to drain the hematoma prevents avascular necrosis of the septum and secondary infections of the hematoma. A saddle-nose deformity can develop from untreated nasal septal hematomas.

93. **What are signs and symptoms of a mandibular fracture?**
- Change in occlusion
- A step-off at the occlusal plane
- Fracture mobility on bimanual palpation
- Floor of mouth hematoma or ecchymosis
- Change in sensation to the lower lip or chin
- Chin deviation on opening
- Anterior open bite or unilateral posterior open bite

94. **What is meant by an unfavorable fracture pattern for a mandible fracture?**

An unfavorable fracture pattern occurs when forces from the muscles on either side of the fracture pull the bony segments apart. This occurs when the mandibular fracture parallels the attached muscles. In contrast, a fracture perpendicular to surrounding muscle pull will bring the segments together and is consistent with a favorable fracture pattern.

95. **What are the contraindications to open reduction internal fixation (ORIF) of mandibular fractures?**
- Comminuted fractures ("Bag of Bones") that are at risk of devitalization with periosteal stripping
- Contaminated wounds
- Unstable medical condition (very high-risk patient)

96. **How are mandibular condylar neck fractures managed in pediatric patients when there is no evidence of malocclusion?**

Soft food diet and observation.

97. **When correcting a lip laceration, what landmark is most important to consider at the time of repair?**

Vermillion border. This site marks the transition between the mucosa and the skin. Failure to reapproximate the vermillion border well results in an unaesthetic result.

98. **When are radiographs of the surrounding perioral soft tissues recommended following dental trauma?**

Tooth fragments can puncture and become embedded in surrounding tissue following trauma. Palpation of these fragments is not always possible. If a laceration is present and tooth fragments cannot be accounted for, radiographic evaluation is necessary to confirm they are not lodged in the soft tissue. Chest radiograph may be indicated to rule out aspiration. Larger fragments should be identified and removed to avoid infection or foreign body reactions.

99. **How much of the upper lip can be lost from an avulsion (e.g., dog bite) and still be treated with primary closure?**

An aesthetic result can still be achieved with primary closure when up to 1/3 of the upper lip is avulsed or resected.

TEMPOROMANDIBULAR JOINT SURGERY

100. **What type of joint is the temporomandibular joint (TMJ)?**
The TMJ is a synovial diarthrodial joint, more specifically described as a ginglymoarthrodial joint. It consists of both rotational and translational movements.

101. **What are the two major classifications of temporomandibular joint disorders?**
Extra-articular disorders and intra-articular disorders.

102. **Which type of temporomandibular joint disorder is most common?**
Extra-articular TMJ disorders are far more common and often clustered together as myofascial pain dysfunction (MFD). MFD accounts for 95% of all TMJ disorders. MFD involves the surrounding musculature of the TMJ and includes local myalgia, muscle spasms, tendinopathies, and myositis.

103. **What nerves innervate the TMJ?**
The auriculotemporal nerve is primarily responsible for the innervation of the TMJ. The masseteric nerve and posterior deep temporal nerve also supply sensation to the TMJ. All nerves are branches of the trigeminal nerve.

104. **What are the main goals of surgical treatment of the TMJ?**
   - Reduce or eliminate inflammation and pain in the joint
   - Improve range of motion of the jaw
   - Decrease adverse loading of the joint

105. **What is the significance of clicking and crepitus sounds at the TMJ?**
Clicking, or sometimes described as a popping, correlates with repositioning of the articular disc in the joint. Crepitus is heard during function when scraping occurs between the articular surface of the condyle and the articular surface of the temporal bone.

106. **What is normal mandibular range of motion?**
A typical adult patient should have a maximal incisal opening (MIO) of 40 to 55 mm, lateral excursion from 8 to 12 mm, and protrusive movements of 8 to 12 mm.

107. **What is internal derangement of the TMJ?**
Internal derangement of the TMJ describes a disturbance in the typical articular function of the joint. The articular disc, which divides the superior and inferior joint spaces, absorbs shock during function and assists with translatory movement of the condyle. When internal derangement is present, the translation of the joint is disturbed from the articular disc being malpositioned or malformed.

108. **What signs and symptoms are consistent with internal derangement of the TMJ?**
   - Pain
   - Headaches
   - Ear pain
   - Clicking or popping sounds
   - Limited opening
   - Mandibular deviation on opening

109. **What imaging studies should be obtained to evaluate the TMJ?**
Panoramic radiographs are great screening tools to assess morphology and position of the mandibular condyles. If temporomandibular joint disease is suspected, CT scans are more sensitive at identifying degenerative or morphologic changes. For soft tissue changes, magnetic resonance imaging (MRI) with contrast in both the open and closed mouth positions is the study of choice.

110. **What findings are observed on MRI consistent with articular joint disease of the TMJ?**
MRIs can be sequenced as T1 (fat, bone marrow enhancing) or T2 (water, edema enhancing). T1 is usually better for identifying anatomy, whereas T2 can often identify pathology better. Early findings of internal derangement show T2 hyperintensity in the bilaminar zone consistent with active inflammation or fluid accumulation in the superior joint space. Disc degeneration such as thickening, folding, or tearing of the articular disc is observed on T1. Anterior positioning of the disc without reduction on opening is also seen well on T1. Cortical erosion, joint space narrowing, subchondral edema, and osteophytes all suggest more advanced disease.

111. **Is orthodontic therapy contraindicated in patients with temporomandibular joint dysfunction?**
Many well-controlled studies have demonstrated it is acceptable to utilize orthodontic therapy when patients have temporomandibular joint dysfunction and some may even benefit from improvement in their masticatory function.

112. **What are some indications for TMJ arthrocentesis?**
   - Anterior disc displacement with reduction plus pain
   - Anterior disc displacement without reduction, acute or chronic
   - Degenerative joint disease

113. **Name some contraindications to TMJ arthrocentesis..**
- Overlying soft tissue infection to the joint
- Severely limited opening
- Fibrous or bony ankylosis

114. **How is a TMJ arthrocentesis performed?**
A single or double port technique can be utilized. The first entry site is 10 mm anterior to the tragus and 2 mm inferior to the canthal-tragal line. An outflow needle is placed 20 mm anterior to the tragus and 10 mm inferior to the canthal-tragal line. The second site functions as a drainage port during lavage of the joint. Approximately 100 cc of lactated ringer solution is used to irrigate the joint. Lysis of adhesions can be achieved by hydraulic pressure in the joint. Steroids (e.g., Depo-Medrol™) can be injected into the joint after lavage.

115. **What is the major benefit of TMJ arthroscopy over arthrocentesis?**
Arthroscopy enables direct visualization of the superior joint space of the TMJ including the synovium and articular disc. This provides enhanced diagnostic ability over arthrocentesis alone. In addition, multiple ports can be inserted into the TMJ and instrumentation can be used to debride the joint, biopsy tissue, inject steroids or sclerosing agents directly, plicate the articular disc, and/or perform lateral pterygoid myotomies.

116. **What is the rationale behind arthroplasty with disc preservation?**
When the articular disc is malpositioned, it can elicit discomfort, inflammation, and reduced function of the joint. If the disc is intact and can be appropriately repositioned, it may normalize function of the joint and reduce retrodiscal tissue inflammation. If the articular disc is malformed or torn, then removal of the disc (partial or full removal) is advised and replacement with an interpositional graft (e.g., temporalis fascia, dermis, or fat) considered.

117. **What is ankylosis of the TMJ? How can it occur?**
TMJ ankylosis refers to a severe limitation in joint mobility due to adherence of the condyle to the articular surface of the skull. The most common cause is trauma. Disturbances in joint function such as prolonged intermaxillary fixation, infection, pathology, and surgery can predispose patients to ankylosis at the TMJ.

118. **Can you describe the serious complications associated with open TMJ arthroplasty?**
- Damage to the facial nerve (temporal or zygomatic branches)
- Injury to the middle ear
- Bleeding from the internal maxillary artery
- Malocclusion
- Condylar degeneration
- Heterotopic bone formation

119. **What are some indications for total joint replacement of the TMJ?**
- Degenerative morphology from osteoarthritis or rheumatoid arthritis
- Avascular necrosis
- Fibrous or bony ankylosis with reduced mobility
- Failed previous operations
- Loss of condylar height due to condylar resorption, pathology, trauma, or congenital deformity

120. **What are some contraindications for total joint replacement of the TMJ?**
- Active infection
- Skeletal immaturity
- Inadequate bone stock for the prosthesis to be inserted
- Metal allergy to prosthesis materials

DENTAL IMPLANTS

121. **What is an endosteal dental implant?**
An endosteal dental implant is fixation screw that is inserted into bone and supports the attachment of a dental prosthesis.

122. **What is osseointegration?**
Osseointegration describes the healing process where the surface of the dental implant forms a direct interface with the surrounding bone. An osseointegrated implant is immobile, unlike a natural tooth, and behaves in a similar manner as an ankylosed tooth.

123. **What criteria is used to define a successful implant?**
- Implant is immobile
- No peri-implant radiolucency seen on radiograph
- Bone loss around the implant is no more than 0.2 mm annually after the first year of implant survival
- No pain, infection, or discomfort
- Able to be restored with a prosthesis

124. **How long does the process of osseointegration take after dental implant placement?**
Typical osseointegration time takes between 3 and 6 months depending on the quality of the bone, forces applied on the implant after insertion, biomaterial of the implant, and implant surface treatment. All these factors should be considered when determining the appropriate time to functionally load an implant.

125. **How is osseointegration tested at the time of implant uncovering?**
There are many different methods for testing implants for osseointegration. The most common method is torque testing. The implant should be able to withstand reverse torque forces of 20 Ncm without any evidence of the implant becoming unscrewed. Percussion testing assesses the acoustic sound of the implant when struck by an instrument. Osseointegrated implants will resonate with a higher-pitched sound while nonintegrated implants produce a dull sound. Resonance frequency analysis (RFA) provides an objective measurement for assessing vibration at the dental implant. This measurement can be repeated to determine the degree of osseointegration over a period of time before a final restoration is placed.

126. **What factors should be considered when evaluating a patient for surgical placement of a dental implant to replace a single missing tooth?**
   - Past medical and dental history
   - Clinical findings (space between teeth, condition of dentition, oral hygiene, quantity of bone, presence of attached gingiva, lip position on repose and smiling, freeway space)
   - Radiographic assessment (quantity and quality of bone, proximity to adjacent structures, presence of pathology, periodontal disease)
   - Patient expectations

127. **What are some contraindications to dental implant placement?**
   - Pathology present at proposed implant site
   - Poor oral health
   - Placement places nearby structures at unavoidable risk (e.g., inferior alveolar nerve)
   - Patient health factors (e.g., uncontrolled diabetes, unstable angina, Immunosuppressed with ANC < 500, psychiatric disorders)
   - Insufficient bone or lack of adequate quality of bone
   - Parafunctional habits or bruxism
   - Unrealistic patient expectations

128. **How much distance is required between a dental implant and an adjacent tooth?**
1.5 mm

129. **How much distance is required between two dental implants?**
3 mm

130. **When placing an implant at a central incisor site, the implant fixture should be placed at what depth in relation to the adjacent central incisor?**
The implant should be placed approximately 3 mm below the level of the cementoenamel junction of the adjacent central incisor and usually no more than 6 mm below the planned contact point with the adjacent tooth. This ensures proper emergence of the restoration and suitable papilla development.

131. **What radiographic studies are necessary prior to implant placement?**
Periapical and panoramic radiographs often provide sufficient information to place a dental implant safely and efficiently. Cone beam computed tomography (CBCT) provides additional data to assess quantity of bone in three dimensions, the quality of bone, and better localization of nearby structures. Additionally, CBCTs can be utilized with virtual implant planning software to aid in preoperative planning and surgical guide fabrication.

132. **Why is irrigation recommended during implant site preparation?**
The implant drilling sequence for implant site preparation involves the use of sequential drills at speeds ranging from 400 to 2000 rotations per minute (RPM) depending on manufacturing recommendations. Heat forms at the bone, and when it exceeds 47°C, can cause cell death. Irrigation helps cool the bone during site preparation and limits primary failure of osseointegration.

133. **Can an implant be placed in an extraction site immediately after a tooth is removed?**
Yes. The implant must demonstrate primary stability upon insertion. This is achieved by engaging apical bone beyond the extraction site. Interradicular bone at molar sites can also provide sufficient bone to achieve primary stability of the implant. Immediate implants should not be placed in actively infected sites. Implants should not be placed when their position comprises optimal prosthetic design. Immediate implant placement should be aborted and delayed after extraction site heals with sufficient bone fill.

134. **When should dental implants be placed at previously grafted bone sites?**
Implants should be placed 3 to 6 months after bone graft depending on the type of material used, method of grafting, location of graft, and patient healing factors. Implants can be placed at the time of bone grafting if there

is sufficient bone to achieve primary stability of the implant. Unfortunately, if the graft is not successful, this can leave a compromised dental implant that may require removal or be predisposed to early failure.

135. **What is an acceptable implant insertion torque to allow for immediate loading of a dental implant?**
    >35 Ncm^2

136. **What materials are used to augment the alveolar ridge prior to dental implant placement?**
    When there is a deficiency in alveolar bone height or width, bone grafting is necessary to achieve an acceptable foundation for implant placement. Autogenous bone remains the gold standard; however, given the morbidity associated with harvesting autogenous bone, alloplastic and synthetic materials are widely accepted. These include allografts (cadaver), xenografts (e.g., bovine, porcine), synthetics (e.g., hydroxyapatite, bioactive glass), and factor-based grafts (e.g., rhBMP-2). Bone graft materials are combined with resorbable or nonresorbable membranes to contain graft materials and prevent ingrowth of epithelial tissue at the graft site.

137. **What are the anatomic considerations for placing a dental implant in the maxilla and the mandible?**
    - Anterior maxilla: There is often a buccal concavity in the anterior maxilla. If implants are placed too upright, apical fenestration of the implant is possible. The incisive foramen is also positioned in the midline on the palate and should be factored into placement.
    - Posterior maxilla: Pneumatization of the maxillary sinus can occur in older patients, particularly those who are missing maxillary first molars for extended periods of time. This decreases available bone in this area and may necessitate a sinus lift to achieve sufficient bone.
    - Anterior mandible: A lingual concavity can be observed at the anterior mandible and lingual perforation is possible if not careful. A CBCT can be attained to confirm anatomy at this location.
    - Posterior mandible: The inferior alveolar nerve (IAN) enters the mandible at the ramus, travels through the mandible in the inferior alveolar canal, and exits at the mental foramen just apical to the mandibular premolars. The path of the canal varies among patients and at least 2 mm should be maintained between the IAN and the implant to avoid nerve injury. When placing implants near the premolar region, the most anterior portion of the inferior alveolar nerve can loop anterior and above the mental foramen. Lingual concavities are also observed in the posterior mandible, particularly near the second molar site.

138. **Why is it controversial to connect dental implants with natural teeth in a fixed partial denture?**
    - Natural teeth are attached to the surrounding bone by its periodontal ligament allowing for physiologic tooth movement up to 0.25 mm. Dental implants on the other hand are osseointegrated and have no physiologic tooth mobility. This leads to overloading of the implant upon function. Intrusion of the natural tooth has also been observed during this relationship.

139. **How much attached gingiva is required around dental implants and why is it necessary?**
    Usually, 2 mm or more of attached gingiva is recommended around all surfaces of dental implants. This ensures ideal hygiene and helps prevent the development of peri-implantitis. When attached gingiva is lacking, a vestibuloplasty or free gingival graft may be necessary to optimize peri-implant health.

140. **What are some radiographic findings suggestive of implant failure?**
    Loss of crestal bone is the most useful sign of impending implant failure. Early bone loss is a sign of implant stress and should not exceed greater than 1.5 mm in the first year following implant placement and less than 0.2 mm annually thereafter.

141. **What are the long-term success rates of dental implants?**
    Implant studies frequently report "success" rates around 95% for single-unit implants at 3 years and 90% at 10 years. However, success in some of these studies still includes compromised esthetic outcomes and "ailing" implants as successes. Success rates are typically higher in the mandible than in the maxilla. Posterior maxilla yields the most failures.

142. **Can dental implants be inserted at an angle?**
    Yes. Dental implants can be inserted at an angle and the functional load does not need to be aligned with an implant. When multiple implants are inserted to restore complete arch edentulism, the posterior implants can be angled away from the anterior implants to increase the anterior-posterior spread for a full arch prosthesis design. This allows for the use of a cantilever while minimizing the strain at the crestal bone.

143. **How much space between the bone and the occlusal margin is required for an implant-supported hybrid prosthesis?**
    A minimum of 13 to 16 mm is required to fabricate a prosthesis. This is usually broken down as soft tissue/abutment (2-3 mm), space (1-2 mm), hybrid bar (4-5 mm), acrylic (2 mm), and the teeth (4 mm).

144. What is a zygomatic implant?

A zygomatic implant is an extended-length implant (30-55 mm) that is inserted into the malar prominence of the zygomatic bone with emergence of the fixture head just palatal to the alveolar ridge or at the alveolar crest. The middle portion of the implant passes through the maxillary sinus or outside the maxillary sinus depending on the path of insertion into the zygoma. Zygomatic implants are used when there is a significant deficiency in maxillary bone and standard implant placement is not possible. They must be placed bilaterally and require cross-arch stabilization. Typically, one zygomatic implant is placed on each side with two standard dental implants inserted in the anterior region. When anterior implant placement is not possible, two zygomatic implants can be placed on each side, in a pattern sometimes referred to as "quad zygoma."

BIBLIOGRAPHY

Abubaker A, Lam D, Benson K. *Oral and Maxillofacial Surgery Secrets*. 3rd ed. St. Louis: Elsevier; 2016.

Bagheri S. *Clinical Review of Oral and Maxillofacial Surgery: A Case-Based Approach*. 2nd ed. St. Louis: Elsevier Mosby; 2014.

Bourguignon C, Cohenca N, Lauridsen E, et al. International Association of Dental Traumatology guidelines for the management of traumatic dental injuries: 1. Fractures and luxations. *Dent Traumatol*. 2020;36(4):314–330.

Brook I. Microbiology and principles of antimicrobial therapy for head and neck infections. *Infect Dis Clin North Am*. 2007;21(2):355–391.

Chung DM, Oh TJ, Lee J, Misch CE, Wang HL. Factors affecting late implant bone loss: a retrospective analysis. *Int J Oral Maxillofac Implants*. 2007;22(1):117–126.

Doonquah L, Holmes PJ, Ranganathan LK, Robertson H. Bone grafting for implant surgery. *Oral Maxillofac Surg Clin North Am*. 2021;33(2):211–229.

Fouad AF, Abbott PV, Tsilingaridis G, et al. International Association of Dental Traumatology guidelines for the management of traumatic dental injuries: 2. Avulsion of permanent teeth. *Dent Traumatol*. 2020;36(4):331–342.

Griggs JA. Dental implants. *Dent Clin North Am*. 2017;61(4):857–871.

Houle A, Markiewicz MR, Callahan N. Soft tissue trauma: management of lip injury. *Oral Maxillofac Surg Clin North Am*. 2021;33(3):351–357.

Hupp J, Tucker M, Ellis E. *Contemporary Oral and Maxillofacial Surgery*. 7th ed. Philadelphia: Elsevier; 2019.

Lam D, Laskin D. *Oral & Maxillofacial Surgery Review*. Quintessence: Batavia; 2020.

Laskin D. *Clinician's Handbook of Oral and Maxillofacial Surgery*. 1st ed. Chicago: Quintessence; 2010.

Louis PJ. Complications of dentoalveolar surgery. *Oral Maxillofac Surg Clin North Am*. 2020;32(4):649–674.

McKenzie WS. Principles of exodontia. *Oral Maxillofac Surg Clin North Am*. 2020;32(4):511–517.

Miloro M, Peterson L. *Peterson's Principles of Oral and Maxillofacial Surgery*. 3rd ed. Shelton: People's Medical Publishing House; 2012.

Quinn PD, Eric JG. *Atlas of Temporomandibular Joint Surgery*. 2nd ed. Ames: John Wiley Sons; 2015.

Ruggiero SL, Dodson TB, Fantasia J, et al. American Association of Oral and Maxillofacial Surgeons position paper on medication-related osteonecrosis of the jaw. *J Oral Maxillofac Surg*. 2014;72(10):1938–1956.

Wilson WR, Gewitz M, Lockhart PB, et al. Prevention of viridans group streptococcal infective endocarditis: a scientific statement from the American Heart Association. *Circulation*. 2021;143(20):e963–e978.

CHAPTER 12

OROFACIAL PAIN

Jeffry Rowland Shaefer, Adam Omar Shafik

1. **What is orofacial pain (OFP)?**
   OFP is the specialty of dentistry that encompasses the diagnosis, management, and treatment of pain disorders of the jaw, mouth, face, and associated regions. The specialty of OFP is dedicated to the evidenced-based understanding of the underlying pathophysiology, etiology, prevention, and treatment of these disorders and improving access to interdisciplinary patient care. These disorders as they relate to orofacial pain include but are not limited to temporomandibular muscle and joint (TMJ) disorders, jaw movement disorders, neuropathic and neurovascular pain disorders, headache, and sleep disorders.

2. **Is OFP a new ADA specialty? And how does one become an OFP specialist?**
   In May 2020, OFP was approved as the ADA's 12th dental specialty. The American Academy of Orofacial Pain (AAOP) was appointed to be the sponsoring organization of the specialty. In March 2022, the American Board of Orofacial Pain (ABOP) was accepted by the Council of Dental Accreditation (CODA) to be the certifying board for the specialty. For one to be considered a specialist, they are required to be a Diplomate of the ABOP which requires one to complete the ABOP examination process involving, first a written exam, and then an oral examination. At this time, one must complete one of the 12 CODA–accredited Orofacial Pain programs to be eligible to take the ABOP examination.

3. **What is typical differential for an orofacial pain problem?**
   From a dentist's viewpoint, one must first, after ruling out odontogenic causes, decide if the patient has a temporomandibular joint disorder (TMD) problem. Then, based on the characteristics of the patient's symptoms, one needs to rule out an intracranial problem such as tumor or aneurysm, and then consider headache, neuralgia, neuropathic pain, and cervicogenic pain.

4. **How does one define neuropathic pain?**
   Neuropathic pain is caused by a lesion or disease of the somatosensory nervous system. Painful neuropathy is characterized by pain of burning, prickling, electrical, and/or sharp nature. One considers that a pain is of a neuropathic nature when it is spontaneous and exhibits allodynia (painful response to nonpainful stimulus) and hyperalgesia (exaggerated response to painful stimulus).

5. **What neuropathic pain disorders affect the jaw function?**
   Trigeminal neuralgia, glossopharyngeal neuralgia, nervus intermedius neuralgia, burning mouth syndrome (BMS), persistent idiopathic facial pain (PIFP), persistent idiopathic dentoalveolar pain (PIDP), post-traumatic trigeminal Neuralgia (PTTN), postherpetic neuralgia are neuropathic pain disorders that can present as extraoral and/or intraoral facial pain.

6. **Is there a new TMD CODA accreditation standard for predoctoral dental education?**
   Yes, CODA standard 2-24e for predoctoral dentistry requires a dental graduate to be competent in diagnosing and managing a patient with TMD.

7. **What is TMD?**
   TMD is a collection of clinical problems that involve the muscles of mastication, the TMJ, or both. Temporomandibular joint disorder (TMD) is a term used to describe disorders affecting the temporomandibular joint (TMJ), masticatory, and associated head and neck musculoskeletal structures. The overall incidence rate of TMD is 3.5% per year, with a slightly higher incidence in females and significantly higher in older age groups. A systematic review has suggested the prevalence of TMDs to be as high as 31% in adults and 11% in children.

8. **What is the typical differential for a TMD problem?**
   When a patient presents with a jaw function problem (limited range-of-motion (ROM)) and /or pain with jaw function, one needs to decide if the problem is joint or muscle based, or both. Somatic problems are classified in the RC/TMD classification system under the Axis I category while psychosocial factors are referred to as Axis II disorders when using the RC/TMD classification system. Axis 1 include TMJ arthralgia, OA of TMJ, disc displacements, myofascial pain with and without referral, myalgia while Axis II disorders include anxiety, and depression.

9. **What are the diagnostic criteria for TMJ arthralgia, myofascial pain of masticatory muscles, TMJ disc displacement with reduction, and disc displacement without reduction?**
   - **TMJ arthralgia**—joint pain with ROM or lateral palpation

- **Myofascial pain of masticatory muscles**—somewhat limited ROM, dull aching pain, familiar pain with palpation, referral with palpation
- **TMJ disc displacement with reduction**—reproducible click which vertical ROM, can also have a click with contralateral ROM, the mandible deviates to affected side until the click and then after the click(reduction), the mandible moves to midline as it opens further, and the click can be eliminated with protrusive opening
- **TMJ disc displacement without reduction**—history of TMJ click that no longer is present, the mandible deflects to the affected side and has limited lateral ROM to the contralateral side

10. How does one define occlusal stability?

   Occlusal stability is present when a patient has reproducible contacts on their teeth. Generally, this best provides even muscle and TMJ function when reproducible tooth contact occurs bilaterally on the posterior teeth. Occlusal instability can occur when bilateral posterior contacts are not present. Posterior teeth contacts are determined by using shimstock to determine "holding" tooth contacts. For instance, if the patient only had contact on one side of their posterior teeth, one could consider their occlusion unstable leading to hyperactivity of the masticatory muscles or uneven pressure on the TMJs. This can lead to TMD dysfunction in some cases.

11. What type of conditions can be related to occlusal instability?

   TMJ OA, acute disc displacement, trauma, and iatrogenic dentistry

12. What are reversible treatments for TMD compared to irreversible treatments?

   Ideally one should use reversible treatments (self-care, exercises, relaxation techniques, occlusal appliance therapy, medications) to create a toolset that the patient can use to manage their problem on their own and not be dependent on healthcare providers. Restorations, equilibration, occlusal adjustments, and surgery are considered irreversible procedures.

13. When would one consider doing an irreversible occlusal treatment on a TMD patient?

   Should a patient present with a dependence on full-time (daytime and nighttime) use of an occlusal appliance, so that when they are not using their appliance, their symptoms return, and they have occlusal instability, one can consider restorative procedures to provide even contact on posterior teeth, i.e., create occlusal stability. Ideally one should choose the least intrusive technique to provide occlusal stability. An equilibration would be less intrusive than fixed partial denture treatment (crown or bridge placement) which is less intrusive than an orthodontic or surgical intervention. One might ask which of these treatments is most precise. An equilibration and/or restoration would be more precise than orthodontics and orthognathic surgery.

14. Should one use different classification systems for TMD versus orofacial pain problems?

   The AAOP classification system, based on the AAOP guidelines, is a clinically oriented list of diagnostic criteria for OFP. The IHS has created the International Classification of Headache Disorders (IHS) which include a category for headaches related to TMD which the AAOP guidelines incorporate. There is the International Classification of Diseases (ICD-10) which one must use when billing under a patient's medical insurance coverage. Most recently, the International Classification of Orofacial Pain (ICOP) was created to better describe neuropathic pain problems presenting as facial pain and to improve our accuracy when making clinical diagnosis.

15. Compare the DC/TMD to the RDC/TMD and both to the ICOP classification systems.

   Different classification systems have been used to diagnose a wide array of orofacial pain conditions. These include International Classification of Headache Disorders (ICHD) (3rd edition), American Academy of Orofacial Pain (AAOP) Classification, International Association for the Study of Pain (IASP) Classification, and Diagnostic Criteria for Temporomandibular Disorders (DC-TMD) (a revised edition of Research Diagnostic Criteria for Temporomandibular Disorders). However, there were potential weaknesses in all of these classification systems when applying them to a diverse orofacial pain population. The diagnostic efficiency of ICHD 2nd edition was 56% in diagnosing orofacial pain conditions. A higher diagnostic efficiency of 92.7% was noted when at least three diagnostic classification systems (AAOP, ICHD, RDC-TMD) were used simultaneously. This finding clarified the need for a comprehensive orofacial pain diagnostic system which is more inclusive of diverse orofacial pain conditions and has a better diagnostic efficiency. To address this issue, the first edition of International Classification of Orofacial Pain (ICOP) was formulated and published in 2020. The diagnostic efficiency of 91% was reached when orofacial pain patients were categorized using the new ICOP classification.

16. Compare the DC/TMD criteria for disc displacement to the Wilkes classification for disc displacement.

   The DC/TMD classification is a validated, research-based classification system for the diagnosis of Axis I and Axis II disorders to include the Axis I disorders involving articular disc displacement disorders. The Wilkes classification is a descriptive classification that is not a validated diagnostic classification but is widely used among oral and maxillofacial surgeons to describe the symptoms and clinical and radiographic findings associated with the diagnosis of an articular disc disorder. The clinical findings for both the DC/TMD and Wilkes classifications are compared in Table 12-1.

Table 12-1. Comparison Between the Wilkes Classification of TMJ Internal Derangement and the DC/TMD

WILKES CLASSIFICATION	DC/TMD AXIS I	COMMENTS
Stage 1 early: initial joint sounds without pain	**Disc displacement with reduction (ICD-10 M26.63):** reproducible joint sounds in 2 of 3 trials	The Wilkes classification is based on the concept that the TMJ undergoes deterioration thru stages. The DC/RDC is adapted/developed for diagnosis to allow comparison of research findings between studies
Early DD with arthralgia	**TMJ arthralgia:** pain to TMJ palpation and with ROM with joint sounds	DC/TMD considers TMJ arthralgia (ICD-10 M26.62) as a separate diagnosis that can accompany any stage of arthropathy
Stage 2: early/intermediate: reproducible reciprocal clicking	**Disc displacement with reduction (ICD-10 M26.63):** reproducible click in 2 of 3 trials in vertical ROM	This stage has S curved opening and closing pattern, jaw deviates to affected side
Stage 3 intermediate/late: soft tissue changes reproducible clicking with locking	**Disc displacement with reduction with intermittent locking (ICD-10 M26.63:** reproducible click with occasional locking	Locking is the key characteristic that identifies a worsening or progressing functional disability
Stage 4 intermediate/late: DD w/o Red (locked) with hard tissue changes	**Disc displacement without reduction with limited opening (ICD-10 M26.63):** DD without reduction with limited ROM but then: **Disc displacement without reduction without limited opening (ICD-10 M26.63)** DD without reduction without limited ROM	Jaw deviates the affected side when ROM is limited
Stage 5: late DD w/o reduction: bone changes on condylar head and articular eminence/fossa	**Degenerative joint disease (ICD-10 19.91):** DD w/o reduction boney changes	Possible occlusal instability (bite changes, speech changes)

Adapted from Burris BJ, Bavarian R, Shaefer JR. Nonsurgical management of temporomandibular joint arthropathy. Dent Clin North Am. 2023;67(1):27–47. https://doi.org/10.1016/j.cden.2022.07.003. PMID: 36404079.

17. **How do you tell a TMJ joint pain patient from a myalgia pain TMD patient?**
    TMJ arthralgia is localized preauricular pain aggravated with palpation or jaw movement, chewing on the contralateral side, and can be sharp, intermittent with jaw function, and characterized by limited opening. Often pain in the TMJ with lateral ROM can feel better when the patient moves side to side on a tongue blade as this separates the inflamed tissues. Myalgia presents as dull aching pain with somewhat limited ROM and has a tendency to persist as a constant moderate pain.

18. **How does the treatment plan for a TMJ arthralgia patient differ from that of a TMD myalgia patient?**
    Both should include self-care, the use of exercises to promote increased jaw ROM and function, medications for control of acute symptoms, and occlusal appliance therapy. One would generally consider anti-inflammatory medications, exercises to increase lateral ROM, and a stabilization appliance for the arthralgia patient. For a myalgia patient, one should provide a muscle relaxer, an exercise regimen oriented toward increasing vertical ROM, and an anterior bite plane. If one suspects a possibility of a systemic problem affecting joint function (the patient has a history of symptoms in other joints or a familial history of immune-mediated or inflammatory arthritis), such a finding can be ruled out or in by ordering a lab panel to include: a rheumatoid factor and anti-cyclic citrullinated peptide (anti-CCP). Less specific screening tests like the anti-nuclear antibody and HLA-B27 may suggest the presence of an immune-mediated arthritis, psoriatic arthritis, ankylosing spondylitis, or mixed connective tissue disease. Referral to a rheumatologist may be appropriate for a definitive diagnosis and subsequent medical management for patients testing positive for these lab tests.

19. **What exercises should one give to TMD patients?**
    One should tailor the exercises a patient is given to their specific diagnosis so as to improve compliance. Patients who do their exercises to improve pain-free ROM will get better. One of the indications for PT is to allow the use

of modalities (heat, cold, ultrasound, iontophoresis) to decrease pain to promote increased ROM thru exercise therapy. Also, if the patient needs help in understanding how to do the exercises, PT will be helpful. For arthralgia patients, one starts with lateral ROM exercises to promote increased condylar translation before one works on vertical ROM exercises. These lateral exercises can be done on one or two tongue blades which allow some unloading of the joint to reduce pain with lateral movement and also improves coordination of lateral movements as the tongue blades can slide upon one another. A rotational stretch can also unload the joint to reduce joint pressure and associated arthralgia. The rotational stretch is done by having the patient put the tip of their tongue onto their soft palette and opening their jaw, keeping their tongue tip touching the palate, being careful not to allow their condyle to begin to translate, thereby ensuring a vertical stretch to unload the joint and stretch the deep masseter muscle. The patient can place their finger on the tip of their nose and on the chin to feel if the mandible is starting to move forward. If it is, the patient should decrease the amount of opening. This exercise is done for 30 seconds 6 times per day, working up to 60 seconds 6 times per day. For the patient with primarily muscle symptoms, a finger stretching exercise is indicated with, again, the goal of increasing pain-free ROM. The patient uses their fingers to measure the amount of opening with the goal of being able to hold their jaw open a three-fingertip amount of opening and holding that position for 60 seconds. This exercise stretches the masseter, temporalis, and medical pterygoid muscles. The patient can start with whichever number of fingers held vertically between their teeth produces jaw muscle tightness. If they start with just one finger, they would hold that between their teeth six times per day for 30 seconds. Once that amount of opening is comfortable for 30 seconds, they can then progress to 60-second stretches with one fingertip. When that becomes comfortable and easy, the patient moves to one knuckle of opening and gradually progresses over a period of weeks or months to be able to get three fingertips between their anterior teeth and hold it for 60 seconds. Once they reach this amount of pain-free opening, they have developed a normal pain-free ROM.

20. What anti-inflammatory medications are recommended for TMD/OFP?

Common NSAIDs used for TMD patients include COX 1 (ibuprofen, naproxen, meloxicam) and COX 2 (celecoxib) forms (Table 12-2). NSAIDs work by inhibiting the cyclooxygenase enzymes, of which there are two forms (COX-1 and COX-2). The COX-1 enzyme is responsible for producing prostaglandins that protect the gastric lining, and as such, the GI damage associated with nonselective NSAIDs is due to suppression of this enzyme. COX-2 on the other hand plays a key role in the inflammatory process by producing inflammatory prostaglandins which lead to the characteristic symptoms of localized pain, erythema, and tenderness. Although all NSAIDs carry a risk of GI side effects, the risk may be lower with COX-2 selective NSAIDs. However, COX-2 selective NSAIDs carry an increased risk of cardiovascular events. Therefore, providers should select an NSAID with consideration to each patient's risk factors and comorbidities.

Corticosteroids should be limited to episodic interventions as prolonged use can lead to adrenal suppression and fluid retention, among other serious side effects. They should be avoided in patients with active infection and in pregnancy/nursing mothers. Methylprednisolone, commonly administered as a 6-day tapered course known as a Medrol dose pack, is a corticosteroid that can be prescribed when NSAIDs provide insufficient relief from pain.

21. What muscle relaxer medications are recommended for TMD/OFP?

Muscle relaxers such as Flexeril, Klonopin, and diazepam (the last two are both benzodiazepines) can be used at night to promote restful sleep and control parafunctional behavior. Commonly used muscle relaxers for TMD also include Robaxin, tizanidine, and baclofen (Table 12-3).

22. When is occlusal appliance therapy indicated?

To provide a stable, even occlusion to distribute forces from parafunctional behavior such as night-time grinding and/or clenching. Patients with a positive clench test during their clinical exam and then the discomfort from which is lessened after a repeated clench test while the patient clenches on tongue blades placed bilaterally over their

Table 12-2. NSAIDs*		
MEDICATION	**SELECTIVITY**	**DOSAGE/MAX DAILY DOSE**
Ibuprofen	Nonselective	300-600 mg tid-qid; maximum 3200 mg/day
Naproxen	Nonselective	250-500 mg bid; maximum 1025-1375 mg/day
Diclofenac	Nonselective	25-50 mg tid-qid, maximum 150 mg/day
Meloxicam	COX-2 preferential	7.5-15 mg, maximum 15 mg/day
Celecoxib	COX-2 selective	100 mg bid, maximum 400 mg/day

*Note that meloxicam and celecoxib are both listed as Cox-2 selective but celecoxib does not affect Cox-1 enzymes while meloxicam affects both but seems more effective against Cox 2 enzymes.

Table 12-3. Commonly Used Muscles Relaxers in TMD Patients

DRUG	DOSAGES	SPECIAL CONSIDERATIONS
Baclofen	5 mg, 10 mg	Risk for seizures/hallucinations when stopping abruptly; taper slowly
Cyclobenzaprine	5 mg, 10 mg	Similar dosing/side effects to TCAs; anti-cholinergic side effects; avoid in elderly, heart block, glaucoma patients
Carisoprodol	350 mg	Potential for dependence
Metaxalone	400 mg, 800 mg	
Tizanidine	2 mg, 4 mg	Must monitor liver function periodically
Methocarbamol	500 mg, 750 mg	

Note that carisoprodol has been shown to be associated with patients developing dependence when taking it for prolonged periods of time.

posterior teeth (simulating the thickness of a stabilization appliance) or when placed between their anterior teeth (simulating the occlusion of an anterior bite plane appliance) should respond well to occlusal appliance therapy.

23. What causes bruxism?
Bruxism seems to be associated with instability of a central pattern generator (central pattern generator allows CNS function without involvement of the cerebral cortex; chewing food and walking can be directed through a central patterned generator), often affected by medication use, stress, anxiety, and diet. Bruxism (80% of night-time parafunction is associated with clenching, 20% with grinding behavior) has been associated with periods of sleep arousal when one goes from a deeper stage of sleep to a lighter one. Quite often, as someone enters into their third cycle of sleep in the early morning hours, they will have a bruxism event just before they awaken and notice tight jaws, sore teeth, or a morning headache when awake.

24. What is a MORA and when do you use it?
A mandibular orthopedic repositioning appliance (MORA) is used to hold the mandible in a forward position to take pressure off the TMJ. It can be used in cases of TMJ arthralgia but it is best indicated when the patient has disc displacement with reduction (DD w Red) and the forward positioning of the mandible allows reduction of the anteriorly displaced disc. The criteria for using it is that the patient has DD w Red, forward positioning of the mandible recaptures the disc, and the forward position feels more comfortable to the patient. Although some practitioners advocate full-time use of a MORA or repositioning device, this can lead to irreversible bite changes requiring irreversible occlusal treatments to correct. Ideally, MORA use should be limited to part-time use at night only to reduce inflammation and resulting arthralgia so that the patient feels more comfortable during day-time jaw function.

25. When is behavioral therapy indicated for a TMD patient?
Every patient should be evaluated for Axis II contributing factors but clear indications for behavioral therapy include history of anxiety, depression, greater than 7 out of 10 pain, severe parafunction, and controlled medication dependency.

26. What TMD symptoms would be contraindicated for treatment of a sleep apnea patient with a dental device?
TMJ arthralgia is a contraindication for treatment with a dental OSA device. But someone with DD w Red who feels more comfortable with their jaw in a forward position can be treated for sleep apnea with a forward positioning device to treat both their sleep apnea and disc displacement without risking aggravating their TMJ discomfort. Masticatory muscle pain is not a strict contraindication for use of a dental sleep apnea device as exercise therapy can manage the myalgia so that the patient can tolerate the use of the dental sleep apnea device.

27. Are there contraindications for treatment of a patient with an occlusal appliance (night guard)?
Not usually, although if the patient has multiple mobile teeth in the opposing arch, secondary occlusal trauma generated from use of the occlusal appliance could influence the prognosis for the mobile teeth. Even if a patient does not have a positive clench test and does not relate a clenching or grinding habit (both of these findings indicate success for treatment with an occlusal appliance), they could benefit from an occlusal appliance which has an established placebo effect. One must be careful when treating the patient who presents with TMJ OA with degenerative boney changes with an occlusal appliance; a flat plane occlusal appliance could promote the patient to lose their proprioception for their habitual occlusion after which the mandible will close from a more "hinge axis" posterior condylar position resulting in a smaller arch of jaw closure, a second-molar only occlusion, and an anterior open bite. One can prevent such a change by indexing the occlusal surface of the stabilization appliance with ½ mm indentations for the opposing arch cusps tips to ensure the patient maintains their proprioception for their existing occlusion.

28. **What type of imaging is indicated for the TMD/OFP patient?**

The panoramic radiograph is the standard of care for an initial screening image for the OFP patient as it allows one to evaluate for odontogenic problems and pathology of the jaws and sinuses. Should one find indications of boney changes in the TMJ, a CT scan or CBCT is dictated to further evaluate and to establish a baseline for future comparisons. If there is a question of the diagnosis for a disc displacement or if the patient presents as a TMJ surgery candidate, a dedicated TMJ open and closed, sagittal and coronal, MRI is indicated. Should the patient present with CN stages, constant numbness or tingling, or a new intense headache, an MRI of the brain is indicated

BIBLIOGRAPHY

Al-Moraissi EA, Farea R, Qasem KA, Al-Wadeai MS, Al-Sabahi ME, Al-Iryani GM. Effectiveness of occlusal splint therapy in the management of temporomandibular disorders: network meta-analysis of randomized controlled trials. *Int J Oral Maxillofac Surg.* 2020;49(8):1042–1056.

Andre A, Kang J, Dym H. Pharmacologic treatment for temporomandibular and temporomandibular joint disorders. *Oral Maxillofac Surg Clin North Am.* 2022;34(1):49–59.

Armijo-Olivo S, Pitance L, Singh V, Neto F, Thie N, Michelotti A. Effectiveness of manual therapy and therapeutic exercise for temporomandibular disorders: systematic review and meta-analysis. *Phys Ther.* 2016;96(1):9–25.

Asquini G, Pitance L, Michelotti A, Falla D. The effectiveness of manual therapy applied to craniomandibular structures in temporomandibular disorders: a systematic review. *J Oral Rehabil.* 2021;48(12):1690–1700.

Benoliel R, Birman N, Eliav E, Sharav Y. The International Classification of Headache Disorders: accurate diagnosis of orofacial pain? *Cephalalgia.* 2008;28(7):752–762.

Benoliel R, Eliav E, Sharav Y. Classification of chronic orofacial pain: applicability of chronic headache criteria. *Oral Surg Oral Med Oral Pathol Oral Radiol Endod.* 2010;110(6):729–737.

Clark GT, Dionne RA. *Orofacial Pain: A Guide to Medications and Management.* Chichester, England: Wiley-Blackwell; 2012.

Forssell H, Kalso E. Application of principles of evidence-based medicine to occlusal treatment for temporomandibular disorders: are there lessons to be learned?. *J Orofac Pain.* 2004;18(1):9–22; discussion 23–32.

Fouda AAH. No evidence on the effectiveness of oral splints for the management of temporomandibular joint dysfunction pain in both short and long-term follow-up systematic reviews and meta-analysis studies. *J Korean Assoc Oral Maxillofac Surg.* 2020;46(2):87–98.

Fricton J. Current evidence providing clarity in management of temporomandibular disorders: summary of a systematic review of randomized clinical trials for intra-oral appliances and occlusal therapies. *J Evid Based Dent Pract.* 2006;6(1):48–52.

Funk CD, FitzGerald GA. COX-2 inhibitors and cardiovascular risk. *J Cardiovasc Pharmacol.* 2007;50(5):470–479.

Greene CS, Menchel HF. The use of oral appliances in the management of temporomandibular disorders. *Oral Maxillofac Surg Clin North Am.* 2018;30(3):265–277.

Headache Classification Committee of the International Headache Society (IHS). The International Classification of Headache Disorders, 3rd edition. *Cephalalgia.* 2018;38(1):1–211.

Hegab AF, Al Hameed HI, Karam KS. Classification of temporomandibular joint internal derangement based on magnetic resonance imaging and clinical findings of 435 patients contributing to a nonsurgical treatment protocol. *Sci Rep.* 2021;1120917.

Heir GM. The efficacy of pharmacologic treatment of temporomandibular disorders. *Oral Maxillofac Surg Clin North Am.* 2018;30(3):279–285.

International Classification of Orofacial Pain, 1st edition (ICOP). *Cephalalgia.* 2020;40(2):129–221.

Kishi Y. Paroxetine-induced bruxism effectively treated with tandospirone. *J Neuropsychiatry Clin Neurosci.* 2007;19(1):90–91.

Medlicott MS, Harris SR. A systematic review of the effectiveness of exercise, manual therapy, electrotherapy, relaxation training, and biofeedback in the management of temporomandibular disorder. *Phys Ther.* 2006;86(7):955–973.

Milam SB, Zardeneta G, Schmitz JP. Oxidative stress and degenerative temporomandibular joint disease: a proposed hypothesis. *J Oral Maxillofac Surg.* 1998;56(2):214–223.

Mujakperuo HR, Watson M, Morrison R, Macfarlane TV. Pharmacological interventions for pain in patients with temporomandibular disorders. *Cochrane Database Syst Rev.* 2010;10:CD004715.

Nicholas M, Vlaeyen JWS, Rief W, et al. The IASP classification of chronic pain for ICD-11: chronic primary pain. *Pain.* 2019;160(1):28–37.

Nissen SE, Yeomans ND, Solomon DH, et al. Cardiovascular safety of celecoxib, naproxen, or ibuprofen for arthritis. *N Engl J Med.* 2016;375(26):2519–2529.

Ohrbach R., Gonzalez Y.M., List T., Michelotti A., Schiffman E.L. Diagnostic criteria for temporomandibular disorders (DC/TMD) clinical examination protocol; 2014. http://www.rdc-tmdinternational.org/Portals/18/protocol_DC-TMD/DC-TMD%20Protocol%20-%20 2013_06_02.pdf. Accessed July 28, 2018.

Okeson JP. The classification of orofacial pains. *Oral Maxillofac Surg Clin North Am.* 2008;20(2):133–144, v.

Schiffman E, Ohrbach R, Truelove E, et al. Diagnostic criteria for temporomandibular disorders (DC/TMD) for clinical and research applications: recommendations of the International RDC/TMD Consortium Network and Orofacial Pain Special Interest Group. *J Oral Facial Pain Headache.* 2014;28(1):6–27.

Schütz TCB, Andersen ML, Tufik S. Effects of COX-2 inhibitor in temporomandibular joint acute inflammation. *J Dent Res.* 2007;86(5):475–479.

Scrivani SJ, Keith DA, Kaban LB. Temporomandibular disorders. *N Engl J Med.* 2008;359(25):2693–2705.

Silberstein SD, Olesen J, Bousser MG, et al. The International Classification of Headache Disorders, 2nd Edition (ICHD-II)—revision of criteria for 8.2 medication-overuse headache. *Cephalalgia.* 2005;25(6):460–465.

Slade GD, Fillingim RB, Sanders AE, et al. Summary of findings from the OPPERA prospective cohort study of incidence of first-onset temporomandibular disorder: implications and future directions. *J Pain.* 2013;14(12 Suppl):T116–T124.

Ta LE, Dionne RA. Treatment of painful temporomandibular joints with a cyclooxygenase-2 inhibitor: a randomized placebo-controlled comparison of celecoxib to naproxen. *Pain.* 2004;111(1-2):13–21.

Toth PP, Urtis J. Commonly used muscle relaxant therapies for acute low back pain: a review of carisoprodol, cyclobenzaprine hydrochloride, and metaxalone. *Clin Ther.* 2004;26(9):1355–1367.

Wilkes CH. Internal derangements of the temporomandibular joint. Pathological variations. *Arch Otolaryngol Head Neck Surg.* 1989;115(4):469–477.

CHAPTER 13

INFECTION AND HAZARDS CONTROL

Helene Sharon Bednarsh, Eve Cuny

1. **What is the difference between infection control and exposure control?**
   Infection control encompasses all recommendations, policies, and procedures to prevent the spread of infection and/or the potential transmission of disease. Exposure control refers to recommendations, policies, and procedures for preventing exposures to potentially infective microbial agents.

2. **Where do the recommendations come from?**
   These recommendations come from the Centers for Disease Control and Prevention (CDC): The most current recommendation on infection control in dental settings is "Summary of Infection Prevention Practices in Dental Settings: Basic Expectations for Safe Care" (2016).

3. **What is the difference between OSHA and CDC?**
   The U.S. Safety and Health Administration (OSHA) was established in 1970 for the sole purpose of protecting the health and safety of all workers. OSHA mandated through its General Duty Clause that "Each employer must 'furnish to each of his employees, employment and a place of employment, which are free from recognized hazards that are causing or are likely to cause death or serious physical harm to his employees.'"

   In May 1989 OSHA issued draft regulations to address an increasing concern regarding occupational exposure to blood and other infectious body fluids (29 CFR Part 1910.1030; Bloodborne Pathogens Standard) and finalized the rule on December 6, 1991. When issuing the final rule, OSHA's administrator said: "Today we are providing full legal force to universal precautions—employers and employees must treat blood and certain body fluids as if infectious. Meeting these requirements is not optional. It's essential to prevent illness, chronic infection and even death."

   The Needlestick Safety and Prevention Act passed in 2000, requiring revisions to the Bloodborne Pathogens Standard. These revisions required employers to provide engineered sharps injury protection devices when available. The CDC is the public health authority in the United States. The CDC makes recommendations to protect health and safety. These are based on current scientific information and are updated as necessary. The CDC monitors disease trends and investigates them to protect the health of the public.

   CDC is an advisory agency and OSHA is a regulatory agency. OSHA regulations are directed at employers to protect employees, whereas the CDC develops guidelines designed to protect workers and patients.

4. **Why are infection control and prevention important?**
   Dental health care workers and patients are exposed to various pathogens in a dental facility. There is potential contact with blood and other fluids, contaminated surfaces, and items and persons harboring transmissible pathogens. There are appropriate procedures that can minimize the risk of transmission and spread of disease.

5. **What are the principles of infection prevention and control?**
   The CDC has developed four major principles to control the spread of infectious diseases from workers to patients, from patients to workers, and between patients. These principles are:
   1. Take action to stay healthy.
   2. Avoid contact with blood or other body fluids.
   3. Limit the spread of contamination.
   4. Make objects safe for use.

6. **What are the major strategies of infection control?**
   The HealthCare Infection Prevention Advisory Committee (HICPAC) is a federal advisory committee chartered to provide advice and guidance to the CDC and the Department of Health and Human Services regarding the practice of infection control. HICPAC as identified "Core Infection Prevention and Control Practices for Safe Healthcare Delivery in All Settings" (2022). They identified the group of core practices listed below as essential for safe patient care (Table 13-1):
   - Leadership support
   - Education and training of healthcare personnel on infection prevention
   - Patient, family, and caregiver education
   - Performance monitoring and feedback
   - Standard precautions
   - Hand hygiene
   - Environmental cleaning and disinfection

Table 13-1. CDC Core Practices for Infection Control and Prevention in Health Care Settings

CORE PRACTICE CATEGORY	COMMENTS
Leadership support	To be successful, infection prevention programs require visible and tangible support from all levels of the healthcare facility's leadership.
Education and training of healthcare personnel on infection prevention	Training should be adapted to reflect the diversity of the workforce and the type of facility, and tailored to meet the needs of each category of healthcare personnel being trained.
Patient, family, and caregiver education	Include information about how infections are spread, how they can be prevented, and what signs or symptoms should prompt reevaluation and notification of the patient's healthcare provider. Instructional materials and delivery should address varied levels of education, language comprehension, and cultural diversity.
Performance monitoring and feedback	Performance measures should be tailored to the care activities and the population served.
Standard precautions	Standard precautions are the basic practices that apply to all patient care, regardless of the patient's suspected or confirmed infectious state, and apply to all settings where care is delivered. These practices protect healthcare personnel and prevent healthcare personnel or the environment from transmitting infections to other patients.
Hand hygiene	Unless hands are visibly soiled, an alcohol-based hand rub is preferred over soap and water in most clinical situations due to evidence of better compliance compared to soap and water. Hand rubs are generally less irritating to hands and are effective in the absence of a sink.
Environmental cleaning and disinfection	When information from manufacturers is limited regarding selection and use of agents for specific microorganisms, environmental surfaces, or equipment, facility policies regarding cleaning and disinfecting should be guided by the best available evidence and careful consideration of the risks and benefits of the available options.
Infection and medication safety	Refer to "Guideline for Isolation Precautions: Preventing Transmission of Infectious Agents in Healthcare Settings, 2007" for details.
Risk assessment and appropriate use of personal protective equipment	PPE, e.g., gloves, gowns, face masks, respirators, goggles, and face shields, can be effective barriers to transmission of infections but are secondary to the more effective measures such as administrative and engineering controls.
Minimizing potential exposures	Refer to "Guideline for Isolation Precautions: Preventing Transmission of Infectious Agents in Healthcare Settings, 2007" for details.
Reprocessing reusable medical equipment	Manufacturer's instructions for reprocessing reusable medical equipment should be readily available and used to establish clear operating procedures and training content for the facility. Instructions should be posted at the site where equipment reprocessing is performed. Reprocessing personnel should have training in the reprocessing steps and the correct use of PPE necessary for the task. Competencies of those personnel should be documented initially upon assignment of their duties, whenever new equipment is introduced, and periodically (e.g., annually).
Transmission-based precautions	Implementation of transmission-based precautions may differ depending on the patient care settings (e.g., inpatient, outpatient, long-term care), the facility design characteristics, and the type of patient interaction, and should be adapted to the specific healthcare setting.

Continued on following page

Table 13-1. CDC Core Practices for Infection Control and Prevention in Health Care Settings—*(Continued)*

CORE PRACTICE CATEGORY	COMMENTS
Temporary invasive medical devices for clinical management (generally not applicable to most dental settings)	Early and prompt removal of invasive devices should be part of the plan of care and included in regular assessment. Healthcare personnel should be knowledgeable regarding risks of the device and infection prevention interventions associated with the individual device and should advocate for the patient by working toward removal of the device as soon as possible.
Occupational health	It is the professional responsibility of all healthcare organizations and individual personnel to ensure adherence to federal, state, and local requirements concerning immunizations; work policies that support safety of healthcare personnel; timely reporting of illness by employees to employers when that illness may represent a risk to patients and other healthcare personnel; and notification to public health authorities when the illness has public health implications or is required to be reported.

Adapted from Healthcare Infection Control Practices Advisory Committee. Core Infection Prevention and Control Practices for Safe Healthcare Delivery in All Settings—Recommendations of the Healthcare Infection Control Practices Advisory Committee (HICPAC) 2022.

- Injection and medication safety
- Risk assessment with appropriate use of personal protective equipment
- Minimizing potential exposure
- Reprocessing of reusable medical equipment
- Transmission-based precautions
- Temporary invasive medical devices for clinical management
- Occupational health

7. What are the major mechanisms whereby diseases are transmitted?

Disease may be transmitted by direct contact with the source of microorganisms (e.g., percutaneous injury, contact with mucous membranes, nonintact skin, or infective fluids, excretions, or secretions) and by indirect contact with contaminated environmental surfaces or medical instruments and aerosols. They may also be transmitted via airborne when exposed to infectious droplets or aerosols.

8. What is aerosolization?

Aerosolization is a process whereby mechanically generated particles (droplet nuclei) remain suspended in the air for prolonged periods and may be capable of contributing to **airborne transmission** of disease, even at considerable distances from the source. Aerosols are airborne particles in the range of 5 to 10 mm in diameter and are capable of being inhaled and penetrating the bronchial tree to the alveoli of the lungs. In contrast, larger particles may be airborne in the sense that they travel through the air, but only for short times and distances; they are too large to be inhaled. They do not play a role in airborne transmission of disease per se, but may contribute to **direct transmission** (e.g., if they are from an infected source and contact a susceptible host in the mucous membranes of the eyes, nose, or mouth) or **indirect transmission** of disease (e.g., when they fall out onto horizontal surfaces and are subsequently transferred to the proper portal of entry into a susceptible host by hand or finger contamination). It is important to recognize the actual meaning of the term *true aerosol* because effective strategies for protecting against aerosol transmission of disease versus diseases transmitted by splash, spatter, and perhaps contaminated surfaces are significantly different.

9. What barriers may be used to block these routes of transmission?

A surgical mask or an appropriate face shield provides some degree of protection from contact with larger airborne particles such as splash and spatter. Surgical masks were neither designed nor intended to protect the worker from true aerosols (see question 8). Surgical masks and protective eyewear help prevent mucous membrane exposures. Clinic attire and gloves offer skin contact protection. The basic idea is to put a barrier between exposed areas of the body and microbe-laden materials.

In regard to tuberculosis (TB) and other airborne transmissible infections such as COVID-19, a surgical mask is not the appropriate barrier for the prevention of transmission of airborne organisms such as *Mycobacterium tuberculosis* found in droplet nuclei. The National Institute for Occupational Safety and Health (NIOSH) recommends several engineering controls when treating patients with active TB or COVID-19, including a negative air pressure room, special air filtration within the room, and use of a personal respirator.

10. What precautions should be taken when treating a patient with suspected or confirmed airborne transmissible disease in a dental office?

    Patients with active airborne transmissible diseases should not be treated in a typical dental setting. Treatment should be deferred until they are no longer infectious or, if emergency treatment must be provided, it should be done in a setting equipped with airborne infection isolation rooms.

11. What does OSHA require in a written exposure control plan?

    OSHA requires at least the following elements:
    1. The employer's "exposure determination," which identifies at-risk employees
    2. An implementation schedule and discussion of specific methods of implementing requirements of the OSHA Bloodborne Pathogens Standard
    3. The method for evaluating and documenting exposure incidents
    4. Noting that consideration was given to the use of safety devices, as evidenced by staff evaluation and determination of whether they were feasible for use in the practice

12. How often must a written exposure control plan be reviewed?

    OSHA's Bloodborne Pathogens Standard requires an annual review of a written exposure control plan. The plan must be reviewed and updated after any changes in knowledge, practice, personnel, guidelines, or regulations that may affect occupational exposure.

13. Are there any revisions to the exposure control plan (ECP)?

    OSHA revised some requirements for the ECP in the Needlestick Safety and Prevention Act of 2000. There has always been a requirement to review and update the ECP annually. This update and review must now include changes in technology that eliminate or reduce exposure to bloodborne pathogens. Therefore, the plan should document consideration and implementation of appropriate safety devices designed to eliminate or minimize occupational exposure. This documentation must include evidence that employees who use the devices have had input into the identification, evaluation, and selection of the devices.

14. What is an exposure incident?

    According to OSHA, an exposure incident is any reasonably anticipated eye, skin, mucous membrane, or parenteral contact with blood or other potentially infectious fluids during the course of one's duties. In more general terms, an exposure incident is an occurrence that puts one at risk of a biomedical or chemical contact or injury on the job.

15. What should be included in the procedure for evaluating an exposure incident?

    At least the following factors should be considered in evaluating an exposure incident:
    1. Where the incident occurred in terms of physical space in the facility
    2. Under what circumstances the exposure occurred
    3. Engineering controls and work practices in place at the time of the exposure, including the use of a safety device
    4. Policies in place at the time of the incident
    5. Type of exposure and severity of the injury
    6. Any information available about the source patient
    7. The presence of visible blood on the device

16. How does OSHA define a "source individual" in the context of an exposure incident?

    The standard defines a source individual as any individual, living or dead, whose blood or other potentially infectious materials may be a source of occupational exposure.

17. Are students covered by OSHA standards?

    In accordance with the Occupational Safety and Health Act of 1970, OSHA jurisdiction extends only to employees and does not cover students if they are not considered to be employees of the institution. If, however, the student is paid by the institution, he or she becomes an employee. Regardless of employee status, most aspects of the OSHA Bloodborne Pathogens Standard are considered to be standards of practice for all health care workers and are designed to prevent the potential transmission of disease. Therefore, the safe practices and procedures outlined in the standard should be followed by all health care workers.

18. How do you determine who is at risk for a bloodborne exposure?

    The first step is to conduct a risk assessment, which begins by evaluating the tasks that are always done, sometimes done, and never done by an employee. If any one task carries with it an opportunity for contact with any potentially infective (blood or blood-derived) fluid or if a person may, even once, be asked to do a task that carries such an exposure risk, that employee is at risk and must be trained to abate or eliminate risk.

19. Can the receptionist help out in the clinic, such as assisting at chairside and reprocessing used instruments?

    The receptionist can help out only if he or she has been trained to work in a manner that reduces risk of an exposure incident, understands the risk, and has received (unless otherwise waived) the hepatitis B vaccine or demonstrates immunity from past infection and completed the annual bloodborne pathogens training. The receptionist must wear appropriate personal protective attire.

20. **What is an *engineering control*?**
    This term refers to industrial hygiene and is used by OSHA for technologically derived devices that isolate or remove hazards from the work environment. The use of engineering controls may reduce the risk of an exposure incident. Examples include ventilation systems, ergonomic design of equipment and furnishings, and safety devices.

21. **What are examples of engineering controls used in dental practice?**
    A self-sheathing needle is an engineering control, as is a sharps container. These items are designed to isolate sharps, wires, and glass. A rubber dam, which serves as a barrier between the operator and potentially infective patient fluids, is also an engineering control because it reduces aerosols and splashing and spattering of large droplets during dental procedures. A newer engineering control in the dental setting is safety devices.

22. **What is an ESIP?**
    ESIP is an acronym for *s*harps with *e*ngineered *s*harps *i*njury *p*rotection. It refers to a non-needle sharp or needle device with a built-in safety feature or mechanism that effectively reduces the risk of an exposure incident. OSHA requires that employers evaluate sharps with ESIP and implement where appropriate.

23. **Where is the most reasonable location for a sharps container?**
    To be most effective in reducing the hazard associated with disposable sharps, the container should be placed in a site near where the sharps are used and not in a separate area that requires transport or additional handling. OSHA states that sharps containers must be as close as feasible to the area where the disposable sharp is being used, rather than transferring it to a central location for disposal.

24. **What needle-recapping devices are acceptable?**
    First, any recapping must be done with either a mechanical device or a technique that uses only one hand (scoop technique). Such techniques ensure that needles are never pointed at or moved toward the practicing health care worker or other workers, either on purpose or accidentally. Newer, self-sheathing anesthetic syringes and needle devices do not require any movements associated with recapping.

25. **What is a work practice control? How does it differ from an engineering control?**
    Work practice controls are determined by behavior, rather than technology. Quite simply, a work practice control is the manner in which a task is performed. Safe work practice controls sometimes require changing the manner in which a task is performed to reduce the likelihood of an exposure incident. For example, in recapping a needle, whether or how you use a device is the work practice. Something as simple as how you wash your hands is also a work practice control.

26. **What is the most appropriate work practice control in cleaning instruments?**
    The best technique for cleaning instruments is to use an ultrasonic cleaner or instrument washer/disinfector because of its potential to reduce percutaneous injuries. If these are not available, the work practice is to select one or two instruments at a time with gloved hands, hold them low in the sink under running water, and scrub them with a long-handled brush. Essentially, the strategy is to clean reusable instruments and items in a manner that minimizes hand contact.

27. **What should a proper handwashing agent be expected to accomplish?**
    At a minimum, it should do the following: (1) provide good mechanical cleansing of skin; (2) have the capacity to kill a variety of microorganisms if used in a surgical setting; (3) have some residual antimicrobial effect to prevent regrowth of resident bacteria and fungi when used for surgical handwashing; and (4) be dispensed without risk of cross-contamination among workers.
    The major concern, exclusive of surgery, is the transient flora on workers' hands. The primary idea is to wash off the flora, not just kill them in situ with an antimicrobial agent. In surgery, antimicrobial products are the standard of care to address the health care worker's resident flora, which multiply under the glove. Surgical handwashing is used when a direct intent of the medical procedure is to break soft tissue.

28. **When should a dental health care worker wash and dry hands before gloving? When should he or she use an antiseptic hand rub agent?**
    CDC Guidelines for hand hygiene are outlined in Table 13-2. Hand hygiene recommendations are specific to the type of procedure to be performed (e.g., clean technique or surgical procedure).

29. **Can dental charts be contaminated? How can you reduce the risk of cross-contaminating dental charts?**
    A dental chart may be contaminated if it is in an area where it may come into contact with potentially infective fluids. This risk may be minimized if the charts are not taken into a patient or clinical area. If, however, they must be accessible during treatment, they should be appropriately handled with noncontaminated gloves. Overgloves worn on top of clinic gloves for handling records are one possibility. Another is to protect the record with a

Table 13-2. Hand-Hygiene Methods and Indications

METHOD	AGENT	PURPOSE	DURATION(MINIMUM)	INDICATION*
Routine handwash	Water and nonantimicrobial soap (e.g., plain soap[†])	Remove soil and transient microorganisms	15 seconds[§]	Before and after treating each patient (e.g., before glove placement and after glove removal). After barehanded touching of inanimate objects likely to be contaminated by blood or saliva. Before leaving the dental operatory or the dental laboratory. When visibly soiled.[¶] Before regloving after removing gloves that are torn, out, or punctured.
Antiseptic handwash	Water and antimicrobial soap (e.g., chlorhexidine, iodine and iodophors, chloroxylenol [PCMX], triclosan)	Remove or destroy transient microorganisms and reduce resident flora	15 seconds[§]	
Antiseptic hand rub	Alcohol-based hand rub[¶]	Remove or destroy transient microorganisms and reduce resident flora	Rub hands until the agent is dry[¶]	
Surgical antisepsis	Water and antimicrobial soap (e.g., chlorhexidine, iodine and iodophors chloroxylenol [PCMX], triclosan)	Remove or destroy transient microorganisms and reduce resident flora (persistent effect)	2-6 minutes	Before donning sterile surgeon's gloves for surgical procedures[††]
	Water and non-antimicrobial soap (e.g., plain soap[†]) followed by an alcohol-based surgical hand-scrub product with persistent activity		Follow manufacturer instructions for surgical hand-scrub product with persistent activity[¶**]	

*(7, 9, 11, 13, 113, 120-123, 125, 126, 136-138).
[†]Pathogenic organisms have been found on or around bar soap during and after use (139). Use of liquid soap with hands-free dispensing controls is preferable.
[§]Time reported as effective in removing most transient flora from the skin. For most procedures, a vigorous rubbing together of all surface of premoistened lathered hands and fingers for ≥15 seconds, followed by rinsing under a stream of cool or tepid water is recommended (9, 120, 123, 140, 141). Hands should always be dried thoroughly before donning gloves.
[¶]Alcohol-based hand rubs should contain 60%-95%, ethanol or isopropanol and should not be used in the presence of visible soil or organic material. If using an alcohol-based hand rub, apply adequate amount to palm of one hand and rub hands together, covering all surfaces of the hands and fingers, until hands are dry. Follow manufacturer's recommendations regarding the volume of product to use. If hands feel dry after rubbing them together for 10 to 15 seconds, an insufficient volume of product likely was applied. The drying effect of alcohol can be reduced or eliminated by adding 1%-3% glycerol or other skin-condition agents (123).
**After application of alcohol-based surgical hand-scrub product with persistent activity as recommended, allow hands and forearms to dry thoroughly and immediately don sterile surgeon's gloves (144, 145). Follow manufacturer instructions (122, 123, 137, 146).
[††]Before beginning surgical hand scrub, remove all arm jewelry and any hand jewelry that may make donning gloves more difficult, cause gloves to tear more readily (142, 143), or interfere with glove usage (e.g., ability to wear the correct sized glove or altered glove integrity).
From Centers for Disease Control and Prevention: Guidelines for Infection Control in Dental Health-Care Settings—2003, *MMWR 2003* 52(No. RR-17):15.

barrier. The use of an electronic health system that includes patient records, radiographs, and other paperwork eliminates the need to be concerned about contaminated patient charts and materials.

PERSONAL PROTECTIVE EQUIPMENT

30. What type of gloves should be worn for different procedures and tasks?
The type of glove must first provide appropriate hand protection for the anticipated exposures, such as biologic, chemical, and/or physical (sharp). Next, within each procedure or exposure category, there are choices of materials based on several factors, including personal health compatibility (allergies and fit).

31. How do you determine what types of personal protective equipment (PPE) you should use?
The selection of PPE should be based on the type of exposure anticipated and the quantity of blood, blood-derived fluids, or other potentially infective materials that might reasonably be expected in the performance of one's duties. With normal use, the material should prevent passage of fluids to skin, undergarments, or mucous membranes of the eyes, nose, or mouth.

32. Do gloves provide protection from a sharps exposure?
They provide protection to a limited degree, at best. Some studies indicate that the mechanical action of a sharp passing through the glove may reduce the microbial load. However, even heavy-duty utility gloves do not block penetration. In addition, blunt instruments pose injury risks for the dental health care worker and patient.

33. Does clinic attire (gowns and lab coats) protect one from potentially infective fluids?
The intent of clinic attire is to prevent potentially infective fluids from reaching skin, especially nonintact skin, which can serve as a portal of entry for pathogenic organisms. Putting an effective barrier, such as a lab coat or clinical gown, between the body and these fluids reduces the risk of infection. Such garments are contaminated and should not be worn outside the clinic area. The attire should prevent patient body fluids from contacting the worker's skin and clothing.

34. Should clinic attire be long- or short-sleeved?
Because most dental procedures can be assumed to generate some spray, splash or spray while the dental personnel's hands and arms are near the patient's mouth, a long-sleeve gown or lab coat is most appropriate for dental personnel.

35. How do you determine whether eyewear is protective?
The best way is to read the standards of the American National Standards Institute (ANSI). These describe protective eyewear as impact-resistant, with coverage from above the eyebrows down to the cheek and solid side shields to provide peripheral protection. The eyewear should protect not only from fluids but also from flying debris that might be generated during a dental procedure. Protective eyewear may consist of either goggles, glasses with side shields, or a chin-length plastic face shield.

36. Is a surgical mask needed under a face shield?
Yes, it is needed, unless the face shield has full peripheral protection at the sides and under the chin. The mask protects the dental health care worker from splashes and spatters to the nose and mouth. A face shield only replaces the need for other eyewear.

37. What type of protection do most masks used in dental offices offer?
The surgical masks used in dental offices do not provide definable respiratory protection; their primary design is to protect the patient. However, the physical barrier certainly protects the worker's nose and mouth from droplet spatter generated during treatment. If respiratory protection is indicated, masks must be certified for respiratory protection. Read the product label. During the COVID-19 pandemic, the CDC recommends the use of N95 or equivalent respirators when performing aerosol-generating procedures instead of a surgical mask. N95 respirators are disposable and considered single patient use.

38. How long can a mask be worn?
One can wear a mask until it becomes wet, torn, or somehow compromised. At a minimum, a new mask must be worn for each patient. Limited research indicates that the duration for use is about 1 hour for a dry field and 20 minutes for a wet field. However, no specific guidelines exist for how often to change a mask during a procedure.

39. What is the purpose of heavy-duty utility gloves?
Heavy-duty utility gloves, such as those made of nitrile rubber, should be worn whenever contaminated sharps are handled. They are worn for safe pickup, transport, cleaning, and packing of contaminated instruments. They also should be used for housekeeping procedures such as surface cleaning and disinfection. Routine cleaning and disinfection are necessary because the gloves also become contaminated. They should not be worn when handling or contacting clean surfaces or items.
NOTE: Examination gloves are not appropriate for instrument cleaning or reprocessing or any housekeeping procedure (Table 13-3).

Table 13-3. How to Select Task-Appropriate Gloves

FOR THIS TASK:	USE THIS GLOVE:
Contact with body, as during surgery	Sterile surgical gloves
Routine intraoral procedures, routine contact with mucous membranes	Nonsterile examination gloves
Nonclinical care or treatment procedures, such as processing radiographs and writing in a patient record	Copolymer gloves or overgloves
Contact with chemical agents, contaminated sharps, and other potential exposure incidents not related to patient treatment	Heavy-duty utility gloves

40. **What is irritant dermatitis?**
It is a nonallergic process that damages superficial layers of skin. It is mainly caused by contact that challenges the skin tissue.

41. **What are the symptoms of irritant dermatitis?**
In general, the top layer of the skin becomes reddened, dry, irritated, or cracked.

42. **What causes of dermatitis are associated with health care workers' hands?**
Nonallergic irritant dermatitis is the most common form of adverse reaction. It is often caused by the following: (1) contact with a substance that physically or chemically damages the skin, such as frequent antimicrobial handwashing agents on sensitive skin; (2) failure to rinse off chemical antiseptic completely; (3) excessive exposure to water; and (4) failure to dry hands properly and thoroughly.

43. **What common types of hypersensitivity symptoms are caused by latex gloves and other latex items?**
    1. **Cutaneous anaphylactic reaction** (type I hypersensitivity) typically develops within minutes after an allergic individual comes into direct contact with allergens via tissues or mucous membranes (donning latex examination or surgical gloves) or is exposed via aerosolization of allergens. Natural rubber latex proteins adhering to glove powder particles can remain suspended in the air for prolonged periods after gloves are placed on the hands and when new boxes of gloves are opened. Wheal and flare reactions (e.g., urticaria, hives) may develop, along with itching and localized edema. Coughing, wheezing, shortness of breath, and/or respiratory distress may occur, depending on the person's degree of sensitization. Type I hypersensitivity can be life-threatening; appropriate medical supplies (e.g., epinephrine) should always be immediately available.
    2. **Contact dermatitis** (delayed type IV hypersensitivity) is characterized by a several-hour delay in the onset of symptoms and a reaction that peaks in 24 to 48 hours. This slow-forming, chronic inflammatory reaction is well demarcated on the skin and is surrounded by localized erythema. Healing may take up to 4 days, with scabbing and sloughing of affected epithelial sites.

44. **What should be done for health care workers who develop symptoms or reactions that may be caused by latex hypersensitivity?**
The first step is to determine that you are dealing with a true reaction to latex. The most common type of hand dermatitis is actually nonspecific irritation and not an immunologic response. Nonspecific irritation can have a similar appearance to a type I or IV reaction but often results from improper hand care, such as not drying hands completely before putting on gloves. In addition, allowing dry hands to go untreated, especially during colder seasons, may lead to development of chapped broken areas in the epithelium.

Definitive diagnosis through clinical and laboratory tests by a qualified health care professional is necessary. Specific treatment and latex avoidance recommendations must be followed by the latex-sensitive or allergic health care worker. Accommodations in products selection and work environment may be required in order for the health care worker to return to work safely. In an alert to health professionals in 1991, the U.S. Food and Drug Administration (FDA) also suggested that persons with severe latex sensitivity should wear a medical identification bracelet in case they require emergency medical care and are unable to alert hospital personnel.

45. **What risk factors are associated with latex allergy?**
    - Frequent exposure to latex
    - Frequent catheterization
    - History of surgery
    - Spina bifida
    - Allergies to certain food, such as bananas, avocados, kiwi fruit, and chestnuts

46. **What are the official recommendations for protection of health care workers with ongoing exposure to latex?**
NIOSH recommends the following steps for worker protection:

1. Use nonlatex gloves for activities that are not likely to involve contact with infectious materials (e.g., food preparation, routine housekeeping, and maintenance).
2. When appropriate barrier protection is necessary, choose powder-free latex gloves with reduced protein content.
3. When wearing latex gloves, do not use oil-based hand creams or lotions unless they have been shown to reduce latex-related problems.
4. Frequently clean work areas contaminated with latex dust.
5. Frequently change the ventilation filters and vacuum bags in latex-contaminated areas.
6. Learn to recognize the symptoms of latex allergy—skin rashes and hives; flushing and itching; nasal, eye, or sinus symptoms; asthma; and shock.
7. If you develop symptoms of latex allergy, avoid direct contact with latex gloves and products until you see a physician experienced in treating latex allergy.
8. Consult your physician about the following precautions:
   - Avoid contact with latex gloves and products.
   - Avoid areas in which you may inhale the powder from latex gloves worn by others.
   - Wear a medical alert bracelet.
9. Take advantage of all latex allergy education and training provided by your employer.
   See the NIOSH website (https://www.cdc.gov/niosh/index.htm) for updated information.

47. **A patient reports a latex allergy and says that if a glove touches her, she will break out. What type of glove should be used in place of latex?**
There are nonlatex (synthetic) gloves that provide appropriate barrier protection and reduce concern for an allergic response. However, depending on the severity of the allergy, more serious responses may occur merely in the presence of latex. You may wish to consult with the patient's allergist for additional recommendations.

48. **Why are lanolin hand creams contraindicated with glove use?**
The fatty acids in lanolin break down the latex, causing wicking. This same process can cause a buildup of film on the hands.

BLOODBORNE INFECTIONS AND VACCINATION

49. **What are Standard Precautions?**
In 1996, the CDC developed new guidelines that combined the major components of universal precautions and body substance isolation into one set of precautions known as Standard Precautions. According to the Oral Health Division of the CDC, they are similar to universal precautions in that they are designed to reduce the risk of transmission of pathogens from recognized and unrecognized sources of infection to other patients and to health care workers. Standard Precautions apply to blood, body fluids, secretions, and excretions (except sweat), regardless of whether they contain blood, to nonintact skin and mucous membranes. Standard Precautions should be used in the care of all patients, regardless of their infectious status. This expanded set of precautions teaches simply that "if it's a wet body substance and it doesn't belong to you, wear your gloves and other PPE as appropriate to avoid direct contact with it while delivering health care to the patient."

50. **What is the chain of infection?**
The chain of infection refers to the prerequisites for infection (by direct or indirect contact). The chain of infection must include the following:
- A susceptible host
- A pathogen with sufficient infectivity and numbers to cause infection
- An appropriate portal of entry to the host (e.g., a bloodborne agent must gain access to the bloodstream, whereas an enteric agent must enter the mouth [digestive tract])
- A reasonably efficient physical mode of pathogen transfer from source to host

51. **Which factor is easiest to control—agent, host, or transmission?**
Agent and host are more difficult to control than transmission. Standard Precautions are directed toward interrupting the transfer of microorganisms from patient to health care worker, and vice versa.

52. **What is one of the single most important measures to reduce the risk of transmission of microorganisms?**
Hand hygiene, such as handwashing, is one of the most important measures in reducing the risk of transmission of microorganisms. Hands should *always* be thoroughly washed between patients, after contact with blood or other potentially infective fluids, after contact with contaminated instruments or items, and after removal of gloves. Gloves also play an important role as a protective barrier against cross-contamination and reduce the likelihood of transferring microorganisms from health care workers to patients and from environmental surfaces to patients. A cardinal rule for safety is never to touch a surface with contaminated gloves that will subsequently be touched with ungloved hands.

53. **Is exposure synonymous with infection?**
No. An exposure is a contact that has a reasonable potential to complete the chain of infection and result in disease of the host. Infection occurs when the exposure leads to transmission of the pathogen.

54. **What are hepatitis B and delta hepatitis?**
Hepatitis B is one of the most common reportable diseases in the United States. HBV is transmitted through blood or blood-contaminated body fluids. It is highly transmissible because of the large numbers of virus in the blood of infected persons (about 100 million/mL). Delta hepatitis is caused by a defective virus (hepatitis D virus [HDV]) that relies on HBV for its pathogenicity and can infect only in the presence of HBV. HBV and HDV co-infection, however, results in a fulminant course of liver disease. Hepatitis D is very rarely seen in the United States but may be encountered when traveling to certain countries. If successfully vaccinated against HBV, one cannot contract HDV.

55. **Why is hepatitis B vaccination so important?**
HBV was the major infectious occupational hazard to health care workers prior to the development of effective vaccines. Transmission has been documented from providers to patients, patient to provider, and patient to patient in healthcare settings. In 1982, a vaccine became available to provide protection from HBV infection. The first-generation vaccine was plasma-derived, but the vaccine in current use is genetically engineered. The safety and efficacy of the vaccine are well established, and there is no current recommendation for booster doses. Furthermore, protection from HBV also confers protection from HDV.

56. **If you are employed in a dental practice, who pays for the HBV vaccine—you or your employer?**
If an employee may be exposed to blood or other potentially infectious fluids during the course of work, it is the obligation of the employer to offer and pay for the series of vaccinations. According to OSHA regulations, the vaccine series must be offered to all at-risk employees within 10 working days of hire or reassignment to the position with occupational exposure to blood. A hepatitis B surface antibody titer test (referred to as anti-Hbs or HBsAb) is recommended 1 to 2 months after completion of the vaccine series to verify that the health care worker is protected. Because this is a U.S. Public Health Service (USPHS) recommendation, the employer is expected to pay the cost of the titer test.

57. **What if I refuse the vaccination?**
In most states, you have a right to refuse the vaccination. You should realize, however, that without the HBV vaccination series or evidence of previous infection, you remain at risk for acquiring HBV infection. Because OSHA considers the HBV vaccination one of the most important protections that a health care worker can have, the agency requires the employee to sign a waiver if the vaccination is refused. Only after the employee has been informed of the safety and efficacy of the vaccine and the potential consequences of not receiving the vaccine can they sign the declination form. The language used in the declination must be that which is specified in the OSHA Bloodborne Pathogens Standard. If an employee with occupational exposure to blood declines the vaccine and later decides to accept it, the employer must still pay the cost of the vaccination series.

58. **What is the risk of acquiring HBV infection from a percutaneous exposure to blood known to be infected with HBV?**
The risk of becoming infected with HBV varies with the presence or absence of HBeAg. If the source is e antigen-positive, the risk of 22% to 30%; if the source is e antigen-negative, the risk is 1% to 6%. This risk is for an unprotected, nonvaccinated health care worker.

59. **What is the risk of HIV transmission associated with percutaneous and/or mucous membrane exposures to blood known to be HIV-positive?**
The risk is about 0.3% (1/300) for percutaneous and about 0.09% (1/900) for mucous membrane exposures. Many factors, however, influence the likelihood of transmission (see question 66). Accumulated data from studies involving health care worker exposures suggest a 0.2% to 0.4% risk of HIV infection, with the worst-case scenario of a severe percutaneous injury involving exposure to blood from a terminal HIV patient.

60. **How can percutaneous injuries be prevented?**
Use devices with engineered safety features designed to prevent injuries such as self-sheathing needles, blunt suture blades, other safe disposable needle systems, and the use of appropriate sharps containers.
Use safer work practices that avoid hand contact with sharps, such as not debriding an instrument by hand with gauze but rather by using a single-hand technique, such as cotton rolls taped to a bracket tray or use of a commercial safe wipe device. Also, when handling sharps, use caution not to come into contact with the sharp instrument, such as not recapping a syringe or disengaging needles from a reusable syringe by hand.

61. **What are the elements of a postexposure management program?**
1. Wound management
2. Exposure reporting and documentation
3. Medical follow-up

62. **How do you assess the risk of infection?**
The risk of infection is assessed by type of exposure, body substance involved, and source evaluation. Assessing the type of exposure determines whether it is percutaneous, mucous membrane, nonintact skin, or a bite resulting in blood exposure. Risk also depends on the type of body fluid, with blood or bloody fluid being a higher risk. Caution should also be used for potentially infectious fluid or tissue. In terms of the source evaluation, consideration must be given to the presence of HBsAg, presence of HCV antibody, and/or the presence of HIV antibody. The risk assessment should be performed by a qualified health care professional, such as an occupational health professional.

63. **What is appropriate wound management?**
    1. Cleaning the wound with soap and water—do not attempt to squeeze or "milk" the wound
    2. Flushing mucous membranes with water

64. **Are any of these injuries preventable?**
Yes. Data indicates that many reported injuries were preventable. In the event of a device failure, an injury may not have been preventable. Device failures should be reported to the FDA MedWatch program. The MedWatch program forms are available at https://www.fda.gov/safety/medi cal-product-safety-information/medwatch-forms-fda-safety-reporting.

65. **What is the major factor in the prevention of bloodborne pathogen transmission in health care settings?**
Although engineering controls are a major factor in reducing the risk of an exposure, work practice controls have the greatest impact on preventing bloodborne disease transmission. Over 90% of the injuries leading to disease transmission have been associated with syringes and sharp instruments. Injuries also may be prevented by engineering controls, particularly the use of safer medical devices. A safe device will not prevent an injury unless it is properly used. The overall message is to maintain consistent levels of attention and take personal care (Box 13-1).

66. **If I injure myself while working on a patient or using contaminated instruments from an identifiable patient, can someone call the patient's personal physician for additional medical history information?**
In almost all states, a written informed consent is necessary before a physician can release information on a patient. Obtaining information without this consent may be a violation of the Health Insurance Portability and Accountability Act (HIPAA) or other state laws. The situation may be discussed with the source patient to ask for consent to obtain additional information about his or her health. Regardless of the answer, an appropriate health care professional should evaluate you as soon as feasible if the injury warrants this.

BOX 13-1 Recommendations for Managing Occupational Blood Exposures

Establish written protocols for management of occupational exposures (these are based on the most current USPHS guidelines):
- Review periodically.
- Provide training to personnel—prevention and response to occupational exposures.
- Identify a qualified healthcare provider who is familiar with the most current USPHS postexposure management recommendations, antiretroviral therapy, bloodborne disease transmission, and the OSHA Bloodborne Pathogens Standard; will ensure prompt evaluation, treatment, management, and follow-up of occupational exposures; and will provide necessary counseling.

Provide immediate care to the exposure site:
- Wash wounds and skin with soap and water.
- Flush mucous membranes with water.

Immediately report the exposure to the infection control coordinator who should:
- Initiate referral to a qualified health care professional.
- Complete necessary reports.

Include the following information in the postexposure report:
- Date and time of exposure.
- Details of the procedure being performed: where and how the exposure occurred; type of device involved; how and when during its handling the exposure occurred.
- Details of the exposure: type and amount of fluid or material; severity of the exposure.
- Details about the exposure source (HBV, HCV, HIV): if the source was infected with HIV—note the stage of disease, history of antiretroviral therapy, and viral load, if known.
- Details about the exposed person (e.g., hepatitis B vaccination, vaccine-response status).
- Details about counseling, postexposure management, and follow-up.

67. **What treatment options are available to a health care worker who has been exposed to HBV?**
Individuals who are vaccinated for HBV and had post-vaccination testing that confirmed they developed antibodies will likely need no treatment. If the health care worker was not vaccinated against HBV or did not develop detectable antibody titer against hepatitis B surface antigen (anti-HBs) after vaccination, hepatitis B immunoglobulin (HBIG) should be administered as soon as possible. The HBV vaccination series should be initiated at the same time. An exposed health care worker may also need to consider the possibility that HIV and/or HCV exposure may have occurred simultaneously.
    The efficacy of HBV postexposure prophylaxis (PEP) is based on perinatal data. These data indicate that if multiple doses of HBIG alone or the vaccine series alone is given within 1 week, the prevention of HBV infection is 70% to 75%. If a combination of HBIG and the vaccine series is administered, the efficacy increases to 85% to 95%.

68. **How effective is the HBV vaccine?**
Anti-HBs titers decline in 30% to 50% of adults within 8 to 10 years after vaccination. However, it is believed that the immune memory remains intact indefinitely after immunization. Chronic infection has rarely been documented in vaccine responders.

69. **Describe postexposure follow-up for HBV.**
The major elements are baseline evaluation and testing of the exposed health care worker, consideration of treatment options, and follow-up testing and counseling, as indicated. If the exposed person has been vaccinated but the vaccine response is unknown, test for anti-HBs. If, however, the exposed health care worker has not been vaccinated, or if the response is known, baseline testing is not necessary.
    For health care workers who receive the HBV vaccine, follow-up testing for anti-HBs is indicated at 1 to 2 months after the last dose. If, however, HBIG was also administered, the vaccine response cannot be ascertained until 3 to 4 months. If the source is not infected, follow-up is not necessary.

70. **When must a percutaneous exposure (e.g., needlestick) be reported to OSHA?**
Any occupational exposure or injury must be recorded on OSHA or the practice's forms if it is work-related, required medical evaluation and/or follow-up, or resulted in seroconversion. There are some specific exceptions for small employers. Seroconversion as the result of occupational exposure also should be reported to the appropriate state agencies and the CDC.

71. **If I am a hepatitis B carrier, can I continue work that involves patient contact?**
You may continue clinical care as long as you adhere strictly to Standard Precautions.

72. **What is hepatitis C?**
HCV is a single-stranded RNA virus isolated in 1989. Much like hepatitis B, HCV may be transmitted via contact with HCV-infected blood. There are major differences between HCV and HBV. A large majority of individuals who contract HCV will develop chronic HCV infection. HCV is rarely implicated in health care–related transmissions, but there have been some cases documented in which HCV was transmitted to patients or clinicians. Cases of patient-to-patient transmission have been associated with a lack of good infection control practices, including improper instrument sterilization and mishandling of multidose medications.

73. **How is HCV transmitted? What are the implications for health care workers?**
HCV is a bloodborne disease and is spread primarily via a parenteral route; sexual and maternal-fetal (vertical) transmission are minor modes of viral passage. Health care workers should follow Standard Precautions, as indicated. HCV has not been found to be efficiently transmitted by occupational exposure, although it has been documented. The prevalence among health care workers is about 1% to 2% (less than in the adult general population) and 10 times lower than for HBV infection. The average risk is 1.8% after a percutaneous injury from an HCV-positive source.

74. **What other information about HCV is important for health care workers?**
    - No postexposure prophylaxis is available. However, medical follow-up for an exposure is important and should be considered an immediate medical concern. The exposed worker can be tested for possible prior exposure to HCV and monitored for early signs of seroconversion.
    - No vaccine is available.
    - Health care workers should be educated about risk and prevention.
    - Policies about testing and follow-up should be established.
    - There are no current recommendations for restriction of practice for HCV-infected health care workers.
    - Risk of transmission from health care worker to patient appears low.
    - Appropriate control recommendations for the prevention of bloodborne disease transmission should be followed.

75. **Does the CDC have specific policy recommendations for follow-up after percutaneous or permucosal exposure to HCV-positive blood?**
The CDC recommended that minimal policies should include the following:
    1. For the source, perform testing for anti-HCV.

2. For the person exposed to an HCV-positive source
   a. perform baseline testing for anti-HCV and ALT activity; and
   b. perform follow-up testing (e.g., at 4-6 months) for anti-HCV and ALT activity (if earlier diagnosis of HCV infection is desired, testing for HCV RNA may be performed at 4-6 weeks).
3. Confirm all anti-HCV results reported positive by enzyme immunoassay using supplemental anti-HCV testing (e.g., recombinant immunoblot assay [RIBA™]).
4. Education of health care workers about the risk for and prevention of bloodborne infections, with routine updates to ensure accuracy.

76. In the absence of postexposure prophylaxis, what other issues should be considered?
The CDC recommends consideration of at least six issues in defining a protocol for the follow-up of health care workers occupationally exposed to HCV:
1. Limited data suggest that the risk of transmission after a needlestick is between that for HBV and HIV. Data for other routes of exposure are limited or nonexistent.
2. Newer generation tests, including rapid tests, are available and have a higher sensitivity and specificity than earlier tests.
3. The risk of transmission by sexual and other exposures is not well defined; all anti-HCV-positive persons should be considered potentially infectious.
4. There are new therapies for treating acute and chronic HCV that have proven to be effective. Therefore, monitoring for disease is important so that if transmission has occurred, treatment can be instituted at an early stage. There is evidence that newer treatment protocols have cleared HCV, but the long-term outcomes have not been established.
5. Costs associated with follow-up are a consideration.
6. A postexposure protocol should address medical and legal implications, such as counseling about an infected health care worker's risk of transmitting HCV to others, therapy decisions, and individual worker concerns.

77. What are the elements of postexposure management for HCV?
As with other bloodborne exposures, baseline testing and follow-up testing and counseling are necessary. If the source patient is HCV-positive, the exposed health care worker should be tested for anti-HCV and ALT. If the source is not infected, baseline testing is not necessary. However, if the source is unknown, the risk of infection must be assessed to determine the indicated follow-up.

78. What if the source is HCV-positive?
If the source is HCV-positive, test for anti-HCV and ALT at baseline and 4 to 6 months after the exposure. For earlier diagnosis of HCV infection, an HCV-RNA test may be done at 4 to 6 weeks. Positive results should be confirmed with a supplemental Western blot confirmatory test. Note that there is a rapid test (screening) for HCV.

79. What is the relationship between viral load and potential rate of transmission to health care workers for HBV, HIV, and HCV?
Detailed information about postexposure management for HIV is available at https://www.cdc.gov/hiv/workplace /healthcareworkers.html.

80. Have there been reports of transmission of HCV from health care workers to patients?
There have recently been reports of transmission in dental facilities. Past reports in the United States involved transmission from a cardiac surgeon to at least three patients. According to the CDC, the genetic match was "almost perfect" between the surgeon and the patients. The CDC further indicated that such transmissions are "exceedingly rare."

81. What are the guidelines for postexposure management for occupational exposure to bloodborne pathogens?
In June 2001, the CDC updated and revised recommendations for HIV (2013) and the guidelines for HIV postexposure management (PEM) to occupational bloodborne exposures to reflect new information and considerations. This document also consolidated recommendations for postexposure prophylaxis (PEP) for HBV and follow-up monitoring guidance for HCV.
 Since 1998, the FDA has approved new antiretroviral (ARV) agents, and more is known of the safety and efficacy of PEP. In light of the newer classes of drugs and new drugs within classes, the CDC updated their guidelines in 2005 to discuss other PEM options. There was also concern over increased resistance, as well as when not to use PEP, such as for low-risk exposures. In 2013, the Society for Healthcare Epidemiology of America (SHEA) issued updated USPHS guidelines for the treatment of occupational exposures to HIV including recommendations for postexposure prophylaxis (PEP). This updates all previous guidelines, but the principles of management remain the same. In December 2013, CDC published updated guidance for Hepatitis B postexposure management, *CDC Guidance for Evaluating Health-Care Personnel for Hepatitis B Virus Protection and for Administering Postexposure Management*.

82. What is included in their summary of recommendations?
    - PEP is recommended when occupational exposures to HIV occur.
    - The source patient status should be determined, when possible.
    - PEP should be started as soon as possible and continued for 4 weeks.
    - PEP regimens should include three or more ARV drugs.
    - There are situations for which expert consultation is indicated.
    - Follow-up should include counseling, baseline testing, and monitoring for drug toxicity and begin at 72 hours postexposure. This is especially important if additional information becomes known about the source patient.
    - The use of the newer fourth-generation combination HIV–p24 antibody test allows for testing to be concluded at 4 months, rather than 6 months.

83. What factors are associated with an increased risk of HIV transmission after a percutaneous injury?
    The risk for HIV infection after an exposure to blood known to be infected with HIV is increased if the exposure is to a larger quantity from the source, as indicated by either or both of the following:
    1. Visible blood on the device
    2. A procedure that involved a needle being directly placed into a vein or artery
        Risk is also increased if the source has terminal illness, possibly meaning a higher titer of virus in the blood. Studies have demonstrated that more blood is transferred if the injury is deep and if hollow bore needles are used.

84. What is the rationale for HIV PEP?
    The rationale behind the use of PEP is based on the concept that infection can be prevented or ameliorated by the use of ARVs. There are indications that if ARVs are given early, the pathogenesis may be affected because systemic infection does not occur immediately. There is a window of opportunity during which ARVs may modify or prevent replication. There is also evidence from human and animal studies that specific agents may work if used appropriately. In addition, retrospective studies of exposed health care workers demonstrated that the use of zidovudine (ZDV; Retrovir) after an occupational exposure was associated with an 81% reduction in risk of seroconversion. Early treatment is most effective; therefore, an occupational exposure to HIV is an urgent medical concern.

85. What is the primary recommendation from SHEA for PEP after an HIV exposure?
    Of primary importance is that the regimen can be tolerated, which eliminates the need to determine the number of drugs; it also expands the possible range of the regimen of ARVs to consider. Furthermore, monitoring the exposed worker for toxicity allows for earlier treatment of side effects or modification in the regimen.

86. What ARVs are FDA-approved and appropriate for HIV PEP under the new guidelines?
    Currently, there are six classes of ARVs approved to treat HIV infection. The choice of an ARV from these classes is based on the knowledge of HIV infection and on which are most appropriate for PEP, with considerations for tolerability, toxicity, and source experience. It is important to note again that regardless of the regimen, the duration of PEP is 4 weeks.

87. What is the most frequently recommended PEP regimen in the new guidelines?
    The USPHS now recommends emtricitabine (FTC) plus tenofovir, which can be taken as a combination (Truvada). Raltegravir (RAL) should be the other agent in the regimen, thereby constituting a three-drug regimen. Again, a qualified health care provider (QHP) would make the decision of what to offer as PEP. There are alternatives available that a QHP might recommend.

88. Have adverse effects been reported about the use of ARVs?
    Studies indicate that about 50% of health care workers report some adverse symptoms, such as nausea, malaise, and headache, and about 33% discontinue use because of adverse symptoms. This consideration is important in designing a regimen that can be tolerable. More serious side effects have been reported, but are rare. The new guidelines emphasize the importance of a regimen that can be adhered to, and tolerability is one aspect. It is critical that the full 4-week course be completed.

89. What is the concern about resistance?
    Resistance remains a concern in the use of ARVs because of source information about resistance or the potential resistance or cross-resistance associated with one or more of the agents used for PEP. There are tests for resistance, as well as more choices for ARVs. Drug resistance is among those issues for which expert consultation is advised. PEP should not be delayed if this consultation is not immediately available because the regimen may be modified if new information becomes available.

90. For what other situations with PEP is expert consultation indicated?
    Pregnancy and breast-feeding are situations for which expert consultation is indicated. However, the decision to offer PEP should be the same as for anyone experiencing an occupational exposure, because HIV transmission is a risk to the mother and fetus. A qualified health care provider should seek expert consultation for ARV selection and monitoring.

91. In what other situations is expert consultation advised?
Expert consultation is advised if there is a delay in medical follow-up (later than 24-36 hours after exposure), if the source is unknown and the injury is significant, if resistance is known or suspected to the recommended drug regimen, and if toxicity or adverse symptoms occur.

92. How long must PEP be taken?
The current recommendation is a 4-week regimen.

93. Do ARVs prevent occupational infection?
PEP does not prevent all occupational infections. There have been at least 21 reports of ARVs failing to prevent infection in health care workers. Factors that may influence failure include ARV resistance, treatment interruption (too short a duration), delayed initiation of treatment, a high titer or inoculum exposure, or host factors. Following current infection control recommendations and using safer needle devices are the primary means of preventing occupationally acquired HIV infection. However, if an exposure occurs, the risk of infection is usually low; when warranted, taking drugs as soon as possible (within 2 hours) after exposure may reduce the risk further.

94. Has the risk of seroconversion increased?
No, the risk remains the same as in previous reports, which is that a low risk may be modified by the use of PEP. The new recommendations, which call for use of rapid testing or fourth-generation testing, allow for prompt treatment by a qualified health care provider. This health care provider should be aware of the classes of ARVs available, risk of drug resistance, the ARVs of choice for PEP, and the follow-up protocol.

95. Are there factors that affect the risk of occupational transmission of HIV?
The CDC has described these factors and the average risk of transmission. The risk after a percutaneous exposure to blood known to contain HIV remains at 0.3%, for mucous membranes it is 0.09%, and for nonintact skin it is estimated to be lower than that for mucous membrane exposures.

96. How does an undetectable viral load affect transmission?
An undetectable viral load may not remove the risk, so PEP (see earlier) and follow-up testing are indicated.

97. Does the severity of exposure determine PEP?
It is no longer recommended that severity determine the number of drugs offered in a PEP regimen. Currently, three or more ARVs are recommended for all occupational exposures. The determination would be made by a qualified health care provider.

98. If I am offered PEP and decide to take it, what type of follow-up should I expect?
Whether or not you choose to accept a PEP regimen, you should at least have medical follow-up, including testing and counseling. In addition, SHEA recommends that follow-up within 72 hours of exposure be provided to afford an opportunity for more counseling and/or explanation of the exposure and PEP regimen and to determine whether PEP is indicated if new information becomes available or if a modification in the regimen should be considered. This is also an opportunity to review and treat any side effects and be aware of possible adverse events.

99. What other type of counseling would be expected?
First, psychological counseling relative to the trauma one may experience from an occupational exposure should be sought. In addition, there should be counseling about avoiding secondary transmission, such as the use of barrier protection during sex, refraining from donations of blood or tissue, and concerns relative to pregnancy and breast-feeding. Other discussions would include drug toxicity reactions, drug interactions with prescribed or over-the-counter medications and supplements and, of utmost importance, the need to adhere to the prescribed regimen. Exposed workers should be made aware of the signs and symptoms of acute HIV infection and should report them immediately.

100. What about follow-up testing?
HIV testing should occur at baseline (time of exposure), 6 weeks, 12 weeks, and 6 months. Testing may be discontinued at 4 months if the fourth-generation combination HIV–p24 antibody test was used. If the source was co-infected with HCV, testing intervals may be prolonged. Other blood assays will also be included.

101. What if I am not exposed, but have questions?
The National Clinicians' Postexposure Prophylaxis hotline (PEPLINE) is an excellent resource (888-448-4911).

102. Does the employer have to pay for ARVs?
OSHA has made no official statement. However, because OSHA relies on the most current USPHS recommendations, the agency may expect the employer to pay for the chemoprophylactic regimen. This rapidly evolving area may change further as the USPHS reviews its recommendations, which are based on surveillance studies demonstrating that ARV therapy is beneficial if taken immediately after a significant exposure incident. PEP may be covered by the employer-provided worker's compensation insurance. This

varies, depending on the carrier, and the worker compensation company should be consulted to determine if coverage is included.

103. **What is a prudent course for postexposure chemoprophylaxis?**

It is important to discuss the postexposure management options in advance of an exposure incident. The discussion should include the potential risk associated with various injuries, source patient factors, selection of a health care professional, and availability of ARVs, if indicated.

104. **Has HIV seroconversion been documented among dental health care workers as the result of an occupational exposure?**

There have been voluntary reports to the CDC of 57 health care workers with documented seroconversion.

105. **Have any dental health care workers possibly seroconverted for HIV as the result of an occupational exposure?**

Yes, about six dental health care workers (of 138 health care workers) have been reported to the CDC as possible cases of occupational transmission.

106. **What is the difference between a documented occupational transmission and a possible occupational transmission of HIV?**

The difference is in the testing. A documented occupational transmission requires that the exposed health care worker be tested for HIV at the time of the incident and that the baseline test be negative. If HIV seroconversion occurs after a designated time, it is considered to be the result of the exposure incident. In the possible category, HIV-positive health care workers have been found to be without identifiable behavioral or transfusion risk. Each reported percutaneous exposure to blood or body fluids or laboratory solutions containing HIV, but HIV seroconversion specifically resulting from an occupational exposure was not documented. There was no baseline testing at the time of the incident to prove that the health care worker was HIV-negative before the incident.

107. **What is the purpose of baseline testing after an occupational exposure incident?**

Baseline HIV antibody, HBV, and/or HCV testing allows the health care professional who evaluates the exposed worker to determine whether any subsequently diagnosed disease was acquired as the result of the exposure incident. Blood is tested soon after the injury has occurred to determine the health care worker's HBV and/or HIV serologic status. Note that the availability of rapid HIV testing (for types 1 and 2) and HCV testing provides results in 20 minutes. Furthermore, there are newer generation HIV tests, which can detect infection in the acute stages.

108. **Can an employee refuse baseline testing?**

An employee may decline testing or choose to delay testing of collected blood for 90 days. If a delay is chosen, the blood must be drawn but not tested until consent is given.

109. **If I consent to baseline blood collection, but not testing, then what?**

If the employee consents to testing of the baseline sample within 90 days, it should be done as soon as possible. If consent is not given within the 90 days, the sample may be discarded.

110. **What is the difference between confidential and anonymous HIV testing?**

Confidential testing with consent means that the test results become part of your confidential medical record and cannot be released without your consent and in accordance with state laws. The test results are linked to your name, even if only in your medical record. Anonymous testing refers to a system whereby test results are linked to a number or code and not to a name. Therefore, you are the only one who will know the results; they will not be part of your medical record. Whether a coded result will suffice as evidence of baseline testing for the purposes of documenting an exposure incident has not been challenged. If you are reluctant to have any HIV test information in your medical record, but are concerned about documenting an incident, you may wish to consider baseline blood collection at an anonymous and confidential test site. Have the anonymous sample tested, and store the confidential sample for not more than the 90 days allowed. Thus, you have time to consider testing and an opportunity to find out whether you are seronegative.

111. **Who pays the cost of HIV testing?**

The employer is responsible for the cost of HIV testing under the obligation to provide medical evaluation and follow-up of an exposure incident, including source patient testing, when indicated. Some of these costs may be covered by worker's compensation insurance.

112. **Is the employer responsible for costs associated with treatment of disease if transmission occurs?**

No. The employer is not expected to pay the costs associated with long-term treatment of disease, only for the immediate evaluation and PEP, as prescribed by OSHA in accordance with USPHS recommendations. Any resulting illness should be reported to the employer's worker compensation insurance carrier.

113. **What is a sharps injury log?**
A sharps injury log is used to record percutaneous injuries from contaminated sharps. The log must be maintained to ensure confidentiality. At a minimum, the log should contain the following:
- Type and brand of device involved
- Work area where the incident occurred
- Explanation of how the incident occurred

114. **How long must an employer maintain employee medical records?**
The employer must maintain employee medical records for the duration of employment plus 30 years in accordance with OSHA's Standard on Access to Employee Exposure and Medical Records (29 CFR 1910.20). An employer may contract with the health care professional to maintain the records as long as they are accessible to OSHA.

115. **Who selects the health care professional for postexposure evaluation and follow-up?**
The employer has the right to choose the health care professional who will treat exposure incidents. This HCP should be qualified to evaluate, treat, counsel, monitor, and test the exposed worker (Table 13-4).

116. **Does the employer have an obligation to former employees?**
OSHA's standard on bloodborne pathogens requires immediate medical evaluation and follow-up of an employee. If an employee leaves the practice, the employer is no longer obligated to meet the obligations in the standard.

117. **Does the employer have any obligation to temporary workers under OSHA standards?**
The responsibility to protect temporary workers from workplace hazards is shared by the agency that supplies a temporary worker. The agency is required to ensure that all workers have been vaccinated and are provided with follow-up evaluations. The contracting employer is not responsible for vaccinations and follow-up unless the contract specifies it. However, the contracting employer is expected to provide gloves, masks, and other PPE.

   Note that this can depend on the nature of the relationship between the temporary worker and referring agency. Some do not have an employee–employer relationship, but act only as a referring agent (receiving some type of fee for the referral), and others employ the temporary workers and assign them to requesting employers. In the first case, the agency has little obligation to provide such things as training or vaccination; in the latter case, the obligation is greater but the person hiring the temporary worker must provide site-specific training. It is prudent before hiring temporary employees to determine the level of obligation by the temporary agency and by the employer hiring the temporary employee.

Table 13-4. Postexposure Evaluation and Follow-up Requirements After Exposure Incident

EMPLOYEE	EMPLOYER	HEALTH CARE PROFESSIONAL (HCP)
Reports incident to employer	Directs employee to HCP—sends to HCP copy of standard	Evaluates exposure incident Arranges for testing of exposed employee and source patient (if not already known)
	Job description of employee	Notifies employee of results of all testing
	Incident report (e.g., route)	Provides counseling
	Source patient's identity and HBV, HIV status (if known), and other relevant medical	Provides postexposure prophylaxis; evaluates reported illnesses (above items are confidential)
	Documents events on OSHA 200 and 101 (if applicable)	
	Receives HCP's written opinion	Sends (only) written opinion to employer—documentation that employee was informed of evaluation results and need for any further follow-up
Receives copy of HCP's written opinion	Provides copy of HCP's written opinion to employee (within 15 days of completed evaluation)	Determines whether HBV vaccine is indicated and if vaccine was received

Adapted from U.S. Safety and Health Administration (OSHA): Enforcement Procedures for the Occupational Exposure to Bloodborne Pathogens, 2001.

118. **How accurate is the HIV antibody test?**
At 6 months after an exposure incident, the current serum test has the ability to detect the presence of HIV antibody with 99.9% accuracy. After 1 year, it is 99.9999% accurate. In addition to the traditional serum test, a saliva collection system is available. The accuracy of the saliva test is reported to be comparable to that of the serum test. The FDA has approved rapid HIV tests that require one drop of blood or a saliva sample and can produce results in 20 minutes. These tests can detect HIV types 1 and 2.

119. **What concerns are raised by the rapid test?**
There were questions about whether the test was to be approved for use in physician's offices and public health clinics rather than laboratories. Because rapid HIV tests are Clinical Laboratory Improvement Amendments of 1988 (CLIA)–waived, they may be used in nonlaboratory settings, such as a dental clinic. However, the dentist must apply for a specific waiver to use the test as a diagnostic tool in the healthcare setting. Information on how to obtain a CLIA certificate of waiver can be found online at https://www.cms.gov/regulations-and-guidance/legislation/clia/downloads/howobtaincertificateofwaiver.pdf.

120. **What should you recommend to a health care worker who has been potentially infected with HIV?**
The first step is to have immediate medical follow-up, including testing and counseling services. Early medical intervention is most important in light of the multidrug combinations for anti-HIV therapy. In addition, it is important to consult state guidelines for HIV-HBV–infected health care workers, your professional association, or a legal advocate.

121. **Have there been any recent reports of HBV transmission from dentists to patients?**
Since 1987, there have been no reports of HBV transmission from a dentist to a patient. From 1970 to 1987, nine clusters were reported, in which HBV infection was associated with dental treatment by an infected dental health care worker. Reasons for the current lack of reports of HBV transmission may include the following:
- Increased adherence to Standard (universal) Precautions
- High compliance with HBV vaccination among dental health care workers
- Reporting bias, incomplete reporting, or failure to correlate HBV transmission with previous dental treatment
  Factors that enhanced the transmission of HBV in the past included failure to use gloves routinely during patient care, failure to receive HBV vaccination, noncompliance with universal precautions, and inability to detect disease in dental health care workers. In at least two of the cases of dentist-to-patient transmission, there were no identifiable breaches in infection control.

INSTRUMENT REPROCESSING AND STERILIZATION

122. **What is a single-use patient care item?**
A single-use patient care item is an item used on one patient and discarded after that use. Many dental products have become available that are labeled as single use. Items labeled as *single use* or *disposable* are not intended to be reprocessed or used for more than one patient. Examples of single-use patient care items include the following:
- Saliva ejector
- Disposable air-water syringe tips
- Disposable impression trays
- Disposable needles
- Carbide and diamond dental burs
  Unless a product has manufacturer's instruction for use for reprocessing, the items should be considered single patient use.

123. **Can a disposable saliva ejector be reprocessed and reused?**
No. It is a single-use item that is impossible to reprocess adequately and should be discarded after a single use.

124. **Can diamond burs be reprocessed for use on more than one patient?**
As of July 2022, there are no diamond burs on the U.S. market that have been cleared by the FDA for reprocessing because the manufacturers have not submitted data to the FDA that these items can be safely cleaned and reprocessed for use on multiple patients. More information on single-use patient devices can be found on the CDC website at https://www.cdc.gov/oralhealth/infectioncontrol/faqs/single-use-devices.html.

125. **How must a reusable air-water syringe tip be reprocessed?**
There are reusable air-water syringe tips and disposable single-use tips. The only acceptable method of reprocessing a reusable tip is first to thoroughly clean the tip, followed by wrapping and packaging, and then sterilizing with steam under pressure, dry heat, or unsaturated chemical vapor. It is important to note that table-top gravity displacement sterilizers are not effective in sterilizing devices that contain lumens, such as air/water syringe tips. Vacuum displacement or steam flush-pressure pulse sterilizers (dynamic air removal) should be effective in sterilizing lumened instruments.

126. Should contaminated reusable patient care items be placed in a holding solution prior to cleaning?
No. A holding solution or presoak is only necessary when items cannot be cleaned in a reasonable time. The purpose of a holding solution is to keep debris moist on the instruments to facilitate cleaning. Holding solutions should consist of a noncorrosive detergent and water. Some holding solutions contain enzymes, which may be useful if surgical instruments contaminated with blood cannot be cleaned before the blood dries on the surface.

127. Why is an automated method of cleaning reusable patient care items recommended, rather than hand scrubbing?
Cleaning should precede all disinfection and sterilization processes; it should involve removal of debris and organic and inorganic contamination. Removal of debris and contamination is achieved by scrubbing with a surfactant, detergent, and water or by use of an automated process (e.g., ultrasonic cleaner, washer disinfector) using chemical agents. If visible debris, inorganic or organic, is not removed, it will interfere with microbial inactivation and can compromise the disinfection or sterilization process. After cleaning, instruments should be rinsed with water to remove chemical or detergent residue. Splashing should be minimized during cleaning and rinsing. Before final disinfection or sterilization, instruments should be handled as though they were contaminated.
   Considerations in selecting cleaning methods and equipment include the following:
- Efficacy of the method, process, and equipment.
- Compatibility with items to be cleaned.
- Occupational health and exposure risks.
   Use of automated cleaning equipment (e.g., ultrasonic cleaner, washer disinfector) does not require presoaking or scrubbing of instruments and can increase productivity, improve cleaning effectiveness, and decrease workers' exposure to blood and body fluids. Use of automated equipment can be safer and more efficient than manually cleaning contaminated instruments.

128. Is a thermal washer disinfector an acceptable substitute for ultrasonic cleaning of dental instruments?
Yes. Washer disinfectors and washer decontaminators that have been cleared for marketing by the FDA are suitable alternatives to ultrasonic cleaning. Household dishwashers, however, are not acceptable for health care applications. Dishwashers and other household appliances have not been evaluated by the FDA to guarantee adherence to the strict operating parameters that health care applications demand.

129. What is the difference between sterilization and disinfection?
Sterilization is a process capable of killing all forms of microorganisms on an instrument or surface, including high numbers of highly resistant bacterial spores, if present. Disinfection is the process of destroying pathogenic organisms, but not necessarily all organisms.

130. What are methods of sterilization common for dentistry?
They include saturated steam, saturated chemical vapor, dry heat—rapid transfer, dry heat—convection, ethylene oxide gas, and chemical immersion.

131. What are the types of heat-based sterilization methods?
1. Steam under pressure, or autoclaving, is the most widely used method. There are two categories of autoclaves: (1) gravity displacement and (2) dynamic air removal (vacuum or steam flush-pressure pulse).
2. Dry heat sterilization involves placing instruments in a dry heat sterilizer cleared for marketing as a medical device by the FDA. Instruments must remain in the unit for a specified period of heating at a required temperature.
3. Unsaturated chemical vapor sterilization uses a proprietary chemical solution, which, when heated under pressure, forms a sterilized vapor phase, with a low concentration of water.
   NOTE: Manufacturer's directions for each sterilizer must be followed closely.

132. What are some considerations in the selection of a sterilizer?
Consider the practice setting size and types of instruments and devices used. You may need more than one type of sterilizer to accommodate needs. The size of the practice, instrument inventory, and space considerations are important factors in the decision-making process.

133. What is an elementary doctrine in choosing a method of sterilization?
Do not disinfect or cold-sterilize what you can sterilize with a heat-based process. "Don't dunk it; cook it." If an item or instrument is heat-stable, it should be heat-sterilized. No other methods (e.g., gases, liquids) have equivalent economy, potency, and safety assurance.

134. According to the Spaulding classification, what are critical, semicritical, and noncritical items?
See Table 13-5.

Table 13-5. Spaulding Classification of Surfaces*

PARAMETER	DESCRIPTION	EXAMPLES	DISEASE TRANSMISSION RISK	REPROCESSING TECHNIQUE†
Critical instruments	Pointed/sharp Penetrates tissue Blood present	Needles Cutting instruments	High	Sterile, disposable Heat sterilization
		Implants		
Semicritical instruments	Mucous membrane or broken skin contact	Medical "scopes" Nonsurgical dental instruments	Moderate	Heat sterilization High-level disinfection
		Specula		
	No tissue penetration	Catheters		
Noncritical instruments	Unbroken skin contact	Face masks Clothing Blood pressure cuffs Diag electrodes	Low	Sanitize (no blood) Intermediate-level disinfection (blood present)
Environmental surfaces	Indirect to no direct patient contact during treatment			Sanitize (no blood) Intermediate-level disinfection
Medical equipment	Indirect contact	Knobs, handles x-ray machine Dental units	Moderate to low	
Housekeeping	No contact	Floors, walls, countertops	Least	

*This table incorporates the expansion of Spaulding's classic "critical, semicritical, noncritical" surface classification.
†Because the vast majority of, if not all, dental instruments are heat-stable, they should be sterilized using a heat-based method (e.g., autoclaving). High-level disinfection using liquid chemical or sterilant germicides is not the current standard of practice in dentistry.
Adapted from Farero MS, Bond WW: Chemical disinfection of medical and surgical instruments. In Block SS, editor: Disinfection, Sterilization, and Preservation, ed 5, Philadelphia, 2001, Lippincott Williams & Wilkins, pp 881–917.

135. **How are critical and semicritical items treated after use?**

If reusable, all heat-stable critical and semicritical instruments should be sterilized with a heat process. In dentistry, almost all reusable patient care items are heat-stable. If a critical item is not heat-stable, it should be replaced with one that is.

136. **To what does the term cold sterilization refer in dentistry?**

In dentistry, cold sterilization refers to the past practice of liquid chemical germicide disinfection by immersion used for reprocessing reusable semicritical instruments or items for patient care. The practice was not sterilization per se and is no longer considered appropriate for reprocessing heat-stable medical instruments. Almost every reusable dental instrument in current use is heat-stable and should be appropriately cleaned, wrapped, and sterilized between uses with a heat-based, biologically monitored process, such as a steam autoclave. Accordingly, the near-universal heat stability of dental instruments creates little justification or economic benefit for the use of other low-temperature sterilization procedures (e.g., with gases, such as ethylene oxide or vapor phase hydrogen peroxide).

137. **Should we still be using our glass bead sterilizer to sterilize endodontic files?**

The glass bead sterilizer has historically been used during endodontic procedures to decontaminate endodontic files while they are used on the same patient. It is not a sterilizer, and this designation is a long-standing misnomer in FDA classification.

Use only FDA-cleared medical devices for sterilization, and follow the manufacturer's instructions for correct use. Glass bead sterilizers should not be used for any instruments or devices that will be used on a patient.

138. **What is flash sterilization?**

In general, the CDC recommends that all reusable patient care items be packaged or wrapped for sterilization and remain packaged until the point of use.

- Flash sterilization, now termed *immediate-use sterilization*, is sterilizing items that are unwrapped or unpackaged.
- Immediate-use sterilization is a method for sterilizing unwrapped patient care items for immediate use.

The time required for an unwrapped sterilization cycle depends on the type of sterilizer and type of item (i.e., porous or nonporous) to be sterilized. The unwrapped cycle in tabletop sterilizers is preprogrammed by the manufacturer to a specific time and temperature setting and can include a drying phase at the end to produce a dry instrument, with much of the heat dissipated. If the drying phase requirements are unclear, the operation manual or manufacturer of the sterilizer should be consulted. If the unwrapped sterilization cycle in a steam sterilizer does not include a drying phase, or has only a minimal drying phase, items retrieved from the sterilizer will be hot and wet, making aseptic transport to the point of use more difficult. For dry heat and chemical vapor sterilizers, a drying phase is not required.

Unwrapped sterilization should be used only under certain conditions:

- Thorough cleaning and drying of instruments precede the unwrapped sterilization cycle.
- Mechanical monitors are checked and chemical indicators used for each cycle.
- Care is taken to avoid thermal injury to dental health care personnel (DHCP) or patients.
- Items are transported aseptically to the point of use to maintain sterility.

Because all implantable devices should be quarantined after sterilization until the results of biologic monitoring are known, unwrapped or flash sterilization of implantable items is not recommended.

Critical instruments that are sterilized unwrapped should be transferred immediately using aseptic technique from the sterilizer to the actual point of use. Critical instruments should not be stored unwrapped. Semicritical instruments that are sterilized unwrapped on a tray or in a container system should be used immediately or within a short time. When sterile items are open to the air, they will eventually become contaminated. Storage, even temporary, of unwrapped semicritical instruments is discouraged because it permits exposure to dust, airborne organisms, and other unnecessary contamination before use on a patient. A carefully written protocol for minimizing the risk of contaminating unwrapped instruments should be prepared and followed.

139. **What is the best way to reprocess a dental handpiece?**

Manufacturer's instructions should be followed. The instructions are specific to the manufacturer and model of the handpiece. The manufacturer's instructions for use verify that a handpiece is heat-stable and should be sterilized between each patient use. The manufacturer's instructions for use should also describe the steps for presterilization maintenance (e.g., cleaning, lubrication) and the most appropriate heat treatment method. All high- and slow-speed dental handpieces manufactured since the late 1980s are heat-stable; older handpieces, if still in working condition, may be modified to withstand heat sterilization. If not so modified, their use should be discontinued, and they should be replaced with heat-stable handpieces.

140. **Which federal agency is responsible for regulating high- and slow-speed dental handpieces?**

The FDA, Center for Devices and Radiological Health, Office of Device Evaluation, Dental and Medical Services Branch, in accordance with the Safe Medical Devices Act, clears medical devices, including sterilizers, for marketing. The user, however, must be aware that clearance to market proves neither efficacy nor manufacturer's claims.

141. **What is the minimal temperature required for sterilization by an autoclave?**

It is 250°F (121°C). Follow the manufacturer's instructions for time, temperature, and pressure parameters.

142. **What are some advantages and disadvantages of sterilization by steam heat under pressure (e.g., an autoclave)?**

Advantages

- Rapid process
- Does not require special ventilation
- Does not involve use or disposal of chemical agents; uses only distilled water
- Highly reliable when properly maintained and used according to manufacturer's instructions

Disadvantages

- Instrument cutting surfaces of carbide steel may become dulled if packages are not thoroughly dry on removal from the sterilizer.
- Carbide steel items may corrode and become dulled if packages are not thoroughly dry on removal from the sterilizer.

143. **In a forced air, dry heat oven preheated to 320° to 338°F (160°C-170°C), how long does it take to sterilize instruments?**

Sterilization is achieved in 2 hours in a properly working unit. However, additional time may be necessary for cool down before metal items can be used.

144. **What are some advantages and disadvantages of dry heat sterilizers?**

Advantages

- They do not dull or otherwise corrode instruments.
- They are equivalent to a steam autoclave in germicidal potency in a completed cycle.

Disadvantages
- The cycle time is long.
- Most plastics, paper, and fabrics char, melt, or burn and cannot be sterilized in this manner.

145. **What packaging material is compatible with autoclaves?**
The most suitable material for use in an autoclave is one that the steam can penetrate—for example, paper or certain plastics. It is best to read the manufacturer's instructions and follow them precisely. Only use packaging intended for use in the type of sterilizer you will be using.

146. **What packaging material cannot be used in dry heat sterilizers?**
The manufacturer's instructions specify that you cannot use most plastic pouches or wraps and paper wraps commonly used for steam autoclaves. They melt or burn at high temperatures.

147. **What packaging material is compatible with unsaturated chemical vapor sterilizers?**
The manufacturer's instructions make clear that perforated metal trays and paper are suitable for use in chemical vapor sterilizers. The vapor must be able to penetrate the material. Chemical vapor sterilizers also rely on high levels of heat and pressure for efficacy.

148. **What is an easy method to demonstrate that sterilization conditions have been reached in a cycle?**
External process indicators (on the outside of the instrument package or wrap) and internal chemical indicators or integrators (inside each package of instruments) demonstrate that some conditions to achieve sterilization were reached.

149. **What is the definition of sterile?**
The state of sterility is an absolute term—an item is sterile or it is not sterile. Sterility is the absence of all viable life forms; the term reflects a carefully designed and monitored process used to ensure that an item has a very low probability of being contaminated with anything at time of use. For surgical instruments, this probability is 1 in 1 million—that is, a sterility assurance level (SAL) of 10^{-6}.

150. **What are the most common reasons for sterilization failure in an autoclave?**
- Inadequate precleaning of instruments
- Improper maintenance of equipment
- Cycle time too short and/or temperature too low
- Improper loading or overloading
- Incompatible packaging material
- Interruption of a cycle to add or remove items

   NOTE: A number of investigations have found that the most frequent cause of sterilizer failure is human error.

151. **What types of sterilization monitoring are available?**
1. Mechanical, electronic
2. Chemical indicators (color change integrators)
3. Biologic indicators (spore tests)

152. **What is a mechanical or electronic monitor?**
These devices involve observation of gauges and indicators on the sterilization equipment (cycle monitors). They measure time, temperature, and pressure, for example.

153. **What is the difference between chemical indicators and biologic indicators (spore) monitors?**
Biologic indicators use nonpathogenic bacterial spores to verify that spore bacteria are killed. They more precisely reflect the potency of the sterilization process by directly measuring death of high numbers of highly resistant, but nonpathogenic, bacterial endospores. Simple chemical indicators merely reflect that the temperature of sterilization has been reached. Other chemical indicators (e.g., integrators) are more sophisticated and demonstrate time and temperature during the process. Chemical indicators, internal and external, use sensitive chemicals to assess physical conditions (e.g., time, temperature) during the sterilization process.

   Although chemical indicators do not prove that sterilization has been achieved, they allow for the detection of certain equipment malfunctions and can help identify procedural errors. External indicators applied to the outside of a package (e.g., chemical indicator tape, special markings) change color rapidly when a specific parameter is reached, and they verify that the package has been exposed to the sterilization process. Internal chemical indicators should be used inside each package to ensure that the sterilizing agent has penetrated the packaging material and has reached the instruments inside. A single-parameter internal chemical indicator provides information regarding only one sterilization parameter (e.g., time or temperature). Multiparameter internal chemical indicators are designed to react to two or more parameters (e.g., time and temperature, or time, temperature, and the presence of steam) and can provide a more reliable indication that sterilization conditions have been met. Multiparameter internal indicators are available only for steam sterilizers (autoclaves).

154. **What are the different types of chemical indicators?**

The CDC recommends a chemical indicator inside each pack of instruments, and on the outside if the indicator cannot be viewed from outside the package. Chemical indicators are usually heat- or chemical-sensitive inks that change color when one or more sterilization parameters (e.g., steam time, temperature, and/or saturated steam) are present. Chemical indicators have been grouped into six classes based on their ability to monitor one or multiple sterilization parameters (see later). If the internal and/or external indicator suggests inadequate processing, the item should not be used. An air removal test (e.g., Bowie-Dick test) must be performed daily in an empty dynamic air removal sterilizer (e.g., class B prevacuum steam sterilizer) to ensure air removal.

Specifically, a comprehensive guide to steam sterilization and sterility assurance in health care facilities Amendment 3 ANSI/AAMI ST79 has described the different classes of chemical indicators as follows:

- Class 1 (process indicators)—chemical indicators intended for use with individual units (e.g., packs, containers) to indicate that the unit has been exposed to the sterilization process and to distinguish between processed and unprocessed units.
- Class 2 (Bowie-Dick test indicators)—chemical indicators intended for use in a specific test procedure (e.g., the Bowie-Dick test used to determine if air removal has been adequate in a steam sterilization process).
- Class 3 (single-variable indicators)—chemical indicators designed to react to one of the critical variables and intended to indicate exposure to a sterilization process at a stated value of the chosen variable.
- Class 4 (multivariable indicators)—chemical indicators designed to react to two or more of the critical variables and intended to indicate exposure to a sterilization process at stated values of the chosen variables.
- Class 5 (integrating indicators)—chemical indicators designed to react to all critical variables, with the stated values having been generated to be equivalent to, or exceed, the performance requirements given in the ISO 11138 series for Biological Indicators (BIs), which are also sometimes referred to as biologic spore tests.
- Class 6 (emulating indicators)—chemical indicators designed to react to all critical variables of specified sterilization cycles, with the stated values having been generated from the critical variables of the specified sterilization process.

ANSI/AAMI/ISO 11140-1 refers to these indicators as cycle verification indicators. See Table 13-6.

155. **What should be done if the spore test is positive?**

The CDC Guidelines for Infection Control in Dental Health Care Settings (2003) recommended the following in the case of a positive spore test:

1. Remove the sterilizer from service and review sterilization procedures (e.g., work practices, use of mechanical and chemical indicators) to determine whether operator error could be responsible.
2. Retest the sterilizer by using biologic, mechanical, and chemical indicators after correcting any identified procedural problems.
3. If the repeat spore test is negative, and mechanical and chemical indicators are within normal limits, put the sterilizer back in service.

The following are recommended if the repeat spore test is positive:

1. Do not use the sterilizer until it has been inspected or repaired or the exact reason for the positive test has been determined.
2. Recall, to the extent possible, and reprocess all items processed since the last negative spore test.
3. Before placing the sterilizer back in service, rechallenge the sterilizer with biologic indicator tests in three consecutive empty chamber sterilization cycles after the cause of the sterilizer failure has been determined and corrected.

Maintain sterilization records (mechanical, and chemical, biologic) in compliance with state and local regulations.

156. **Which nonpathogenic organisms are used for biologic monitoring sterilization for each type of sterilization method?**

For autoclaves and chemical vapor sterilizers, *Geobacillus stearothermophilus* (formerly *Bacillus stearothermophilus*) spores are used. For dry heat and ethylene oxide units, *Bacillus atrophaeus* (formerly *Bacillus subtilis*) is used. Placement of the monitor in a load is critical; the manufacturer's instructions should be followed closely.

157. **How often should biologic monitoring of sterilization units be performed?**

- The 2008 CDC guidelines recommended use of "biologic indicators to monitor the effectiveness of sterilizers at least weekly with an FDA-cleared commercial preparation of spores intended specifically for the type and cycle parameters of the sterilizer."

Also, if a sterilizer is used frequently (e.g., several loads per day), daily use of biologic indicators allows earlier discovery of equipment malfunctions or procedural errors and thus minimizes the extent of patient surveillance and product recall needed in the event of a positive biologic indicator. Each load should be monitored if it contains implantable objects. If feasible, implantable items should not be used until the results of spore tests are known to be negative.

Table 13-6.

ANSI/AAMI/ ISO11140-1:2005	FDA GUIDANCE FOR INDUSTRY AND FDA STAFF*	FDA CONSENSUS STANDARD RECOGNITION	COMMENTS
Class 1—process indicators	Process indicators	Process indicators	Considered equivalent
Class 2—indicators for use in specific tests	Air removal indicators	Indicators for use in specific tests	No differences
Class 3—single-variable indicators	Not included	Class not part of consensus standard recognition by FDA	N/A
Class 4—multivariable indicators	Process indicators or chemical integrators	Not included	Some class 4 devices that can meet the recommended performance standards of the FDA and demonstrate substantial equivalence to a legally marketed chemical indicator may also be able to meet the performance requirements of a class 4 multivariable indicator.[†]
Class 5—integrating indicators	Chemical integrators	Class not part of consensus standard recognition by FDA	Some class 5 devices that can meet the recommended performance standards of the FDA and demonstrate substantial equivalence to a legally marketed chemical indicator may also be able to meet the performance requirements of a class 5 integrating indicator.[†]
Class 6—emulating indicators	Chemical integrators	Emulating indicators	Some class 6 devices that can meet the recommended performance standards of the FDA and demonstrate substantial equivalence to a legally marketed chemical indicator may also be able to meet the performance requirements of a class 6 emulating indicator.[†]

Also see ANSI/AAMI/ISO 15882 for information on the selection, use, and interpretation of chemical indicators. See also 10.5.2.

*At the date of this publication, FDA recognition of chemical indicators is limited to class 1 process indicators, class 2 indicators for use with special tests, and chemical integrators, which have resistance characteristics consistent with guidelines from the U.S. Food and Drug Administration (FDA): Premarket notification [510(k)] submissions for chemical indicators, 2003.

[†]As defined in ANSI/AAMI/ISO 11140-1:2005. Sterilization of health care products—chemical indicators. Part 1: general requirements, American National Standards Institute.

Adapted from American National Standards Institute (ANSI): Chemical indicator classifications: AAMI/ANSI ST79, amendment 3, ANSI, 2012, pp 233–235.

- ANSI/AAMI ST79 recommended the use of biologic indicators "within process challenge devices for routine sterilizer efficacy monitoring at least weekly, but preferably every day that the sterilizer is in use," along with every load that contains an implantable device.
- ARON recommended that "biological indicators should be used to monitor sterilizer efficacy. Efficacy monitoring should be performed at least weekly and preferably daily."

At a minimum, according to the CDC, biologic monitoring of sterilization units should be done on a weekly basis (Box 13-2).

158. **How should sterile packs of patient care items be stored?**
All sterile and disposable patient care items should be in enclosed storage areas that are clean and dry. Packages containing sterile supplies should be inspected before use to verify barrier integrity and dryness. Although some health care facilities continue to date every sterilized package and use shelf-life practices, other facilities have switched to event-related practices. This approach recognizes that the product should remain sterile indefinitely unless an event causes it to become contaminated (e.g., torn or wet packaging).

Even for event-related packaging, at a minimum, the date of sterilization should be placed on the package and, if multiple sterilizers are used in the facility, the sterilizer used should be indicated on the outside of the packaging material to facilitate the retrieval of processed items in the event of a sterilization failure. If packaging is compromised, the instruments should be recleaned, packaged in new wrap, and sterilized again.

HANDLING AND DISPOSAL OF DENTAL WASTE

159. **What constitutes regulated medical waste?**
Regulated medical waste includes, but is not limited to, items such as blood-soaked gauze or cotton rolls, tissue, and contaminated sharps. The definition of regulated medical waste varies based on state waste regulations. One should always consult their state regulatory agency for their definition of regulated waste. Contaminated sharps must be segregated and placed into an approved, color-coded or labeled, spillproof, and leakproof container. This container must be puncture-resistant and should be as close as possible to the area where sharps waste is generated. Containers should be considered as full when they are 75% full to avoid injury in overfilled containers. Regulated waste must be in labeled containers (biohazard label), and the transport and disposal must be by a licensed medical waste hauler. Again, a log of waste removal and receipts should be part of the record keeping.

160. **What are the categories of medical waste?**
There are two categories—nonregulated medical waste, which is not assumed to be infectious and can be disposed of in the regular trash, and regulated medical waste, which may pose a risk of infection during handling and disposal. Sharps must be handled according to disposal recommendations for sharps. It is important to note that although teeth are biologic waste, they are hazardous waste if they contain amalgam because of the toxic nature of amalgam. Hazardous waste must be managed differently.

161. **How should regulated medical waste be managed?**
There should be a written waste management program that defines regulated waste according to CDC recommendations and federal, state, or local laws. These require that appropriate containers be used that are properly labeled and leakproof. A color-coded (red) or labeled (biohazard warning) container may be used for nonsharp medical waste.

162. **Who regulates dental waste?**
OSHA regulates how the waste is handled in a dental facility by employees to ensure that they are protected from potential hazards associated with the waste. Federal, state, and local laws govern the disposal itself.

BOX 13-2 Indications for More Frequent Biologic Monitoring of Sterilization Units

1. If the equipment is new and being used for the first time
2. During the first operating cycle after a repair
3. If there is a change in packaging material
4. If new employees are using the unit or being trained in use of the equipment or procedure for monitoring
5. After an electrical or power source failure
6. If door seals or gaskets are changed
7. If cycle time and/or temperature is changed
8. Waste not to be processed in an instrument sterilizer
9. For all cycles to render infectious waste as noninfectious, as mandated by state law
10. If the method of biologic monitoring is changed

163. What is the intent of the Resource Conservation and Recovery Act (RCRA) of the U.S. Environmental Protection Agency (EPA)?

The intent of the RCRA is to hold the generator of a hazardous waste responsible for its ultimate disposal or treatment and for any clean-up costs associated with improper disposal. Each dentist, therefore, is responsible for ensuring proper disposal of waste, and improper disposal by an unscrupulous company is ultimately the responsibility of the dentist.

164. What is potentially infective waste?

It is waste contaminated by patient material and should be handled and disposed of accordingly.

165. Does the term contaminated refer to wet or dry materials, or both?

Contaminated refers to both wet and dry materials. For example, HBV can remain viable in dried materials for at least 7 days and perhaps longer. However, HBV is easily killed by moderate levels of heat or by a wide variety of chemical germicides, including low-level germicides.

166. Is all contaminated waste potentially infective waste?

No, but all infective waste is contaminated by definition. Some contaminated waste, although it contains potential pathogens, may not be of sufficient quantity or type to pose a reasonable threat of infection transmission.

167. What is toxic waste?

Toxic waste is capable of causing a poisonous effect.

168. What is hazardous waste?

This is waste that may pose a risk to individuals or the environment; it is regulated according to the type of hazardous waste, such as chemicals and materials. Hazardous waste is not necessarily biologic waste, but it can be. Toxic waste is a type of hazardous waste that may have a poisonous effect.

169. What are some examples of hazardous waste?

Some examples are spent fixer, lead foil, and amalgam. Although each is a hazardous waste and must be handled using proper PPE, their disposal is not the same. Therefore, it is necessary to segregate all waste, including medical waste, at chairside to ensure that it is disposed of properly.

170. If potentially infective waste is autoclaved, must you biologically monitor the cycle?

If you use heat sterilization equipment to treat potentially infective waste, most state regulations mandate that you must biologically monitor each waste load to ensure that the cycle was successfully completed. Each load must be labeled with a date and batch number so that if a sterilization failure occurs, the load can be retreated. Although required by many states, the merits of or necessity for this degree of monitoring is highly controversial among experts.

171. How is waste discarded?

Nonregulated medical waste may be disposed of with the general waste. Regulated medical waste disposal is governed by the EPA and possibly by state or local laws. Hazardous waste requires using a waste hauler with an appropriate license to dispose of or reclaim the materials depending on their nature. The U.S. Department of Transportation also has jurisdiction over waste haulers. All waste transported for disposal should be entered into a specific waste log, and receipts from the hauler should be part of record-keeping procedures.

172. Can blood be discarded in the sewer system?

If it is a sanitary sewer system and allowed by law, then blood can be discarded into the system. As with any other task that carries a risk of exposure, appropriate PPE should be worn.

173. What method should be used to dispose of potentially infective items such as gauze, extracted teeth, masks, and gloves?

Blood-soaked gauze, extracted teeth, and any other material contaminated by patient fluids, saliva, or blood should be considered potentially infective waste and disposed of according to federal, state, or local law.

174. What is the most appropriate method for disposal of used needles and sharps?

Although needles may be recapped by a one-hand technique or mechanical device, they should not be bent or broken or otherwise manipulated by hand. An appropriate sharps container should be used for disposal of all spent sharps and needles.

175. What is household waste?

Household waste is nonregulated and should be disposed of according to local requirements or regulations.

DENTAL WATER QUALITY

176. Is there concern about the microbial biofilm known to populate dental unit water lines?

Biofilm contamination of dental unit water lines (DUWLs), although not a new phenomenon, has received widespread attention from the media and scientific community. Numerous products are available that will control the growth of biofilm and proliferation of microorganisms present in DUWL. There are also test kits available to monitor the water quality of dental units. The American Dental Association has released a statement recognizing the microbial levels in DUWLs are not acceptable for the delivery of health care, and urging improvement of the amplified microbiologic quality of water through research, product development, and training. Other organizations, such as the CDC and Organization for Safety and Asepsis Procedures (OSAP), have issued guidelines for DUWLs. Current CDC guidelines recommend DUWL be maintained to ensure they meet the drinking water standard of no more than 500 colony forming units per mL of water.

177. **Have there been any documented cases of infection or disease in dental health care workers from microorganisms in DUWLs?**
Some published reports have suggested increased exposure of dental health care workers to *Legionella* bacteria from aerosolized DUW. DUW from an unmaintained dental unit may contain literally millions of bacteria and fungi per milliliter, many of them potential clinical pathogens. The lack of specific epidemiologic studies has prevented accurate assessment of the potential effect on public health. There has been one reported death of a patient linked to contaminated DUWL. To date, however, a major public health problem has not been identified.

178. **What is biofilm?**
Microbial biofilms are found almost anywhere that moisture and a suitable solid surface for bacterial attachment exist. Biofilms consist primarily of naturally occurring, slime-producing bacteria and fungi. These form microbial communities in the DUWL along the walls of small-bore plastic tubing in dental units that deliver coolant water from high-speed dental handpieces and air-water syringes. As water flows through the microbial matrix, some microorganisms may be released. Dental plaque is the best-known example of a biofilm.

179. **Where do the microorganisms come from?**
The vast majority are indigenous to house water mains. Patient microorganisms may be transient "tourists" in the biofilm.

180. **What conditions facilitate biofilm formation?**
Low numbers of microbes continually enter the DUWLs. They can be affected by nutrients in the incoming water, stagnation in the tubing, and the low flow rate near tubing walls. In addition, the small inside diameter of DUWLs results in a large surface-to-volume ratio, which presents optimal conditions for the growth of biofilm microorganisms, especially when the water sits stagnant.

181. **What are some suggested control measures?**
You can use independent reservoirs, chemical treatment, filtration, sterile water delivery systems, or combinations of these. The primary and perhaps most effective measure is routine monitoring (culturing), coupled with a regimen of chemical disinfection of the lines. Other strategies include improvement of the incoming water quality (e.g., sterile water in independent water reservoirs, heating, ultraviolet irradiation, filtering, constant low-level chemical treatment of incoming tap water) and controlling the microbial levels in the output water (e.g., filters).

182. **What is the purpose of flushing water lines?**
Current recommendations are to flush water lines for at least 2 minutes at the beginning of the clinic day and for at least 20 seconds between patients. This process does not remove biofilm, but it may transiently lower the levels of free-floating microorganisms in the water. Control of water line contamination requires a number of steps, such as chemical disinfection of the lines, sterile water source, specific filtration system in the water line, or a combination of these treatments. Only a chemical disinfection regimen done on a routine basis will remove or control biofilm formation. Filters, for example, remove only the free-floating microorganisms that originate from the biofilm.

183. **What is the purpose of an antiretraction valve?**
Its purpose is to prevent aspiration of patient material into water lines, thereby reducing the risk of transmission of potentially infective fluids or patient material from one patient to another.

184. **What should be done with the water supply on a dental unit when local health authorities issue a boil water notice after the quality of the public water supply is compromised?**
Use of the dental unit should be stopped if it is attached to the public water supply or if tap water is used to fill the bottle of an isolated water supply to the unit. Immediately contact the unit manufacturer for instructions on flushing and disinfecting the water lines. The use of house water should not resume until the boil water notice is lifted by the local authorities.

ACKNOWLEDGMENT

The authors gratefully acknowledge the contribution of the previous chapter author.

BIBLIOGRAPHY

Adams D, Bagg J, Limaye M, et al. A clinical evaluation of glove washing and re-use in dental practice. *J Hosp Infect.* 1992;20:153–162.
Agolini G, Russo A, Clementi M. Effect of phenolic and chlorine disinfectants on hepatitis C virus binding and infectivity. *Am J Infect Control.* 1999;27:236–239.

Allen AL, Organ RJ. Occult blood accumulation under the fingernails: A mechanism for the spread of blood-borne infection. *J Am Dent Assoc.* 1982;105:455–459.

American Dental Association. Infection control recommendations for the dental office and dental laboratory. *J Am Dent Assoc.* 1988;116:241–248.

Anderson HK, Fiehn NE, Larsen T. Effect of steam sterilization inside the turbine chambers of dental turbines. *Oral Surg Oral Med Oral Pathol Oral Radiol Endod.* 1999;87:184–188.

Association for the Advancement of Medical Instrumentation (AAMI). *American National Standards Institute (ANSI): Comprehensive Guide to Steam Sterilization and Sterility Assurance in Health Care Facilities—ANSI/AAMI ST79.* Arlington, VA: Association for the Advancement of Medical Instrumentation; 2017.

Association for the Advancement of Medical Instrumentation (AAMI). *American National Standards Institute (ANSI): Comprehensive Guide to Steam Sterilization and Sterility Assurance in Health Care Facilities—ANSI/AAMI ST79.* Amendment 3, Arlington, VA: Association for the Advancement of Medical Instrumentation; 2012.

Association of PeriOperative Registered Nurses (AORN). *Recommended Practices for Sterilization in the Perioperative Practice Setting.* Denver: AORN; 2012.

Brown AR, Papasian CJ, Shultz P, et al. Bacteremia and intraoral suture removal: can an antimicrobial rinse help? *J Am Dent Assoc.* 1998;129:1455–1461.

Burke FJT, Baggett FJ, Lomax AM. Assessment of the risk of glove puncture during oral surgery procedures. *Oral Surg Oral Med Oral Pathol Oral Radiol Endod.* 1996;82:18–21.

Burke FJT, Wilson NHF. The incidence of undiagnosed punctures in non-sterile gloves. *Br Dent J.* 1990;168:67–71.

Centers for Disease Control and Prevention (CDC). A comprehensive immunization strategy to eliminate transmission of hepatitis B virus infection in the United States: recommendations of the Advisory Committee on Immunization Practices (ACIP) part II: immunization of adults. *MMWR Recomm Rep.* 2006;55(RR-16). quiz.

Centers for Disease Control and Prevention (CDC). *Alert: Prevention of Needlestick Injuries in Health Care Settings;* 1999. https://www.cdc.gov/niosh/docs/2000-108/default.html.

Centers for Disease Control and Prevention (CDC). Guideline for hand hygiene in health-care settings: recommendations of the Healthcare Infection Control Practices Advisory Committee and the HICPAAC/SHEA/APIC/IDSA 2868 Hand Hygiene Task Force. *MMWR Recomm Rep.* 2002;51(RR-16):1–46,.

Centers for Disease Control and Prevention (CDC). Guidelines for environmental infection control in health-care facilities: recommendations of CDC and the Healthcare Infection Control Practices Advisory Committee (HICPAC). *MMWR Recomm Rep.* 2003;52(RR-10):1–42,.

Centers for Disease Control and Prevention (CDC). Guidelines for infection control in dental health-care settings—2003. *MMWR Recomm Rep.* 2003;52(RR-17):1–66,.

Centers for Disease Control and Prevention (CDC). Guidelines for preventing the transmission of *Mycobacterium tuberculosis* in health-care facilities. *MMWR Recomm Rep.* 1994;43(RR-13):1–132.

Centers for Disease Control and Prevention (CDC). *Hepatitis B Information for Health Professionals.* http://www.cdc.gov/hepatitis/HBV/HBVfaq.htm#overview. Accessed July 18, 2022.

Centers for Disease Control and Prevention (CDC). Hepatitis B virus: a comprehensive strategy for eliminating transmission in the United States through universal childhood vaccination. *MMWR Recomm Rep.* 1991;40(RR-13):1–25.

Centers for Disease Control and Prevention (CDC). *Hepatitis C Information for Health Professionals.* http://www.cdc.gov/hepatitis/HCV/HCVfaq.htm#b1. Accessed July 18, 2022.

Centers for Disease Control and Prevention (CDC). Immunization of health-care workers—recommendations of the Advisory Committee on Immunization Practices (ACIP) and the Hospital Infection Control Advisory Committee (HICPAC). *MMWR Recomm Rep.* 1997;46(RR-18):1–42.

Centers for Disease Control and Prevention (CDC). *Occupational HIV Transmission and Prevention Among Health Care Workers.* https://www.cdc.gov/hiv/pdf/workplace/cdc-hiv-healthcareworkers.pdf. Accessed June 8, 2023.

Centers for Disease Control and Prevention (CDC). *Occupational HIV Transmission and Prevention Among Health Care Workers.* https://www.cdc.gov/hiv/pdf/workplace/cdc-hiv-healthcareworkers.pdf. Accessed June 8, 2023.

Centers for Disease Control and Prevention (CDC). Public Health Service guidelines for the management of health-care worker exposure to HIV and recommendations for post exposure prophylaxis. *MMWR Recomm Rep.* 1998;47(RR-7):1–33.

Centers for Disease Control and Prevention (CDC). Recommendations for preventing transmission of human immunodeficiency virus and hepatitis B virus to patients during exposure-prone invasive procedures. *MMWR Recomm Rep.* 1991;40(RR-8):1–9.

Centers for Disease Control and Prevention (CDC). Recommendations for prevention and control of hepatitis C (HCV) infection and HCV-related chronic disease. *MMWR Recomm Rep.* 1998;47(RR-19):1–38.

Centers for Disease Control and Prevention (CDC). Recommendations for prevention of HIV transmission in health-care settings. *MMWR Morb Mortal Wkly Rep.* 1987;36(Suppl 2S):1S–18S.

Centers for Disease Control and Prevention (CDC). *Selecting, Evaluating, and Using Sharps Disposal Containers.* http://www.cdc.gov/niosh/docs/97-111 accessed 6.8.2023.

Centers for Disease Control and Prevention (CDC). *Summary of infection prevention practices in dental settings: basic expectations for safe care,* 2016.

Centers for Disease Control and Prevention (CDC). Updated U.S. Public Health Service guidelines for the management of occupational exposures to HBV, HCV, and HIV and recommendations for postexposure prophylaxis. *MMWR Recomm Rep.* 2001;50(RR-11):1–52.

Centers for Disease Control and Prevention (CDC). Updated U.S. Public Health Service guidelines for the management of occupational exposures to HIV and recommendations for postexposure prophylaxis. *MMWR Recomm Rep.* 2005;54(RR-09):1–17.

Centers for Disease Control and Prevention (CDC). *Vital Signs, New Hope for Stopping HIV: Testing and Medical Care Save Lives.* http://www.cdc.gov/VitalSigns/HIVtesting/index.html. Accessed July 18, 2022.

Centers for Disease Control and Prevention (CDC). *Guideline for Disinfection and Sterilization in Healthcare Facilities;* 2008. Update: May 2019. https://www.cdc.gov/infectioncontrol/guidelines/disinfection/index.htm. Accessed June 8, 2023.

Centers for Disease Control and Prevention (CDC). *Interim infection prevention and control recommendations for healthcare personnel during the coronavirus disease 2019 (COVID-19) pandemic,* 2022. https://www.cdc.gov/coronavirus/2019-ncov/hcp/infection-control.html. Accessed June 8, 2023.

Centers for Disease Control and Prevention (CDC). *Guidance for evaluating Health-care Personnel for Hepatitis B Virus Protection and for Administering Postexposure Management Recommendations and Reports*, 2013/62(rr10);1–19. http://www.cdc.gov/mmwr/preview/mmwrhtml/rr6210a1.htm?s_cid=rr6210a1_w. Accessed July 18, 2022.

Centers for Disease Control and Prevention (CDC). *Healthcare-associated hepatitis B and C outbreaks reported to the Centers for Disease Control and Prevention (CDC) in 2008–2019*. http://www.cdc.gov/hepatitis/statistics/healthcareoutbreaktable.htm. Accessed July 18, 2022.

Centers for Disease Control and Prevention (CDC), *Division of Healthcare Quality Promotion: Guide to Infection Prevention for Outpatient Settings: Minimum Expectations for Safe Care*. https://www.cdc.gov/infectioncontrol/pdf/outpatient/guide.pdf. Accessed July 18, 2022.

Centers for Disease Control and Prevention (CDC). *Tb screening and testing of health care personnel*. 2022. https://www.cdc.gov/tb/topic/testing/healthcareworkers.htm.

Checchi L, Montebugnoli L, Boschi S, Achille CD. Influence of dental glove type on the penetration of liquid through experimental perforations: a spectrophotometric analysis. *Quintessence Int.* 1994;25:647–649.

Checchi L, Montebugnoli L, Samaritani S. Contamination of the turbine air chamber: a risk of cross infection. *J Clin Periodontal.* 1998;25:607–611.

Chin G, Chong J, Kluczewska A, Lau A, et al. The environmental effects of dental amalgam. *Aust Dent J.* 2000;45:246–249.

Chua KL, Taylor GS, Bagg J. A clinical and laboratory evaluation of three types of operating gloves for use in orthodontic practice. *Br J Orthod.* 1996;23:115–220.

Cleveland JL, Robison VA, Panlilio AL. Tuberculosis epidemiology, diagnosis and infection control recommendations for dental settings. An update on the Centers for Disease Control and Prevention Guidelines. *J Am Dent Assoc.* 2009;140(9):1092–1099.

Conly J, Hill S, Ross J, et al. Handwashing practices in an intensive care unit: The effects of an educational program and its relationship to infection rates. *Am J Infect Control.* 1989;17:330–339.

Cristina ML, Spagnolo AM, Sartini M, et al. Evaluation of the risk of infection through exposure to aerosols and spatters in dentistry. *Am J Infect Control.* 2008;36:304–307.

Danforth D, Nicolle LE, Hume K, et al. Nosocomial infections on nursing units with floors cleaned with a disinfectant compared with detergent. *J Hosp Infect.* 1987;19:515–518.

Dharan S, Mourouga P, Copin P, et al. Routine disinfection of patients' environmental surfaces. Myth or reality? *J Hosp Infect.* 1999;42:113–117.

Epstein JB, Rea G, Sibau L, et al. Assessing viral retention and elimination in rotary dental instruments. *J Am Dent Assoc.* 1995;126:87–92.

Fine DH, Furgang D, et al. Assessing pre-procedural subgingival irrigation and rinsing with an antiseptic mouth rinse to reduce bacteremia. *J Am Dent Assoc.* 1996;127:641–646.

Fine DS, Yip J, Furgang D, et al. Reducing bacteria in dental aerosols: pre-procedural use of an antiseptic mouthrinse. *J Am Dent Assoc.* 1993;124:56–58.

Garner JS. Hospital Infection Control Practices Advisory Committee: Guideline for isolation precautions in hospitals. *Infect Control Hosp Epidemiol.* 1996;17:53–80.

Garner JS, Favero MS. Guideline for handwashing and hospital environmental control. *Infect Control.* 1986;7:231–243.

Giglio JA, Roland RW, Laskin DM, Grenevicki L. The use of sterile versus nonsterile gloves during out-patient exodontia. *Quintessence Int.* 1993;24:543–545.

Gonzalez E, Naleway C. Assessment of the effectiveness of glove use as a barrier technique in the dental operatory. *J Am Dent Assoc.* 1988;117:467–469.

Griffiths PA, Babb JR, Fraise AP. Mycobactericidal activity of selected disinfectants using a quantitative suspension test. *J Hosp Infect.* 1999;41:111–121.

Harrel SK, Barnes JB, Rivera-Hidalgo F. Aerosol and splatter contamination from the operative site during ultrasonic scaling. *J Am Dent Assoc.* 1998;129:1241–1249.

Harrel SK, Molinari J. Aerosols and splatter in dentistry; a brief review of the literature and infection control implications. *J Am Dent Assoc.* 2004;135:429–437.

Harte JA, Molinari JA. In: *Practical Infection Control in Dentistry.* Philadelphia: Lippincott Williams & Wilkins; 2010:221–231.

HCV Guidance. Recommendations for Testing, Managing, and Treating Hepatitis C, *Infectious Diseases Society of America, American Association for the Study of Liver Diseases*. https://www.hcvguidelines.org/. Accessed June 8, 2023.

Healthcare Infection Control Practices Advisory Committee. Guideline for Disinfection and Sterilization in Healthcare Facilities. https://www.cdc.gov/infectioncontrol/pdf/guidelines/disinfection-guidelines-H.pdf.

Healthcare Infection Control Practices Advisory Committee. *Core Infection Prevention and Control Practices for Safe Healthcare Delivery in All Settings—Recommendations of the Healthcare Infection Control Practices Advisory Committee (HICPAC)*; 2017. Reviewed December 27, 2018.

Hedderwick SA, McNeil SA, Lyons MJ, Kauffman CA. Pathogenic organisms associated with artificial fingernails worn by healthcare workers. *Infect Control Hosp Epidemiol.* 2000;21:505–509.

Hokett SD, Honey JY, Ruiz F, et al. Assessing the effectiveness of direct digital radiography barrier sheaths and finger cots. *J Am Dent Assoc.* 2000;131:463–467.

Hubar JS, Oeschger MP. Optimizing efficiency of radiograph disinfection. *Gen Dent Jul.* 1995;43:360–362.

Huntley DE, Campbell J. Bacterial contamination of scrub jackets during dental hygiene procedures. *J Dent Hyg.* 1998;72:19–23.

Jordan SLP, Stowers MF, Trawick EG, Theis AB. Glutaraldehyde permeation: choosing the proper glove. *Am J Infect Control.* 1996;24:67–69.

Klyn SL, Cummings DE, Richardson BW, Davis RD. Reduction of bacteria-containing spray produced during ultrasonic scaling. *Gen Dent.* 2001;49:648–652.

Kolstad RA. How well does the Chemiclave sterilize handpieces? *J Am Dent Assoc.* 1998;129:985–991.

Kuhar DT, Henderson DK, Struble KA, et al. US Public Health Service Working Group: Updated US Public Health Service guidelines for the management of occupational exposures to human immunodeficiency virus and recommendations for postexposure prophylaxis. *Infect Control Hosp Epidemiol.* 2013;34:875–892.

Larsen PE. The effect of chlorhexidine rinse on the incidence of alveolar osteitis following the surgical removal of impacted mandibular third molars. *J Oral Maxillofac Surg.* 1991;49:932–937.

Larson EL. APIC guideline for hand washing and hand antisepsis in health care settings. *Am J Infect Control*. 1995;23:251–269.

Leonard DL, Charlton DG. Performance of high-speed dental handpieces subjected to simulated clinical use and sterilization. *J Am Dent Assoc*. 1999;130:1301–1311.

Lewis DL, Arens M. Resistance of microorganisms to disinfection in dental and medical devices. *Nat Med*. 1995;1:956–958.

Lewis DL, Boe RK. Cross-infection risks associated with current procedures for using high-speed dental handpieces. *J Clin Microbiol*. 1992;30:401–406.

Litsky BY, Mascis JD, Litsky W. Use of an antimicrobial mouthwash to minimize the bacterial aerosol contamination generated by the high-speed drill. *Oral Surg Oral Med Oral Pathol*. 1970;29:25–30.

Lockhart PB. An analysis of bacteremias during dental extractions: a double-blind, placebo-controlled study of chlorhexidine. *Arch Intern Med*. 1995;156:513–520.

Logothetis DD, Martinez-Welles JM. Reducing bacterial aerosol contamination with a chlorhexidine gluconate pre-rinse. *J Am Dent Assoc*. 1995;126:1634–1639.

Macdonald G. Can the thermal disinfector outperform the ultrasonic cleaner? *J Am Dent Assoc*. 1996;127:1787–1788.

Mangram A, Horan T, Pearson M, et al. Guideline for prevention of surgical site infection, 1999. Hospital Infection Control Practices Advisory Committee. *Infect Control Hosp Epidemiol*. 1999;20:247–278.

Mann GLB, Campbell TL, Crawford JJ. Backflow in low-volume suction lines: the impact of pressure changes. *J Am Dent Assoc*. 1996;127:611–615.

Martin MV, Dunn HM, Field EA, et al. A physical and microbiological evaluation of the re-use of non-sterile gloves. *Br Dent J*. 1988;165:321–324.

Miller CH, Palenik CJ. *Infection Control and Management of Hazardous Materials for the Dental Team*. 4th ed. St. Louis: Mosby; 2010.

Miller CH, Palenik CJ. Sterilization, Disinfection, and Asepsis in Dentistry. In: Block SS, ed. *Disinfection, Sterilization, and Preservation*. 5th ed. Philadelphia: Lippincott Williams & Wilkins; 2001.

Miller CH, Waskow JR, Rigen SD, Gaines DJ. Justification for heat-sterilizing air-driven slow-speed handpiece motors between patients. *J Dent Res*. 1996;75:415.

Monticello MV, Gaber DJ. Glove resistance to permeation by a 7.5% hydrogen peroxide sterilizing and disinfecting solution. *Am J Infect Control*. 1999;27:364–366.

Morrison A, Conrod S. Dental burs and endodontic files: are routine sterilization procedures effective? *J Can Dent Assoc*. 2009;75(1):39.

Olsen RJ, Lynch P, Coyle MB, et al. Examination gloves as barriers to hand contamination in clinical practice. *JAMA*. 1993;270:350–353.

Parker HH. 4th, Johnson RB. Effectiveness of ethylene oxide for sterilization of dental handpieces. *J Dent*. 1995;23:113–115.

Patton L, Campbell TL, Evers SP. Prevalence of glove perforations during double-gloving for dental procedures. *Gen Dent*. 1995;43:22–26.

Perkaki K, Mellor AC, Qualtrough AJE. Comparison of an ultrasonic cleaner and a washer disinfector in the cleaning of endodontic files. *J Hosp Infect*. 2007;67:355–359.

Pippin DJ, Verderame RA, Weber KK. Efficacy of face masks in preventing inhalation of airborne contaminants. *J Oral Maxillofac Surg*. 1987;45:319–323.

Pratt LH, Smith DG, Thornton RH, et al. The effectiveness of two sterilization methods when different pre-cleaning techniques are employed. *J Dent*. 1999;27:247–248.

Redd JT, Baumbach J, Kohn W, et al. Patient-to-patient transmission of hepatitis B virus associated with oral surgery. *J Infect Dis*. 2007;195:1311–1314.

Rego A, Roley L. In-use barrier integrity of gloves: Latex and nitrile superior to vinyl. *Am J Infect Control*. 1999;27:405–410.

Richards JM, Sydiskis RJ, Davidson WM, et al. Permeability of latex gloves after contact with dental materials. *Am J Orthod Dentofac Orthop*. 1993;103:224–229.

Richter FL, Cords BR. Formulation of sanitizers and disinfectants. In: Block SS, ed. *Disinfection, sterilization and preservation*. 5th ed. Philadelphia: Lippincott Williams & Wilkins; 2001:473–487.

Rutala WA, Weber DJ. Healthcare Infection Control Practices Advisory Committee: Guideline for disinfection and sterilization in healthcare facilities, 2008. *Am J Infect Control*. 2013;41(5 Suppl):S67–S71.

Sagripanti JL, Eklund CA, Trost PA, et al. Comparative sensitivity of 13 species of pathogenic bacteria to seven chemical germicides. *Am J Infect Control*. 1997;25:335–339.

Salisbury DM, et al. The effect of rings on microbial load of health care workers' hands. *Am J Infect Control*. 1997;25:24–27.

Sanchez E, Macdonald G. Decontaminating dental instruments: testing the effectiveness of selected methods. *J Am Dent Assoc*. 1995;126:359–362.

Schwimmer A, Massoumi M, Barr C. Efficacy of double gloving to prevent inner glove perforation during outpatient oral surgical procedures. *J Am Dent Assoc*. 1994;125:196–198.

Sehulster L, Chinn R, CDC. HICPAC: Guidelines for environmental infection control in health-care facilities. Recommendations of CDC and the Healthcare Infection Control Practices Advisory Committee (HICPAC). *MMWR Recomm Rep*. 2003;52(RR-10):1–42.

Siegel JD, Rhinehart E, Jackson M, Chiarello L; Healthcare Infection Control Practices Advisory Committee. *2007 Guideline for Isolation Precautions: Preventing Transmission of Infectious Agents in Healthcare Settings*. https://www.cdc.gov/infectioncontrol/pdf/guidelines/isolation-guidelines-H.pdf.

Silverstone SE, Hill DE. Evaluation of sterilization of dental handpieces by heating in synthetic compressor lubricant. *Gen Dent*. 1999;47:158–160.

Spaulding EH. Chemical disinfection and antisepsis in the hospital. *J Hosp Res*. 1972;9:5–31.

Strausbaugh L, Jackson M, Rhinehart E, Siegel J. *HICPAC: Guideline to Prevent Transmission of Infectious Agents in Healthcare Settings*; 2002. https://www.osha.gov/laws-regs/regulations/standardnumber/1910/1910.1030. Accessed June 8, 2023.

Toledo-Pereyra LH. Joseph Lister's surgical revolution. *J Invest Surg*. 2010;23:241–243.

Tzukert AA, Leviner E, Sela M. Prevention of infective endocarditis: not by antibiotics alone. *Oral Surg Oral Med Oral Pathol Oral Radiol Endod*. 1986;62:385–388.

U.S Safety and Health Administration (OSHA). *How to Prevent Needlestick Injuries: Answers to Some Important Questions,* Washington, DC, U.S. Safety and Health Administration. https://www.cdc.gov/niosh/newsroom/feature/needlestick_disposal.html#:~:text=Using%20devices%20with%20safety%20features%20provided%20by%20your%20employer,and%20appropriate%20sharps%20disposal%20containers. Accessed June 8, 2023.

U.S Safety and Health Administration (OSHA). *Occupational Exposure to Bloodborne Pathogens; Needlesticks and Other Sharps Injuries; final rule.* https://www.osha.gov/laws-regs/regulations/standardnumber/1910/1910.1030; https://www.osha.gov/personal-protective-equipment.

U.S. Food and Drug Administration (FDA). *Evaluation of Automatic Class III Designation (de novo) Summaries*; 2013. http://www.fda.gov/aboutfda/centersoffices/officeofmedicalproductsandtobacco/cdrh/cdrhtransparency/ucm232269.html.

U.S. Food and Drug Administration (FDA). *FDA News Release—FDA Permits Marketing of Quicker Method for Checking Effectiveness of Medical Device Steam Sterilization.* https://www.osha.gov/laws-regs/standardinterpretations/2016-05-09.

U.S. Food and Drug Administration (FDA). *FDA Supplementary Guidance on the Content of Premarket Notification [510(k)] Submissions for Medical Devices With Sharps Injury Prevention Features.* Rockville, MD: U.S. Food and Drug Administration; 1995.

U.S. Safety and Health Administration (OSHA). *Enforcement procedures for the occupational exposure to bloodborne pathogens.* 2001. https://www.osha.gov/sites/default/files/enforcement/directives/CPL_02-02-069.pdf.

Upton LG, Barber HD. Double-gloving and the incidence of perforations during specific oral and maxillofacial surgical procedures. *J Oral Maxillofac Surg.* 1993;51:261–263.

Wasley A, Kruszon-Moran D, Kuhnert W, et al. The prevalence of hepatitis B virus infection in the United States in the era of vaccination. *J Infect Dis.* 2010;202:192–201.

Watson CM, Whitehouse RLS. Possibility of cross-contamination between dental patients by means of the saliva ejector. *J Am Dent Assoc.* 1993;124:77–80.

Weber DJ, Barbee SL, Sobsey MD, Rutala WA. The effect of blood on the antiviral activity of sodium hypochlorite, a phenolic, and a quaternary ammonium compound. *Infect Control Hosp Epidemiol.* 1999;20:821–827.

Williams GT, Denyer SP, Hosein IK, et al. Limitations of the efficacy of surface disinfection in the healthcare setting. *Infect Control Hosp Epidemiol.* 2009;30:570–573.

Zaragoza M, Salles M, Gomez J, et al. Handwashing with soap or alcoholic solutions? A randomized clinical trial of its effectiveness. *Am J Infect Control.* 1999;27:258–261.

CHAPTER 14

DENTAL PUBLIC HEALTH

Athanasios Zavras, Edward S. Peters

If you do not have oral health, you're simply not healthy.
—C. Everett Koop, former U.S. Surgeon General

THE ART AND SCIENCE OF PUBLIC HEALTH

1. **What is the definition of public health and what are the core sciences of public health?**
   The World Health Organization defines public health as "all organized measures (whether public or private) to prevent disease, promote health, and prolong life among the population as a whole." The core sciences of public health are:
   - Epidemiology, the science of measuring disease levels in the population and identifying determinants of health and risk factors for disease
   - Biostatistics, the science of designing research and analyzing data to extract actionable, impactful knowledge
   - Environmental Health, the science of identifying how the environment, natural or built, affects health
   - Behavioral Sciences, the science of how we make decisions and how to achieve behavioral change at the population level
   - Health care Management and Economics, the science of "building" and maintaining an effective, efficient, and sustainable health care system that is able to serve everyone as well as contribute positively to the economy

2. **What are the 12 principles of the ethical practice of public health?**
   1. Public health should address principally the fundamental causes of disease and requirements for health, aiming to prevent adverse health outcomes.
   2. Public health should achieve community health in a way that respects the rights of individuals in the community.
   3. Public health policies, programs, and priorities should be developed and evaluated through processes that ensure an opportunity for input from community members.
   4. Public health should advocate and work for the empowerment of disenfranchised community members, aiming to ensure that the basic resources and conditions necessary for health are accessible to all.
   5. Public health should seek the information needed to implement effective policies and programs that protect and promote health.
   6. Public health institutions should provide communities with the information they have that is needed for decisions on policies or programs and should obtain the community's consent for their implementation.
   7. Public health institutions should act in a timely manner on the information they have within the resources and the mandate given to them by the public.
   8. Public health programs and policies should incorporate a variety of approaches that anticipate and respect diverse values, beliefs, and cultures in the community.
   9. Public health programs and policies should be implemented in a manner that most enhances the physical and social environment.
   10. Public health institutions should protect the confidentiality of information that can bring harm to an individual or community if made public. Exceptions must be justified on the basis of the high likelihood of significant harm to the individual or others.
   11. Public health institutions should ensure the professional competence of their employees.
   12. Public health institutions and their employees should engage in collaborations and affiliations in ways that build the public's trust and the institution's effectiveness.

3. **Is access to health care a universal human right?**
   Depending on the part of the world that one resides, the answer differs. For most countries, access to needed health care services is indeed a basic human right, similar to access to free education. In the United States, this topic is controversial and constantly debated. For some, it is a privilege reserved for those who contribute financially to the economy via taxes or other direct health insurance contributions. For others, it is a basic human right irrespective of ability to pay. The Declaration of Human Rights, first published in 1948 under the auspices of the United Nations mentions health in Article 25, as follows:

UN Declaration of Human Rights Article 25

1. Everyone has the right to a standard of living adequate for the health and well-being of himself and of his family, including food, clothing, housing and medical care and necessary social services, and the right to security in the event of unemployment, sickness, disability, widowhood, old age or other lack of livelihood in circumstances beyond his control.
2. Motherhood and childhood are entitled to special care and assistance. All children, whether born in or out of wedlock, shall enjoy the same social protection.

4. **What is the WHO International Classification of Functioning, Disability and Health (ICF)? Why is the ICF important for public health?**

   ICF belongs to the "family" of international classifications developed by the World Health Organization (WHO) aimed to provide a framework to code a wide range of information about health (e.g., diagnosis, functioning and disability, reasons for contact with health services).

   The overall goal of the ICF classification is to provide a unified and standard language and framework for the description of health and health-related states. It defines components of health and some health-related components of well-being (such as education and labor). The domains contained in ICF can, therefore, be seen as health domains and health-related domains. These domains are described from the perspective of the body, the individual, and society in two basic lists: (1) Body Functions and Structures; and (2) Activities and Participation. As a classification, ICF systematically groups different domains for a person in a given health condition (e.g., what a person with a disease or disorder does or can do). Functioning is an umbrella term encompassing all body functions, activities, and participation; similarly, disability serves as an umbrella term for impairments, activity limitations, or participation restrictions. ICF also lists environmental factors that interact with all these constructs. In this way, it enables the user to record useful profiles of individuals' functioning, disability, and health in various domains.

   ICF redefines the concepts of health and health-related abilities. It introduces the social model of disability as a replacement of the surgical model that was based primarily and brings to light conditions that affect one's ability to function as an individual and member of society.

5. **What are the two global public health treaties that have been ratified by the majority of country members of the United Nations?**

   a. **Framework Convention on Tobacco Control.** The WHO Framework Convention on Tobacco Control (WHO FCTC) is the first international treaty negotiated under the auspices of WHO. It was adopted by the World Health Assembly on May 21, 2003 and entered into force on February 27, 2005. It has since become one of the most rapidly and widely embraced treaties in United Nations history. It aims to tackle some of the causes of that epidemic, including complex factors with cross-border effects, such as trade liberalization and direct foreign investment, tobacco advertising, promotion and sponsorship beyond national borders, and illicit trade in tobacco products. The WHO FCTC was developed in response to the globalization of the tobacco epidemic and is an evidence-based treaty that reaffirms the right of all people to the highest standard of health. The Convention represents a milestone for the promotion of public health and provides new legal dimensions for international health cooperation.

   b. **Minamata Convention on Mercury.** Established in 2013 and entered into force on August 16, 2017, on the 90th day after the date of deposit of the 50th instrument of ratification, acceptance, approval, or accession. The Minamata Convention on Mercury is a global treaty to protect human health and the environment from the adverse effects of mercury. The Convention includes a ban on new mercury mines, the phase-out of existing ones, the phase-out and phase-down of mercury use in a number of products and processes, control measures on emissions to air and on releases to land and water, and the regulation of the informal sector of artisanal and small-scale gold mining. The Convention also addresses interim storage of mercury and its disposal once it becomes waste, sites contaminated by mercury as well as health issues.

6. **Describe the U.S. Occupational Safety and Health Administration (OSHA) and its role in dental practice.**

   The mission of OSHA is to ensure the safety and health of U.S. workers. As part of the Department of Labor, OSHA and the states that operate OSHA-approved state plans establish guidelines and standards to promote worker safety and health that apply to every workplace, including medical and dental offices. The work practice control, engineering control, and personal protective equipment regulations are examples of OSHA safety topics that have a direct impact on dental infection control. The regulations designed to protect the dental health care worker often translate into increased safety for the dental patient.

7. **What are primary, secondary, and tertiary prevention?**

   Primary prevention involves health services that provide health promotion and protection, with the goal of preventing the development of disease. Examples are community-based fluoridation for caries prevention and smoking cessation programs.

   Secondary prevention includes services that are provided once the disease is present to prevent further progression. These services include dental restorations and oral cancer screening.

Tertiary prevention services are provided when disease has advanced to the point where loss of function or life may occur. Definitive surgery or radiation therapy to treat oral cancer and extractions of diseased teeth to eliminate infection are examples.

8. **What is oral health promotion?**

Health promotion is a set of educational, economic, and environmental incentives to support behavioral changes that lead to better health. On the individual level, oral health promotion involves improvements in oral hygiene practices, achieving a healthy diet and balanced nutrition, and abstaining from high-risk activities. Examples of health-promoting activities in the community include community water fluoridation, salt fluoridation, supervised oral hygiene programs at schools, and sealant programs.

9. **Define health disparities..**

The National Institutes of Health has defined health disparities as the "differences in the incidence, prevalence, mortality, and burden of diseases and other adverse health conditions that exist among specific population groups in the United States." Health disparities may occur because of various reasons, such as poverty, unequal access to health care, lower educational attainment, racism, social networks, geographic location (neighborhoods), and social stigma.

10. **How do disparities affect oral health?**

There are substantial differences in oral health concerning clinical conditions, awareness of treatment options, treatment recommendations, access to care, and treatment received by different socioeconomic, racial, and ethnic groups. In general, individuals from higher socioeconomic strata tend to have better oral health outcomes and better access to care. Individuals belonging to minority populations or those living in poverty tend to have higher rates of disease, access impediments, and lower dental service utilization. Social determinants of health (SDOH) such as low employment levels, neighborhood level of violence, and lack of nutritious foods in food deserts complicate the individual's health behavior and often prove more difficult to tackle.

One of the success stories of dental public health in reducing health disparities is the reduction of childhood dental caries across all racial and socioeconomic groups in the 2000s, along with significant improvements in access. This success has been linked to universal expansion of dental insurance coverage for children via the Affordable Care Act (ACA), proving a cause-and-effect between ability to pay and health. However, as ACA did not address funding for adult dental care, disparity statistics in adults continue to rise.

11. **How do you define social determinants of health and what are some examples?**

SDOH are conditions in the places where people live, learn, work, and play that affect a wide range of health risks and outcomes. While traditional epidemiology has focused on identifying and controlling individual risk factors for disease, such as smoking or heavy alcohol consumption, social epidemiology focuses on risk factors beyond the individual's immediate control. For example, food deserts are areas where access to quality food such as fruits and vegetables is limited. Individuals that live in food deserts may have poor diet, such as consumption of processed food, as a result of such limited access and not as a personal choice.

Another example of a social determinant of health is institutionalized racial discrimination. Research suggests that conditions of exclusion and discrimination cause increased stress for the excluded individual that eventually lead to biological response as increased inflammatory markers that are associated with obesity or heart disease.

Healthy People 2030 uses a place-based framework that outlines five key areas of SDOH:
- Health care access and quality
- Education access and quality
- Social and community context
- Economic stability
- Neighborhood and built environment

Realizing the strong biological consequences of unchecked social determinants of health has led medical and dental schools to adopt innovations in the curriculum to focus on SDOH control. A dentist able to perform technical procedures must be equally comfortable in advocating and exercising leadership in the implementation of the Healthy People 2030 objectives in their community. One such objective is NWS-01, which reduces household food insecurity and hunger from the current 11% of households (with food insecurity or hunger) to a target of 6%.

12. **Before the implementation of any community-based program, the process of planning and evaluation is necessary. What are the basic steps involved in planning for a program?**

Planning involves making choices to achieve specific objectives. Thus, a planner should perform needs assessment, review and prioritize alternative programs and solutions, assess the effectiveness and feasibility of the program under consideration, examine the community to determine if the program is needed, involve key stakeholders, secure financial and human resources and initiate the process to implement the program. Program evaluation should be designed prior to implementation based on SMART metrics. SMART stands for **S**pecific, **M**easurable, **A**chievable, **R**elevant, and **T**ime-bound. During program implementation, the evaluation process must be ongoing in real time and able to address problems rapidly.

13. **What skills must someone have before managing dental public health programs?**
    The implementation of a public health program requires such skills as strategic planning, needs assessment, negotiating with key stakeholders, operational acumen, social marketing, communications, human resources management, financial planning and management, evaluation, and quality assurance.

14. **What is Dental Public Health?**
    Dental Public Health is the science and art of preventing and controlling dental diseases and promoting dental health through organized community efforts. It is that form of dental practice that serves the community as a patient rather than the individual. It is concerned with the dental health education of the public, with applied dental research, and with the administration of group dental care programs, as well as the prevention and control of dental diseases on a community basis. Implicit in this definition is the requirement that the specialist has broad knowledge and skills in public health administration, research methodology, the prevention and control of oral diseases, and the delivery and financing of oral health care.

15. **What basic knowledge should general dentists have in dental public health?**
    According to the American Association of Public Health Dentistry (AAPHD), a dental public health curriculum during dental education has the potential to increase the number of providers who can respond to the public's unmet needs and challenges, both in private practices and publicly supported clinics.
       AAPHD-listed eight dental public health competencies (HRSA-funded project):
    1. Demonstrate the ability to incorporate ethical reasoning and actions that promote culturally competent oral health care to individuals and populations.
    2. Critique, synthesize and apply information from scientific and lay sources to improve the public's oral health.
    3. Describe social and health care systems and determinants of health and their impact on the oral health of the individual and population.
    4. Assess risk for oral diseases and select appropriate, evidence-based preventive interventions and strategies to promote health and control oral diseases at the individual and population level.
    5. Demonstrate the ability to access and describe the use of population-based health data for health promotion, patient care, and quality improvement.
    6. Demonstrate the ability to communicate and collaborate with relevant stakeholders to advocate for policies that impact oral and general health for individuals or populations.
    7. Develop a capacity for lifelong learning and professional growth in order to provide leadership that utilizes principles of dental public health.
    8. Demonstrate the ability to participate in inter-professional care across the lifespan of people from diverse communities and cultures.

16. **What are the core competencies of the Dental Public Health Specialty?**
    Dental Public Health is one of the twelve recognized specialties of Dentistry. The practice of Dental Public Health focuses on the oral health needs of populations and communities. The specialty includes activities such as public health surveillance, conducting research in epidemiology or health services research, development and administration of public health programs, program evaluation, and health policy development.
       To become a specialist in Dental Public Health, a dentist must enroll and successfully complete 2 years of postgraduate education.
       The most traditional educational path includes the completion of a Masters in Public Health degree (MPH) from a US or Canadian School of Public Health followed by 1 year of a Dental Public Health residency. The MPH provides theoretical knowledge in general public health sciences, whereas the residency provides the application of public health into the dental health system. Other models exist that integrate the didactic part of the MPH and the practical aspect of the residency into combined 2-year or 3-year programs. Upon graduation, educationally qualified dental public health dentists are eligible for certification from the American Board of Dental Public Health (ABDPH).
       There are currently 15 active and accredited dental public health programs in the United States and Canada. Educational programs are reviewed every 7 years and obtain accreditation status from Commission on Dental Accreditation (CODA) and must address the following ten core competencies:
    1. Manage oral health programs for population health
    2. Demonstrate ethical decision-making in the practice of dental public health
    3. Evaluate systems of care that impact oral health
    4. Design surveillance systems to measure oral health status and its determinants
    5. Communicate on oral and public health issues
    6. Lead collaborations on oral and public health issues
    7. Advocate for public health policy, legislation, and regulations to protect and promote the public's oral health, and overall health
    8. Critically appraise evidence to address oral health issues for individuals and populations
    9. Conduct research to address oral and public health problems
    10. Integrate the social determinants of health into dental public health practice

17. **What are some of the major concerns related to the oral health workforce in the United States?**

With 329 million people, the United States has an estimated 200,000 active dentists. The crude dentist-to-population ratio is 1 dentist for every 1645 individuals. Dentists tend to work in urban areas. While major metropolitan areas are well covered, the maldistribution of the workforce away from rural areas and areas where the working poor reside is well documented. According to a recent report from the Health Resources and Services Administration (HRSA, HHS) on health workforce shortage areas (HPSAs), there are *64 million people living in dental underserved areas*, representing 19% percent of the population, and less than 40% percent of the dental needs have been met in these areas. As of January 1, 2022, the number of HPSAs has increased to 6812, which corresponds to a need for 11,218 additional practitioners.

There are currently over 5500 full-time dental faculty positions in the United States. The greying of the dental faculty workforce presents another challenge. According to ADEA, the aging of the faculty has led to an acceleration of open and unfilled faculty positions. Currently over 43% of vacancies are attributed to aging, up from 29% in 2014-2015. According to the 2018-2019 ADEA Survey of Dental School Faculty, over 5.5% of the 5506 full-time U.S. dental school faculty FTEs stand open, and the length of time it takes to fill those positions is increasing as well.

Left unchecked, this alarming trend will only worsen in the future. Over 40% of current full-time dental faculty are over 60 years old, but data from the 2020 ADEA Survey of Dental School Seniors show that, upon graduation, only 0.3% of dental school seniors planned to enter academia at a dental school, nowhere near enough to fill the anticipated vacancies, and perhaps even more disturbingly, down 25% from just 3 years before.

FLUORIDE IN PREVENTION

18. **Water fluoridation is one of the few public health measures that save more money than they cost. Why is water fluoridation so cost effective?**

Fluoridation is a low-cost, low-technology procedure that benefits an entire community. It requires no patient compliance and is therefore easy to administer. The major costs are associated with the initial equipment purchase; later costs are for maintenance and fluoride supplies. The average cost for a community to fluoridate its water is estimated to range from approximately $0.50/year/person in large communities to approximately $3.00/year/person in small communities. For most cities, every $1 invested in water fluoridation saves $38 in dental treatment costs.

19. **What are the major mechanisms of action for fluoride in caries inhibition?**
    1. The topical effect of constant infusion of a low concentration of fluoride into the oral cavity is thought to increase remineralization of enamel.
    2. Fluoride inhibits glycolysis in which sugar is converted to acid by bacteria.
    3. During tooth development, fluoride is incorporated into the developing enamel hydroxyapatite crystal, which reduces enamel solubility.

20. **What is the recommended level of fluoride in the water supply?**
    The U.S. Public Health Service sets the optimal fluoride level at 0.7 to 1.2 ppm.

21. **A parent of a 6-year-old child asks about fluoride supplementation. The child weighs 20 kg and lives in a fluoride-deficient area, with 0.8 ppm of fluoride ion in the drinking water. What do you recommend?**
    Systemic fluoride should not be prescribed, as it is >0.6 ppm minimum recommendation, therefore water fluoridation is adequate.

22. **What are alternatives to systemic fluoride supplementation (e.g., tablets)?**
    - Topically applied gels of 2.0% NaF, 0.4% SnF, 1.23% acidulated phosphate fluoride (APF)
    - Varnishes
    - Prophylactic pastes or pumice
    - Mouth rinses of 0.2% NaF weekly, 0.05% NaF daily, 0.1% SnF daily
    - Daily dentifrice
      The fluoride supplementation can be self-applied or professionally applied. The professionally applied fluorides are more concentrated than the self-applied fluorides and therefore are not needed as frequently. For patients with a high caries risk, the American Dental Association (ADA) recommends fluoride varnish applications at 3- to 6-month intervals for those younger than 6 years, fluoride varnish or gel applications at 6-month intervals for those age 6 to 18 years, and fluoride varnish or gel applications at 3- to 6-month intervals for those older than 18 years.

23. **In prescribing fluoride supplementation, what tradeoffs must be considered?**
    The benefit of caries reduction must be considered against the risk of fluorosis. Fluorosis occurs with the presence of excessive fluoride during tooth development and causes discoloration of tooth enamel. Affected teeth appear chalky white on eruption and later turn brown. This risk is especially important during the development of the

incisors in the second to third years. To avoid this problem, you must assess the fluoride content of the drinking water before dispensing fluoride supplementation. The fluoride in water, along with any supplemental fluoride, must not exceed 1 ppm. If 1 ppm is exceeded, the probability that fluorosis may develop increases as the fluoride concentration increases.

24. **Where is ingested fluoride absorbed?**
Eighty percent of absorption occurs in the upper gastrointestinal tract.

25. **What are the manifestations of fluoride toxicity?**
The ingestion of 5 g or more of fluoride in an adult results in death within 2 hours if the person does not receive medical attention. In a child, ingestion of a single dose greater than 400 mg results in death caused by poisoning in about 3 hours. Doses of 100 to 300 mg in children cause nausea and diarrhea.

26. **How much fluoride is contained in an average 4.6-ounce tube of toothpaste?**
Sodium monofluorophosphate or sodium fluoride toothpaste contains approximately 1.0 mg of fluoride/g of paste. Therefore, a 4.6-oz tube of toothpaste contains 130 mg of fluoride. A level of 435 mg of fluoride consumed in a 3-hour period is considered fatal for a 3-year-old child—only a little over three tubes of toothpaste need to be consumed to reach a fatal level.

27. **What is the rationale behind the use of pit and fissure sealants in caries prevention?**
Occlusal surfaces, particularly fissures, have not experienced as rapid a decline in the incidence of caries as proximal surfaces because fluoride's protective effect is confined to smooth surfaces only. It has been observed that sealing the fissures from the oral environment prevents the development of occlusal caries. Sealants should be part of an early preventive program for protecting permanent molars.

28. **Describe evidence-based dentistry (EBD) and its three important domains.**
Evidence-based dentistry is an approach to practice, an approach to making clinical decisions, and the provision of personalized dental care based on the most current scientific knowledge. The practice of EBD is based on the following:
1. The best available scientific evidence
2. A dentist's clinical skill and judgment
3. Individual patient's needs and preferences

29. **What are the recommended sources when searching for clinical evidence?**
- PubMed
- TRIP Database
- DARE (Database of Abstracts of Reviews of Effectiveness)
- National Guideline Clearinghouse
- Cochrane Library
- ADA's EBD website

EPIDEMIOLOGY

30. **Differentiate between incidence and prevalence.**
Incidence is the number of new cases of disease occurring within a population during a given period. It is expressed as a rate, (cases)/(population during time period).
   Prevalence is the proportion of a population affected with a disease at a given point in time—(cases)/(population).
   Example: A dentist counts the number of patients presenting to the office with newly diagnosed periodontal disease in a 6-month period. Of the 100 people who came to the office, 10 had periodontal disease. The incidence rate is calculated as 10/100 in 6 months, or 0.2/year. The range for incidence rates is from 0 to ∞. The prevalence of periodontal disease may be obtained by counting all patients with periodontal disease in the same period—that is, if 50 of 100 patients have periodontal disease, the prevalence is 50%. Remember, incidence is a rate and requires a unit of time, whereas prevalence is a proportion and is expressed as a percentage of the population.

31. **What is relative risk? Odds ratio?**
The **relative risk** measures the association between exposure and disease. It is expressed as a ratio of the rate of disease among exposed persons to the rate among unexposed persons. Relative risk estimates the strength or magnitude of an association. The calculation of relative risk requires incidence rates, which are provided by cohort studies.
   The **odds ratio** provides an estimate of the relative risk in case-control studies; because disease has already occurred, the incidence of disease cannot be determined.

32. **Confidence intervals are often provided when data are reported. What do they indicate?**
Confidence intervals (CIs) represent the range within which the true magnitude of the effect lies with a certain degree of certainty. For example, a relative risk of 2.1 may be reported with a 95% CI (1.5, 2.9). This indicates that

the study determined the relative risk to be 2.1 and that we are 95% certain that the true relative risk is not less than 1.5 or more than 2.9. If the 95% CI includes the null value (1.0), the result is not statistically significant.

33. **Compare cross-sectional, case-control, and cohort studies.**
    Cross-sectional studies are a type of descriptive epidemiologic study in which the exposure and disease status of the population are determined at a given point. For example, the caries status of U.S. adults age 45 to 65 years in 1992 may be determined by a national dental survey and examination.

    Case-control and cohort studies are analytic epidemiologic studies. In **case-control studies,** participants are selected on the basis of disease status. The "cases" are persons who have the disease of interest, and the control group consists of persons similar to the case group except that they do not have the disease of interest. Information about exposure status is then obtained from each group to assess whether an association exists between exposure and disease.

    In **cohort studies,** participants are selected on the basis of exposure status. Study participants must be free of the disease of interest at the time the study begins. Exposed and nonexposed participants are then followed over time to assess the association between exposure and specific diseases.

34. **Define clinical trial, the major types of clinical trials, and their purpose.**
    Clinical trial is a research study to answer specific questions about vaccines or new therapies or new ways of using known treatments. The National Institutes of Health (NIH) has classified clinical trials into five types:
    1. *Treatment trials:* To test experimental treatments, new combinations of drugs, or new approaches to surgery or radiation therapy. For example, in dentistry, treatment trials are commonly used to test new dental restorative materials, implants, and treatment for dry mouth.
    2. *Prevention trials:* To look for better ways to prevent disease in people who have never had the disease or to prevent a disease from returning. These approaches may include medicines, vaccines, vitamins, minerals, or lifestyle changes. Prevention trials are frequently carried out in dental caries prevention.
    3. *Diagnostic trials:* To find better tests or procedures for diagnosing a particular disease or condition. Using different methods to assess the level of the clinical attachment and bone support in the diagnosis of periodontitis is an example of a diagnostic trial.
    4. *Screening trials:* To test the best way to detect certain disease or health conditions. A clinical trial to evaluate the effectiveness of different screening strategies for oral cancer is an example of screening trial.
    5. *Quality of life trials* (or supportive care trials): To explore ways to improve the comfort and quality of life for individuals with chronic illnesses. A dental trial that investigates clinical effectiveness and quality of life for conventional dental treatment compared to an alternative intervention is an example of quality of life trial.

35. **Discuss the importance of blinding and randomization in experimental studies.**
    Randomization and blinding are two methods of reducing bias in research studies. In a **randomized study,** all participants have an equal likelihood of receiving the treatment of interest. For example, patients are randomly assigned to two groups, one of which receives a particular treatment and the other, placebo. Several techniques are available to ensure randomization of the study participants. In a **double-blind study**, both the investigator observing the results and the participants are unaware of which individuals are assigned to which group. One means of achieving a blinded study is the use of placebos.

36. **Distinguish between split-mouth and crossover designs.**
    In **split-mouth studies**, different treatments are applied to different sections of the mouth. The effects of treatment must be localized to the region receiving the treatment. In **crossover studies**, patients serve as their own control and receive treatments in sequence—treatment A and then treatment B—and the disease course is compared between the two periods. The disease under investigation must be assumed to be stable during the period of treatment.

37. **What are some of the important oral health trends in children documented in the most recent NIDCR report of the Oral Health of the Nation that have taken place in the last 20 years since the publication of the first Surgeon's General Report on Oral Health in 2000?**
    - In children younger than 12, untreated tooth decay in primary teeth has significantly decreased from 23% to 15%.
    - This positive change has been greatest for children aged 2 to 5 years, with caries experience decreasing to 10%.
    - Importantly, there is evidence of declining disparities as these positive trends are experienced by preschool children across all racial and ethnic groups and family income levels. Minority and low-income children had the largest declines in untreated caries.
    - The prevalence of at least one sealed permanent molar in children 6 to 8 years has increased significantly from 14% to 31%, with the largest gains experienced among Mexican American children.
    - For children aged 6 to 11 years, the prevalence of dental cavities in permanent teeth also has declined significantly during the past 20 years, from 25% to 18%.
    - The prevalence of dental sealants among children aged 9 to 11 years has increased from 29% to 53%.

- Today the great majority of children (9 in 10) have dental insurance in the United States as a result of the Affordable Care Act and CHIP implementation.

38. **What are some of the important oral health trends in adolescents documented in the most recent NIDCR report of the Oral Health of the Nation that have taken place in the last 20 years since the publication of the first Surgeon's General Report on Oral Health in 2000?**
    - Adolescents between the ages of 12 and 19 years have not seen the same prevention improvements as younger children. In particular, there has been no significant change in dental caries, with three in five adolescents (57%) experiencing cavities. Mexican American adolescents have significantly higher rates of caries (69%) than the general population.
    - Adolescents experienced a slight improvement in the prevalence of untreated tooth decay, with approximately one in six adolescents having untreated caries, a decline of about 3%. Evidence of disparities seems to persist with caries affecting about 23% of those living in poverty.
    - Preventive dental care has increased during the past 20 years in adolescents, with the prevalence of at least one sealed permanent molar nearly tripling from 18% to 48%.

39. **What are some of the important oral health trends in adults documented in the most recent NIDCR report of the Oral Health of the Nation that have taken place in the last 20 years since the publication of the first Surgeon's General Report on Oral Health in 2000?**
    - U.S. adults have not experienced any significant improvements in their oral health in the last 20 years.
    - Untreated dental caries in working-age adults during the past two decades has remained stagnant (28% vs. 29%). The largest contribution to this statistic is due to working-age adults living in poverty (52%). In 2000, the average number of surfaces with untreated caries for those living in poverty was four. In 2021, the average number of surfaces affected by untreated caries has increased by 50% for working-age adults, regardless of poverty status.
    - Among the general population of adults aged 50 to 64, approximately 75% have a functional dentition, defined as sufficient number of natural teeth. However, for adults living in poverty less than half (47%) have a functional dentition.
    - Oral and pharyngeal cancer associated with tobacco and ethanol use is decreasing. However, HPV+-associated oropharyngeal cancers have doubled, especially among men who develop oropharyngeal cancer 3.5 times more than women. Today seven out of ten oral pharyngeal cancers in the United States are caused by HPV, and the number of new cases is increasing each year.
    - Older adults continue to experience high rates of dental caries. However, untreated tooth decay in older adults has declined by 6%, from an estimated 28% to 22%.
    - Since 2000, edentulism has decreased from 32% to 17% for adults ages 65 and older, with the average age of edentulism increasing. Among adults 65 to 74 years of age, 13% are edentulous today, compared with 50% in the 1960s.

HEALTH POLICY

40. **How does the Americans with Disabilities Act affect dentists?**
    - Dentists cannot deny anyone care because of a disability.
    - Offices must undergo architectural changes to allow access for the disabled.
    - Employees are protected against dismissal because of a disability.
    - Offices must accommodate disabled workers so they can perform jobs.

41. **Differentiate between licensure and registration.**
    Licensure is granted through a government agency to those who meet specified qualifications to perform given activities or claim a particular title. Registration is a listing of qualified individuals by a governmental or nongovernmental organization.

42. **What are the types of supervision for allied dental personnel, as defined by the ADA?**
    1. **Indirect:** The dentist diagnoses a condition and then authorizes dental personnel to carry out treatment while the dentist remains in the office.
    2. **Direct:** The dentist diagnoses a condition, authorizes treatment, and evaluates the outcome.
    3. **General:** General supervision is defined by practice acts within each state and may require that the dentist be available but not necessarily on the premise or site where care is delivered.

43. **Define structure, process, and outcome as they relate to quality assurance.**
    Quality assurance is the process of examining physical structures, procedures, and outcome as they affect the delivery of health care. It consists of assessment to identify inadequacies, followed by implementation of improvements to correct the inadequacies.
    Structure refers to the layout and equipment of a facility. Included are items such as the building, equipment, and record forms. **Process** involves the services that the dentist and auxiliary personnel perform for patients and how skillfully they do so. **Outcome** is the change in health status that occurs as a result of the care delivered.

44. **How do cost-benefit and cost-effectiveness analyses differ?**

Cost-effectiveness and cost-benefit analyses are similar yet distinct techniques to help allocate resources to maximize objectives. **Cost-benefit analysis** requires that all costs and benefits be expressed in dollar terms to provide a measure of net benefit. **Cost-effectiveness analysis** uses alternative measures to value effectiveness. Objections to valuing life in terms of dollars led to the use of cases of disease prevented, life-years gained, or quality-adjusted life-years. The result is a cost-effectiveness ratio that expresses the cost per unit of effectiveness.

45. **What is adverse selection?**

Adverse selection occurs when people at high risk for an illness are the predominant purchasers of insurance, especially when the risk for illness and the premium are based on a low-risk population. Thus, high-risk people are attracted to the insurance by its low rates, which allow them to avoid payments for a likely illness.

46. **What is an example of a moral hazard?**

A moral hazard is when someone does not have incentive to avoid risk when they are protected from the consequences. For example, patients with insurance demand more medical care than patients who have to pay the cost themselves.

47. **What is a community rating?**

The premiums charged to all insurance subscribers are the same, regardless of individual risk and who pays for medical care. Community rating spreads the cost out, allowing those who are less healthy to afford medical care, but it can create higher costs for those who are healthy. The cost ultimately falls on the general public.

48. **What are the different financing mechanisms for dental care?**

Dentistry is financed mainly through fee-for-service self-pay; 56% of all dental expenses are paid out of pocket by the patient. Payment to the dentist by an organization other than the patient is called third-party payment. Third-party payers represented by private insurance pay about 33% of total dental expenses, followed by government-financed or public programs (e.g., Medicaid, U.S. Department of Veterans Affairs).

49. **What is capitation payment?**

HMO premiums are usually made on a capitation basis—that is, HMO providers receive a given fee per enrollee, regardless of how much or little care is delivered.

50. **Explain the differences among IPA, PPO, and HMO.**

All three represent managed-care practices. Managed care refers to forms of insurance coverage in which utilization and service patterns are monitored by the insurer, with the aim of containing costs. An HMO (health maintenance organization) is usually a self-contained, staff model practice in which no distinction is made between the providers of insurance and providers of health care. HMO premiums are paid on a capitation basis. In contrast, IPA (independent practice association) and PPO (preferred provider organization) represent groups of doctors who practice in the community and are distinct from the insurance provider. However, the insurance agency contracts with the providers for discounted rates and may refer patients to these providers exclusively. If a patient chooses to go to a different provider from the one recommended by the insurance company, the patient may face a financial penalty, such as an additional charge.

51. **How do managed care arrangements differ from the traditional model of dental care?**

Traditional medical and dental care has been paid on a fee-for-service basis. The patient chooses any provider in the community, and the insurance company usually pays a certain percentage of the charge. In the current era of cost-consciousness, many insurance companies are modifying or eliminating this model altogether. Fee-for-service usually provides no incentive for the patient or provider to contain costs. It is no longer widely in use.

Most people today have some type of managed care insurance. Managed care organizations supervise the financing of medical and dental care delivered to members. To be cost-effective, they buy services in bulk for many members at a time and also provide members with a list of doctors from which to choose and lists of laboratories where tests can be performed. Even doctors are provided with lists of medicines from which to choose. Different plans have different restrictions on choice.

52. **How do Medicaid and Medicare differ?**

Medicare, an entitlement fund, was created to provide health insurance to those 65 years of age and older, certain disabled groups, and people with certain kidney diseases. Medicare has two parts, an institutional or hospital portion (Part A) and a noninstitutional portion, or physician services (Part B). Part A has no premium, but Part B is supplemental and voluntarily purchased. Medicare does not provide dental care.

Medicaid is a means-tested program to provide health insurance to poor people eligible for welfare assistance programs. Medicaid is a joint federal and state program with federal guidelines that allow states some flexibility in which services are provided and who is eligible. The federal government provides states with matching dollars. Medicaid covers hospital and physician costs without a premium or copayment. Medicaid is required by federal law to provide dental services to children. However, adult dental services are optional, and the decision of whether to provide dental care is determined at a state level.

53. **What is the economic impact of oral disease in the United States?**

According to Oral Health in America report issued by the NIDCR in 2021, health and the economy are closely linked. Some of the economic consequences of dental disease that were identified in the report were:
- $45.9 billion of productivity losses in the United States associated with untreated oral disease were estimated in 2015.
- Marginalized groups carry the disproportionate economic burden of untreated oral disease as they experience higher rates of such maladies.
- A Surgeon General's Report on Community Health and Economic Prosperity acknowledged the influence "of structural, cultural, and interpersonal racism and bias on health, wealth, and well-being" (U.S. Department of Health and Human Services 2021).
- 2.4 million Emergency Department visits occurred in 2014 as a result of lack of access to care for nontraumatic dental conditions.
- $1.6 billion were charged for ED visits in the same time period, with Medicaid reportedly being the primary payer for these visits.
- While emergency ED visits lead to increased costs, they fail to address untreated dental disease; an estimated 90% of patients receive only pain medication or antibiotics and a referral to dental providers for treatment.
- Dental care costs per person in the United States have increased by 30% over the past 20 years.

54. **What is the financial burden of head and neck cancers?**

In a recent analysis of economic burden of head and neck cancers in the United States conducted in 2018, the total annual economic loss attributed to head and neck cancer was reported to be $4.4 billion. Costs included treatment costs, rehabilitation, and loss of wages. The cost per individual and total costs were higher for patients with advanced stage head and neck cancer and for those who received more than one treatment, such as surgery and radiotherapy or surgery and chemotherapy.

55. **What percentage of all U.S. health care expenditures is for dental care?**

In 2016, approximately 3.7% of all U.S. health care expenditures was for dental services. While in the 2000s, the predictions were that dental expenditures would surpass $179.8 billion by 2021, the actual spending was significantly less than predicted, $142 billion. The 2021 level of spending was $3 billion less than in 2019 ($145 billion), raising questions about the real causes for such declines in the face of significant inflationary trends in the economy.

ACKNOWLEDGMENT

The authors gratefully acknowledge the contribution of the previous chapter author.

BIBLIOGRAPHY

Altman D, Mascharenhas AK. Competencies for the 21st century dental public health specialist. *J Public Health Dent.* 2016;76:S18–S28.

American Board of Dental Public Health. *Informational Brochure.* Available at https://aaphd.memberclicks.net/assets/ABDPH/Updated%20ABDPH_Informational_Brochure_2021-2022.pdf.

American Dental Association. *Principles of Ethics and Code of Professional Conduct.* Chicago: American Dental Association; 1992.

American Dental Association. Professionally applied topical fluoride: Evidence-based clinical recommendations. *J Am Dent Assoc.* 2006;137:1151–1159.

American Dental Education Association. *Trends in Dental Education;* 2020–2021. https://adea.org/snapshot/.

American Association of Public Health Dentistry: *Competencies for the Predoctoral Curriculum.* https://www.aaphd.org/dph-curriculum.

Antczak-Bouckoms A, Tulloch JFC, Bouckoms AJ, et al. Diagnostic decision making. *Anesth Prog.* 1990;37:161–165.

Basquill LC, Govoni M, Bednarsh H. OSHA—what is its role in dentistry and how do we provide training? *Compend Contin Educ Dent.* 2005;26(Suppl):10–13.

Burt BA, Eklund SA. *Dentistry, Dental Practice and the Community.* Philadelphia: WB Saunders; 1992.

Centers for Disease Control and Prevention (CDC). Current tobacco use among middle and high school students—United States, 2011. *MMWR Morb Mortal Wkly Rep.* 2012;61:581–585.

Centers for Disease Control and Prevention (CDC). Guidelines for infection control in dental health-care settings—2003. *MMWR Recomm Rep.* 2003;52(RR-17):1–66.

Centers for Disease Control and Prevention (CDC). *National Center for Health Statistics (NCHS): National Health and Nutrition Examination Survey data.* Hyattsville, MD: U.S. Department of Health and Human Services, Centers for Disease Control and Prevention, Centers for Disease Control and Prevention (CDC), National Center for Chronic Disease and Health Promotion: Oral Health Resources. Synopses of State and Territorial Dental Public Health Programs: trends; 2009–2010. https://www.cdc.gov/chronicdisease/.

Centers for Disease Control: *About Social Determinants of Health.* https://www.cdc.gov/socialdeterminants/about.html.

Centers for Disease Control and Prevention (CDC): *Water Fluoridation Reporting System (WFRS). 2010 Water Fluoridation Statistics.* http://water.epa.gov/infrastructure/drinkingwater/pws/factoids.cfm.

Centers for Medicare and Medicaid Services. Office of the Actuary, National Health Statistics Group, *National Health Expenditure Accounts: National Health Expenditures.* http://www.cms.hhs.gov/NationalHealthExpendData. See Appendix I, National Health Expenditure Accounts (NHEA).

Chattopadhyay A. *Oral Health Epidemiology: Principles and Practice.* Sudbury, MA: Jones and Bartlett; 2011.

Cleveland JL, Junger ML, Saraiya M, et al. The connection between human papillomavirus and oropharyngeal squamous cell carcinomas in the United States: Implications for dentistry. *J Am Dent Assoc.* 2011;142:915–924.

Contreras OA, et al.: *Our Future Faculty—The Importance of Recruiting Students and Residents to Academic Dentistry ADEA 2018 Data Brief.* https://www.adea.org/.

Detels R, Holland WW, McEwen J, Omen GS: *Textbook of Public Health*, vols. 1, 2, 3, 3rd ed. New York, 1997, Oxford University Press.

Division of Oral Health. *National Center for Chronic Disease Prevention and Health Promotion July 10*; 2013. http://www.cdc.gov/OralHealth/index.html.

Dye BA, Tan S, Smith V, Lewis BG, Barker LK, Thornton-Evans G, et al. Trends in oral health status: United States, 1988–1994 and 1999–2004. National Center for Health Statistics. *Vital Health Stat.* 2007;11(248).

Eaton DK, Kann L, Kinchen S, et al. Centers for Disease Control and Prevention (CDC): Youth risk behavior surveillance—United States, 2011. *MMWR Surveill Summ.* 2012;61(SS04):1–162.

Feldstein PJ. *Health Care Economics.* Albany, NY: Delmar; 1988.

Gift HC, Drury TF, Nowjack-Raymer RE, Selwitz RH. The state of the nation's oral health: Mid-decade assessment of Healthy People 2000. *J Public Health Dent.* 1996;56:84–91.

Health and Human Services (HHS): *Healthy People 2030.* https://health.gov/healthypeople/objectives-and-data/browse-objectives/nutrition-and-healthy-eating/reduce-household-food-insecurity-and-hunger-nws-01.

Health Resources and Services Administration: *Shortage Areas.* https://data.hrsa.gov/topics/health-workforce/shortage-areas.

Hennekens CH, Buring JE. *Epidemiology in Medicine.* In: Mayrent SL, ed. Boston: Little Brown; 1987.

Howlader N, Noone AM, Krapcho M, et al., eds. *SEER Cancer Statistics Review.* Bethesda, MD: National Cancer Institute; 1975–2011. http://seer.cancer.gov/csr/1975_2011/. based on November 2013 SEER data submission, posted to the SEER website, April 2014.

Jacobs P. *The Economics of Health and Medical Care.* Gaithersburg, MD: Aspen; 1991.

Jong A. *Dental Public Health and Community Dentistry.* St. Louis: Mosby; 1981.

Kofman M, Pollitz K. *Health Insurance Regulation by State and the Federal Government: A Review of Current Approaches and Proposals for Change.* Georgetown Health Policy Institute; 2006.

Kression NR. Racial/ethnic disparities in health care: lessons from medicine for dentistry. *J Dent Educ.* 2005;69:998–1002.

Pagano M, Gauvreau K. *Principles of Biostatistics.* Boston: Harvard School of Public Health; 1991.

Pagano M, Gauvreau K. Two Distributions With Identical Means, Medians, and Modes. In: *Principles of Biostatistics.* Boston: Harvard School of Public Health; 1991.

Public Health Leadership Society. *Principles of the Ethical Practice of Public Health*; 2002. version 2.2. https://www.apha.org/-/media/files/pdf/membergroups/ethics/ethics_brochure.ashx.

Quality Assurance Advisory Committee. A quality assurance primer for dentistry. *J Am Dent Assoc.* 1988;117:239–242.

Riordan PJ. Fluoride supplements in caries prevention: a literature review and proposal for a new dosage schedule. *J Public Health Dent.* 1993;53:174–189.

Ripa LW. A half century of community water fluoridation in the United States: review and commentary. *J Public Health Dent.* 1993;53:17–44.

Rozier RG, Beck JD. Epidemiology of oral disease. *Curr Opin Dent.* 1991;1:308–315.

Silverman S. *Oral Cancer.* Atlanta: American Cancer Society; 1990.

United Nations. *Declaration of Human Rights*: https://www.un.org/en/about-us/universal-declaration-of-human-rights.

Weinstein MC, Fineberg HV. *Clinical Decision Analysis.* Philadelphia: WB Saunders; 1980.

Weintraub JA, Douglass CW, Gillings DB. *Biostatistics: Data Analysis for Dental Health Professionals.* Chapel Hill, NC: Cavco; 1985.

World Health Organization: *Framework Convention on Tobacco Control.* https://fctc.who.int/who-fctc/overview.

World Health Organization. Introduction. In: *International Classification of Functioning, Disability and Health: ICF.* Geneva, Switzerland: WHO; 2001:3.

World Health Organization: *Trade, Foreign Policy, Diplomacy and Health.* https://apps.who.int/iris/handle/10665/269844.

World Health Organization: *World Health Statistics.* https://www.who.int/data/gho/publications/world-health-statistics.

World Health Organization: *Minamata Convention information.* https://www.mercuryconvention.org/en/about.

Zavras AI, Shanmugham JR. Measurement and Distribution of Oral Cancer. In: Mascarenhas AK, Okunseri C, Dye BA, eds. *Burt and Eklund's Dentistry, Dental Practice, and the Community.* 7th ed. St Louis, MO: Elsevier; 2020:189–201.

CHAPTER 15

LEGAL AND ETHICAL ISSUES

Bernard Friedland

LEGAL ISSUES

1. What are the sources of American law?
   In the United States, there are three primary sources of law:
   1. The federal and state constitutions.
   2. Statutes and administrative regulations. Statutes are created by legislatures. Legislatures also authorize agencies to issue regulations that help interpret and clarify what a statute means.
   3. The common law.
      Today, much, if not the overwhelming majority of laws are administrative in nature, such that some people who believe that Congress and state legislatures may not constitutionally delegate so much rule-making power to administrative agencies refer derisively to modern America as The Administrative State (https://www.nationalaffair s.com/publications/detail/confronting-the-administrative-state).

2. What are administrative agencies?
   An administrative agency is a government body established by Congress or a state legislature and is empowered to implement legislative directives by developing more precise and technical rules than is feasible in a legislative setting. To put it colloquially, an administrative agency puts meat (rules and regulations) on the bones (statutes).

3. Name some administrative agencies whose rules and regulations apply to dentists.
   Some apply to dentists by virtue of them owning a place of employment and some apply by virtue of the fact that they are dentists.
   1. The Occupational Safety and Health Administration (OSHA; https://www.osha.gov/)
   2. Dental boards in all states in which dentists are licensed, even if they do not practice in a state
   3. The National Practitioner Data Bank (https://www.npdb.hrsa.gov/)
   4. The state radiation control authority

4. Which government agencies set standards for the manufacture and approval of x-ray machines and for their use?
   The manufacturing and approval of x-ray machines are overseen by the federal Food and Drug Administration under the Electronic Product Radiation Control Program (https://www.fda.gov/radiation-emitting-products/electronic-product-radiation-control-program). The *use* of x-ray machines is governed by state law. While most states regulate the use of dental x-rays similarly, there are differences. For example, some states mandate the use of lead aprons for every dental x-ray, while others do not. The website of the American Society of Radiologic Technologists (https://www.asrt.org/main/standards-and-regulations/legislation-regulations-and-advocacy/radiation-control-program-offices) has links to the states' radiation control agencies.

5. How does a dentist get to serve on a dental board?
   States differ on exactly who may serve and how they are appointed to a dental board, but the appointments to dental boards are generally political in nature. For example, in Arkansas, members are appointed by the Governor (https://www.healthy.arkansas.gov/programs-services/topics/arkansas-state-board-of-dental-examiners/legal-files). In California, the dentists, hygienists, dental assistants, and three public members are appointed by the Governor. Of the remaining two public members, one is appointed by the Speaker of the Assembly and one by the Senate Rules Committee (https://www.dbc.ca.gov/formspubs/sunset_report_2018vol1.pdf).

6. You purchase a cone-beam CT (CBCT) scanner for use on your patients. An orthodontist and a periodontist, both of whom recently opened a practice in your building, would like to refer their patients who need a CBCT to you. What considerations should you take into account concerning the use of the scanner both on your own patients and on patients referred for a CT scan from other practices?
   There are a number of important considerations to take into account:
   1. First and foremost, contact your malpractice carrier. Malpractice carriers generally cover you for any legal/ malpractice issues related to scans taken on your own patients. Even then, it is a good idea to inform your carrier that you have acquired a CT machine and to confirm that your malpractice indeed covers you under these circumstances. It is possible that some may require you to purchase a rider. A rider is a provision that adds benefits to or amends the terms of your malpractice policy. Riders may provide additional coverage

options, or they may restrict or limit coverage. Typically, there is an additional cost if your carrier requires you to purchase a rider.

2. Matters may be more complicated if you choose to accept outside referrals for scans. Your first step should again be to check with your malpractice carrier concerning coverage in cases involving "outside" patients. Some insurers may not cover you at all for such patients, not even allowing you to purchase a rider. Even if the company does cover you, with or without a rider, you may wish to take additional precautions to limit your exposure to the extent permitted by law. There is nothing in the law (or ethics) that requires the person taking the scan to be responsible for interpreting or reading it, only that it be read by *someone* competent to do so. It would be prudent to have a written, signed contract with each outside referring dentist that states clearly that they and not you will be responsible for reading the scan or to have someone competent read it. You would also be well advised to obtain patients' informed consent prior to taking the image that explains that you are performing only the technical service of taking the scan and that their dentists are responsible for reading the scan. Your malpractice carrier can help you draft the above-mentioned documents.

3. While the aforementioned precautions should be upheld by courts, others will not be. Among the latter are having patients sign a waiver of liability for the interpretation of the films or giving them the choice of whether to have the films read by someone competent to do so.

7. **You purchase a cone-beam CT (CBCT) scanner for use on your patients, but you are not comfortable or competent to read scans and you decide to use the services of an individual radiologist or a group that employs a panel of radiologists. What considerations should enter into your decision as to whom to use?**
Aside from the obvious matter of using a competent radiologist, you also need to consider licensing issues. Assume that you live in state X and that the radiologist is licensed in state Y. May you use her services? The answer depends on your own state's licensing laws. Your state's dental board may permit the radiologist to read scans of patients taken in State X as long as she is licensed in *a* state, *any* state. Or State X's dental board may permit the radiologist to read scans of patients taken in its state as long as she is licensed in *one of certain* states approved by your dental board. Alternatively, State X's dental board may require the radiologist to have a full or perhaps a limited State X license. If the latter is the case and you are using a group that employs radiologists, you should tell them that your scans should be read only by radiologists licensed in your state. While it is no doubt true that many dentists use the services of radiologists not licensed in the dentists' states, practitioners should be aware that doing so could open them up to a range of unwanted ramifications, such as a charge of facilitating the illegal practice of dentistry, which could have criminal implications, as well as actions by the dental board against the dentist's license. The most prudent course of action is to ask your dental board whether a radiologist who reads your scans must be licensed in your state before employing her services and to follow that advice.

8. **May dentists lose their license for criminal actions not involving the practice of dentistry?**
Yes, they may. Dental boards may deny initial licensure, renewal of a license, may revoke a license, or may impose restrictions on a license for offenses that appear to be unrelated to dentistry. For example, the North Carolina Dental Board may refuse to issue a license to anyone who

"Has been convicted of any of the criminal provisions of this Article or has entered a plea of guilty or nolo contendere to any charge or charges arising therefrom"

or "Has been convicted of or entered a plea of guilty or nolo contendere to any felony charge or to any misdemeanor charge involving moral turpitude" (North Carolina General Statutes Chapter 90, §229). In some states, the Board may be allowed to rely and act upon the criminal conviction without holding a hearing itself, but in others, the law may require it to hold a hearing. California follows the latter rule.

State license applications ask applicants the following question or variations thereof:

"Have you ever been arrested, charged, arraigned, indicted, prosecuted, convicted or been the subject of any criminal investigation or any court proceeding in relation to any criminal violation? Do not report minor traffic violations for which a fine of $100 or less was imposed." (https://www.mass.gov/doc/dental-licensure-by-credential/download (Accessed on June 15, 2023)).

9. **What elements must a patient prove by a preponderance of the evidence in order to prevail in a malpractice lawsuit?**
Four elements are necessary to prove negligence and win a malpractice suit. The patient must establish the following: (1) a dentist-patient relationship existed (i.e., the dentist owed the patient the care and skill of the average qualified practitioner); (2) the dentist breached his or her duty by failing to exercise the level of care and skill of the average qualified practitioner; (3) the patient suffered injury; and (4) a connection exists between the dentist's breach of duty and the patient's injury (causation) (Fig. 15-1).

Causation in the law is a complicated concept. What a layperson might think is an obvious connection, e.g., A caused B, may not be so clear cut in the law and the two might in fact not be related at all in the legal sense.

10. **What issues may constitute a defense against malpractice?**
In theory, a dentist need not introduce any evidence to prevail in a lawsuit brought by a patient. This is because the patient has the burden of proof. In reality, a dentist will often introduce evidence to refute a

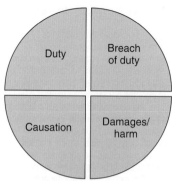

Fig. 15-1. The elements that a patient must prove in order to prevail in a malpractice lawsuit.

patient's assertions. If a dentist is able to refute any of the four elements that a plaintiff patient must prove, the dentist will prevail. In practice, the most hotly contested issue usually revolves around the standard of care. Typically, the plaintiff has an expert witness testify on his or her behalf and the dentist has one testify on her or his behalf. The matter of causation is another area that may be hotly contested. Even if a dentist breached the standard of care, that does not mean that the breach resulted in harm to the patient. For example, assume that a patient complains to a dentist that he has had an ulcer for 6 weeks that is not healing and that the dentist responds by saying "Let's wait another month and see what happens." The patient happens to see another dentist a week later who does a biopsy, and the histology shows the lesion to be squamous cell carcinoma. The first dentist should certainly have biopsied an ulcer that has been present for 6 weeks and, by failing to do so, breached the standard of care. However, the 1-week delay in diagnosis would not affect the progress; hence, there are no damages, and the plaintiff is unable to prove all four of the required elements to win a tort suit.

11. **People sometimes joke, saying "Lawyers always say 'never admit (to) anything.'" Why do lawyers advise this?**
    In any trial, be it civil or criminal, not all evidence is permitted to be introduced. All state courts, as well as federal courts, follow rules of evidence. These rules arise from the legislatures in the form of statutes, or from common law or the rules of the court (Massachusetts Guide to Evidence. Section 102. Purpose and construction; https://www.lexisnexis.com/supp/lawschool/resources/federal-rules-of-evidence.pdf). Among other reasons for excluding certain evidence is that courts want to include only evidence that is reliable. Since people rarely admit to doing something bad or wrong, courts deem such admissions to be reliable. Thus, if a dentist says to a patient "I'm sorry, but I just messed up," that admission would be admissible. It may be that the dentist had not in fact "messed up" or that her actions made no difference to the outcome. Consider, for example, that a file separates during an endodontic procedure such that the tooth is no longer salvageable and that when the file separated, the dentist said to the patient "I just messed up. I broke the file in your tooth." Upon your lawyer sending the case to an endodontist for an expert opinion, the endodontist's report states that due to an extreme curvature of one of the roots, the tooth was not amenable to endodontic treatment and would have been lost in any event. While the latter can be explained to the jury, the facts are highly technical and the jury may simply not understand them or may think that the endodontist is simply a hired hack trying to get you off the hook and decide "if the dentists said she messed up, that's good enough for us" and find the dentist liable.

12. **What is the Occupational Safety and Health Administration (OSHA) and what is its purpose?**
    OSHA is a regulatory agency of the United States Department of Labor. While OSHA's regulations may incidentally benefit patients, its mandate is to protect employees in the work setting, including in health care settings (https://www.osha.gov/lawsregs/oshact/completeoshact; 29 U.S.C. §§ 651–678).

13. **Who may report a dentist on suspicion of violating an OSHA standard and must such persons identify themselves to OSHA? When is a complaint most likely to be filed against a dentist?**
    Any employee may lodge a complaint with OSHA. Furthermore, persons reporting a dentist may do so confidentially. If employees give OSHA their name, they may ask OSHA to not disclose their name to their employer (https://www.osha.gov/workers/file-complaint).
    Dentists are most likely to be reported to patients by disgruntled employees, especially if they are fired from their job. A dentist may not condition any payment (e.g., a month or 3 months' severance salary) to a fired employee upon a promise by the employee not to report the dentist to OSHA.

14. **Does a treatment plan need to be in writing and signed by the patient?**
    The relationship between a dentist and a patient is a contractual one, where the dentist promises to provide certain services that meet the standard of care and the patient promises to pay for those services. State laws may differ on which contracts must be in writing, but as a general rule, even though most dentists present a written treatment plan to patients and have them sign the one they agree to undertake, the contract between dentist and patient, like most contractual relationships, need not be memorialized in writing. It is nevertheless prudent to put a treatment plan in writing because if there is any dispute as to the treatment rendered or the fees to be charged, the written contract is some evidence of what was agreed upon. This chapter is not a legal treatise, but it is worth noting that patients contract with the dentist for services and not for goods. Thus, a dentist is not selling a denture, an implant, or a crown, even though each of these is good, but rather is selling his/her service and expertise.
    The Uniform Commercial Code § 2-201 specifies those contracts which must be in writing. Most states follow this code, but there may be deviations from it.

15. **How may a dentist terminate a dentist-patient relationship after beginning treatment?**
    There are four ways to terminate the dentist-patient relationship: (1) the patient may inform the dentist that he or she no longer wishes to be cared for by the dentist; (2) the treatment has run its course; (3) the dentist and patient mutually agree that the patient will no longer be treated by the dentist; and (4) the dentist terminates the relationship.
    Perhaps an example best clarifies the second way. Suppose a patient is referred to an endodontist for treatment of tooth #9. Once the endodontist has completed treatment and any necessary follow-up, the dentist-patient relationship is terminated. In this case, the dentist is under no obligation to treat the patient at any time in the future. A possible exception may be if future treatment is needed for tooth #9. In cases involving 3 and 4, the dentist should avoid the risk of being liable for abandonment by notifying the patient of his or her decision in writing, providing the telephone number of the local dental society that the patient may call for a referral, and offering to provide emergency treatment for a reasonable (depending on the circumstances) period of time. The dentist is obligated to provide a copy of the patient's record to any person designated by the patient to receive it. The dentist is permitted to charge a reasonable fee for duplicating the record.

ETHICAL ISSUES

16. **How is the ethical practice of dentistry broadly governed?**
    The ethical rules and principles of professional conduct for the practice of dentistry are set forth in the American Dental Association's Principles of Ethics and Code of Professional Conduct, which describes the ethical obligations of dentists. Additionally, many dental boards incorporate the ADA Code into their regulations, either explicitly or implicitly, effectively making it the code of ethics in almost every state. (California Dental Association. CDA Code of Ethics. https://www.cda.org/Portals/0/pdfs/code_of_ethics/code-of-ethics-2020.pdf (Accessed on June 15, 2023); Ethics. Washington State Dental Association; https://www.wsda.org/public/ethics (Accessed on June 15, 2023); https://www.dentalboard.ms.gov/laws-and-codes (Mississippi) (Accessed on June 15, 2023))

17. **List the five fundamental principles that underpin the ADA Code?**
    Nonmaleficence (do no harm)
    Beneficence (do good)
    Autonomy (respect the right of competent adults to make informed decisions about their medical care)
    Justice (be fair in your dealings with patients, colleagues, and society)
    Veracity (be honest and truthful)

18. **The principles enumerated in the ADA Code have their origin in the "4-principles" approach to medical ethics—respect for patient autonomy, nonmaleficence, beneficence, and justice—popularized by Beauchamp and Childress and to which the ADA added the principle of veracity. List three other ethical theories.**
    1. Teleological (Utilitarian) ethics
       Actions are judged to be morally good if they achieve a good goal or outcome; consequences, not intentions, are important.
    2. Deontological ethics
       The consequences of an action are generally irrelevant to the moral assessment; there are rights that must not be violated.
    3. Casuistry (case-based reasoning; This is colloquially referred to as the four boxes approach.

19. **May a dentist refuse to care for certain patients?**
    It is unethical for a dentist to refuse to accept patients because of their race, creed, color, gender, religion, national origin, or because of a disability. In some cases, it may be not only unethical but also illegal. For example, the Americans with Disabilities Act makes it illegal to discriminate against persons with disabilities.
    While most prohibitions against discrimination apply to so-called immutable characteristics such as race and ethnicity, prohibitions against discrimination also include characteristics that are susceptible to change. Among

the latter are religion and even gender, with persons nowadays being able to undergo gender reassignment surgery. Dentists should be careful not to use characteristics that are not explicitly protected as a way of turning away prospective patients. For example, refusing to treat patients who wear a hair covering or specific clothing of some sort as part of their religious belief because the dentist wants to treat only Christians, is not permissible as the dentist is using the hair covering or clothing as a pretext to discriminate.

A dentist may also not remain deliberately ignorant to avoid treating certain groups of patients. For example, in the early days of the HIV epidemic, some dentists were afraid to care for HIV-infected patients and predicated their refusal to do so on the fact that they did not know how to practice infection control properly. These arguments did not prevail; dental boards acted against them, and these dentists were told to acquire the education and skills required.

20. You are undertaking a comprehensive treatment plan on a patient. She has good dental insurance, but has difficulty paying the copayments required by her insurer. Since the insurance coverage is more than sufficient to adequately compensate you for the work and in order to "help her out," you decide not to collect any copayments from her. Is this permissible?

Under the ADA Code, it is impermissible to waive a copayment. Section 5.B.1. Waiver of Copayment says: A dentist who accepts a third-party payment under a copayment plan as payment in full without disclosing to the third party that the patient's payment portion will not be collected, is engaged in overbilling. The essence of this ethical impropriety is deception and misrepresentation; an overbilling dentist makes it appear to the third party that the charge to the patient for services rendered is higher than it actually is.

At first glance, waiving a copayment may not seem to mislead or be a fraud upon the insurer – after all, the company is paying the same dollar amount. However, it is misleading with respect to the percentage of the bill that the company is paying. When you forego collecting a copayment, the insurer is paying 100% of the bill, when it may have contractually agreed to pay only 80% for the particular service.

The American Medical Association is more forgiving toward providers. AMA Opinion 6.12—Forgiveness or Waiver of Insurance Copayments says "*Physicians commonly forgive or waive copayments to facilitate patient access to needed medical care. When a copayment is a barrier to needed care because of financial hardship, physicians should forgive or waive the copayment.*" (American Medical Association. Opinion 6.12—forgiveness or waiver of insurance copayments. Code of Medical Ethics).

21. May you ethically undertake treatment that is "outside"* the standard of care? For example, a patient requests that you reimplant an avulsed tooth that has been out of the mouth for 6 hours.

Note: I use the words "'outside' the standard of care" rather than "'below' the standard of care" as the latter reflexively implies an element of wrongdoing or poor care.

Many ethicists are of the opinion that treatment that deviates from the standard of care is permissible under some circumstances. Some authorities argue that there are no limits to patient autonomy as long as there is no risk of harming others. Others though express the view that a patient's autonomy may be restricted if there is a threat of severe harm to the patient's or others' well-being or for other reasons, including, but not limited to, futility. The practitioner should carefully weigh the risks and benefits of such treatment and obtain what some commentators refer to as enhanced consent. A full discussion of this topic is beyond the scope of this text, but readers are encouraged to read the publications referenced.

While no guarantees concerning the legal ramifications of performing treatments that are outside the standard of care can be made, practitioners who abide by getting enhanced informed consent should feel comfortable that they have a defensible position, ethically, morally, and legally.

22. While going through your patient schedule in order to prepare for the following day, you realize that you need to obtain some medical information from one patient's physician in order to know whether you can proceed with treatment. You are unable to reach the patient. Are you allowed to contact the patient's physician without her consent?

Yes, you may. The Health Insurance Portability and Accountability Act's (HIPAA's) Privacy Rule says: *The Privacy Rule allows covered health care providers to share protected health information for treatment purposes without patient authorization, as long as they use reasonable safeguards when doing so. These treatment communications may occur orally or in writing, by phone, fax, e-mail, or otherwise* (45 CFR Part 160 and Subparts A and E of Part 164). (https://www.hhs.gov/hipaa/for-professionals/faq/482/does-hipaa-permit-a-doctor-to-share-patient-information-for-treatment-over-the-phone/index.html).

23. A patient's fixed partial denture/bridge is ready and you have appointments available on December 18, 20, and 23. He says he doesn't want it cemented until the new year so that his dental insurance, which he has exhausted for this year, will cover most of the cost of the bridge. Is this permitted?

There are no laws covering when you may or must bill for services. Instead, the matter is governed by contract, and specifically the master contract you have with each insurance company. Be aware that contract language may differ between insurers. Typically, insurance contracts either mandate or allow one of two choices with respect to when one may or must bill. These choices are: (1) you may or must bill at the time of prepping and temping or (2) you may or must bill upon completion of the treatment. Some insurance companies permit you to choose one of the aforementioned options for when you wish to bill. If you choose one method, then you are obligated to follow that rule for all patients and all treatments with that insurance company, that is, you must be consistent. In the example above, if you selected in your contract to bill at the time of prepping and temping, you should have submitted the insurance claim prior even to December 18. Even if you did do this, you may not actually receive payment until the next calendar year, but the payment will count toward the insured's calendar year allowance for the year in which prepping and temping were completed. If you elected to bill upon completion of the treatment, then you may submit the claim only once the bridge has been cemented.

24. A patient's anterior fixed partial denture/bridge is ready and you have appointments available on December 18, 20, and 27. He says he wants you to put it in on the 23rd because his daughter is getting married on the 30th and he wants to look good at her wedding, but he wants you to cement it with temporary cement until the new year so that his dental insurance, which he has exhausted for this year, will cover most of the cost of the bridge. Is this permitted?

If you selected to bill at the time of prepping and temping, then you are contractually obligated to submit the insurance claim at the time those procedures were completed. Even if you did do this, you may not actually receive payment until the next calendar year, but the payment will count toward the insured's calendar year allowance for the year in which prepping and temping were completed. If you elected to bill upon completion of the treatment, then the scenario painted above is a little more nuanced. Although you cemented the bridge only with temporary cement and will cement it only permanently in the new year, an insurance company will almost certainly look askance at this practice as an attempt to get around the contract and will in all likelihood look upon the date of temporary cementation as the date of service.

With respect to the two preceding questions, it is instructive to look at the ADA's Dental Claim Form (https://www.ada.org/-/media/project/ada-organization/ada/ada-org/files/publications/cdt/2019adadentalclaim -form_2019may.pdf (Accessed on June 15, 2023).

In one section, the ADA Dental Claim Form states:

> I hereby certify that the procedures as indicated by date are in progress (for procedures that require multiple visits) or have been completed.

25. You are a general dentist and have a good friend who is a prosthodontist and who belongs to a country club that permits her to invite one guest a month at no additional expense. You are her regular monthly invitee. You refer all your patients who require substantial prosthodontic treatment to her. Are there any potential red flags that you should be aware of?

One concern is that by accepting the golfing invitation, you may open yourself up to action by the dental board. In Section 5.F.4. Referral Services, the ADA Principles of Ethics & Code of Professional Conduct states "*A dentist is allowed to pay for any advertising permitted by the Code, but is generally not permitted to make payments to another person or entity for the referral of a patient for professional services.*" Almost all state dental boards incorporate this prohibition into their regulations in one form or another. For example, Massachusetts' regulations say *Licensees are prohibited from engaging in the following practices:*

(2) Paying or accepting fees in any form or manner as compensation for referring patients to any person for professional services, written work orders, or other services or articles supplied to the patient. (234 CMR §5.20)

Thus, your acceptance of the golfing invitations may be construed as accepting compensation for your referrals.

As long as the prosthodontist is competent, there is probably little risk of your being on the receiving end of a lawsuit by a patient whom you referred to her. If, however, her reputation in the dental community is that her work is satisfactory at best and questionable on occasion, you may open yourself up to a suit by a patient who received substandard care from her. While such lawsuits are rare, a patient may sue you under the doctrine of negligent referral even though you did not undertake the work. The basis of the suit is that your *referral* was negligent.

26. In their text on ethics in dentistry, Ozar and Sokol elucidate what they refer to as the central values of dental practice. List them.

In order of importance, from the greatest to the least important, they are:
1. A patient's life and general health
2. A patient's oral health
3. A patient's autonomy
4. A dentist's preferred patterns of practice
5. Esthetic values
6. Efficient use of resources

Note that the patient's life and general health take precedence over a patient's oral health. This is the ethical underpinning for not performing dental procedures on patients that may endanger or aggravate their health. For example, the ADA's standard of care requires that elective dental care be delayed if the patient's blood pressure is greater 160/100 mm Hg and that even emergency dental treatment be delayed if a patient's systolic blood pressure is greater than 180 mm Hg and/or a patient's diastolic pressure is greater than 109 mm Hg (https://www.ada.org/en/member-center/oral-health-topics/hypertension (Accessed on June 15, 2023). Dentists may feel pressured, especially by VIP or celebrity patients, to undertake treatment that is medically contra-indicated, but they should not depart from their normal protocols. There is evidence that suggests that departing from normal protocols may lead to less optimal outcomes.

ACKNOWLEDGMENT

The author gratefully acknowledges the contribution of the previous chapter author.

BIBLIOGRAPHY

Beauchamp T, Childress J. *Principles of Biomedical Ethics*. 8th ed. New York: Oxford University Press; 2019.
Diekema DS. The preferential treatment of VIPs in the emergency department. *Am J Emerg Med*. 1996;14(2):226–229.
Drane JF, Coulehan JL. The concept of futility. Patients do not have a right to demand medically useless treatment. Counterpoint. *Health Prog*. 1993;74(10):28–32.
Friedland B. Medicolegal issues related to conebeam CT. *Semin Orthod*. 2009;15(1):77–84.
Harris J. Consent and end of life decisions. *J Med Ethics*. 2003;29(1):10–15.
Lantos J, Matlock AM, Wendler D. Clinician integrity and limits to patient autonomy. *JAMA*. 2011;305(5):495–499.
Solak v. *Dental Board of California*, No. B222438 (Cal. Ct. App. Nov. 19, 2010).
Teven CM, Gottlieb LJ. The four-quadrant approach to ethical issues in burn care. *AMA J Ethics*. 2018;20(6):595–601.

INDEX

Page numbers followed by *f, t,* and *b* indicate figures, tables, and boxes, respectively.